1998
YEAR BOOK OF
CRITICAL CARE
MEDICINE®

Statement of Purpose

The YEAR BOOK Service

The YEAR BOOK series was devised in 1901 by practicing health professionals who observed that the literature of medicine and related disciplines had become so voluminous that no one individual could read and place in perspective every potential advance in a major specialty. In the final decade of the 20th century, this recognition is more acutely true than it was in 1901.

More than merely a series of books, YEAR BOOK volumes are the tangible results of a unique service designed to accomplish the following:

- to *survey* a wide range of journals of proven value
- to *select* from those journals papers representing significant advances and statements of important clinical principles
- to provide *abstracts* of those articles that are readable, convenient summaries of their key points
- to provide *commentary* about those articles to place them in perspective

These publications grow out of a unique process that calls on the talents of outstanding authorities in clinical and fundamental disciplines, trained literature specialists, and professional writers, all supported by the resources of Mosby, the world's preeminent publisher for the health professions.

The Literature Base

Mosby and its Editors survey more than 1,000 journals published worldwide, covering the full range of the health professions. On an annual basis, the publisher examines usage patterns and polls its expert authorities to add new journals to the literature base and to delete journals that are no longer useful as potential YEAR BOOK sources.

The Literature Survey

The publisher's team of literature specialists, all of whom are trained and experienced health professionals, examines every original, peer-reviewed article in each journal issue. More than 250,000 articles per year are scanned systematically, including title, text, illustrations, tables, and references. Each scan is compared, article by article, to the search strategies that the publisher has developed in consultation with the 270 outside experts who form the pool of YEAR BOOK editors. A given article may be reviewed by any number of editors, from one to a dozen or more, regardless of the discipline for which the paper was originally published. In turn, each editor who receives the article reviews it to determine whether or not the article should be included in the YEAR BOOK. This decision is based on the article's inherent quality, its probable usefulness to readers of that YEAR BOOK, and the editor's goal to represent a balanced picture of a given field in each volume of the YEAR BOOK. In addition, the editor indicates when to include figures and tables from the article to help the YEAR BOOK reader better understand the information.

Of the quarter million articles scanned each year, only 5% are selected for detailed analysis within the YEAR BOOK series, thereby assuring readers of the high value of every selection.

The Abstract

The publisher's abstracting staff is headed by a seasoned medical professional and includes individuals with training in the life sciences, medicine, and other areas, plus extensive experience in writing for the health professions and related industries. Each selected article is assigned to a specific writer on this abstracting staff. The abstracter, guided in many cases by notations supplied by the expert editor, writes a structured, condensed summary designed so that the reader can rapidly acquire the essential information contained in the article.

The Commentary

The YEAR BOOK editorial boards, sometimes assisted by guest commentators, write comments that place each article in perspective for the reader. This provides the reader with the equivalent of a personal consultation with a leading international authority—an opportunity to better understand the value of the article and to benefit from the authority's thought processes in assessing the article.

Additional Editorial Features

The editorial boards of each YEAR BOOK organize the abstracts and comments to provide a logical and satisfying sequence of information. To enhance the organization, editors also provide introductions to sections or individual chapters, comments linking a number of abstracts, citations to additional literature, and other features.

The published YEAR BOOK contains enhanced bibliographic citations for each selected article, including extended listings of multiple authors and identification of author affiliations. Each YEAR BOOK contains a Table of Contents specific to that year's volume. From year to year, the Table of Contents for a given YEAR BOOK will vary depending on developments within the field.

Every YEAR BOOK contains a list of the journals from which papers have been selected. This list represents a subset of the more than 1,000 journals surveyed by the publisher and occasionally reflects a particularly pertinent article from a journal that is not surveyed on a routine basis.

Finally, each volume contains a comprehensive subject index and an index to authors of each selected paper.

The 1998 Year Book Series

Year Book of Allergy, Asthma, and Clinical Immunology: Drs. Rosenwasser, Borish, Boguniewicz, Nelson, Routes, and Spahn

Year Book of Anesthesiology and Pain Management®: Drs. Tinker, Abram, Chestnut, Roizen, Rothenberg, and Wood

Year Book of Cardiology®: Drs. Schlant, Collins, Gersh, Graham, Kaplan, and Waldo

Year Book of Chiropractic®: Dr. Lawrence

Year Book of Critical Care Medicine®: Drs. Parrillo, Balk, Calvin, Franklin, and Shapiro

Year Book of Dentistry®: Drs. Meskin, Berry, Jeffcoat, Leinfelder, Roser, Summitt, and Zakariasen

Year Book of Dermatologic Surgery®: Drs. Greenway, Barrett, Papadopoulos, and Whitaker

Year Book of Dermatology®: Dr. Thiers

Year Book of Diagnostic Radiology®: Drs. Osborn, Groskin, Dalinka, Maynard, Pentecost, Rebner, Ros, Smirniotopoulos, and Young

Year Book of Drug Therapy®: Drs. Lasagna and Weintraub

Year Book of Emergency Medicine®: Drs. Wagner, Dronen, Davidson, King, Niemann, and Roberts

Year Book of Endocrinology®: Drs. Bagdade, Braverman, Horton, Kannan, Landsberg, Molitch, Morley, Nathan, Odell, Poehlman, Rogol, and Ryan

Year Book of Family Practice®: Drs. Berg, Bowman, Davidson, Dexter, and Scherger

Year Book of Gastroenterology®: Drs. Aliperti and Fleshman

Year Book of Geriatrics and Gerontology®: Drs. Burton, Beck, Ostwald, Rabins, Reuben, Roth, Shapiro, and Whitehouse

Year Book of Hand Surgery®: Drs. Amadio and Hentz

Year Book of Hematology®: Drs. Spivak, Bell, Ness, Quesenberry, Wiernik, and Horowitz

Year Book of Infectious Diseases: Drs. Keusch, Barza, Bennish, Poutsiaka, Skolnik, and Snydman

Year Book of Medicine®: Drs. Cline, Frishman, Jett, Klahr, Malawista, Mandell, McCallum, and Utiger

Year Book of Neonatal and Perinatal Medicine®: Drs. Fanaroff, Maisels, and Stevenson

Year Book of Nephrology, Hypertension, and Mineral Metabolism: Drs. Schwab, Bennett, Emmett, Hostetter, Kumar, and Toto

Year Book of Neurology and Neurosurgery®: Drs. Bradley and Gibbs

Year Book of Nuclear Medicine®: Drs. Gottschalk, Blaufox, Neumann, Strauss, and Zubal

Year Book of Obstetrics, Gynecology, and Women's Health: Drs. Mishell, Herbst, and Kirschbaum

Year Book of Occupational and Environmental Medicine®: Drs. Emmett, Frank, Gochfeld, and Hessl

Year Book of Oncology®: Drs. Ozols, Eisenberg, Glatstein, Loehrer, and Tallman

Year Book of Ophthalmology®: Drs. Wilson, Augsburger, Cohen, Eagle, Grossman, Laibson, Maguire, Nelson, Penne, Rapuano, Sergott, Spaeth, Tipperman, Ms. Gosfield, and Ms. Salmon

Year Book of Orthopedics®: Drs. Morrey, Beauchamp, Currier, Tolo, Trigg, and Swiontkowski

Year Book of Otolaryngology–Head and Neck Surgery®: Drs. Paparella and Holt

Year Book of Pathology and Laboratory Medicine®: Drs. Raab, Cohen, Olson, Sirgi, and Stanley

Year Book of Pediatrics®: Dr. Stockman

Year Book of Plastic, Reconstructive, and Aesthetic Surgery®: Drs. Miller, Bartlett, Garner, McKinney, Ruberg, Salisbury, and Smith

Year Book of Psychiatry and Applied Mental Health®: Drs. Talbott, Ballenger, Frances, Lydiard, Meltzer, Schowalter, and Tasman

Year Book of Pulmonary Disease®: Drs. Jett, Maurer, Ryu, Strollo, and Wenzel

Year Book of Rheumatology®: Drs. Panush, Hadler, LeRoy, Liang, Reichlin, Simon, and Weinblatt

Year Book of Sports Medicine®: Drs. Shephard, Drinkwater, Eichner, Torg, Alexander, and Mr. George

Year Book of Surgery®: Drs. Copeland, Bland, Deitch, Eberlein, Howard, Luce, Seeger, Souba, and Sugarbaker

Year Book of Thoracic and Cardiovascular Surgery®: Drs. Ginsberg, Wechsler, and Williams

Year Book of Urology®: Drs. Andriole and Coplen

Year Book of Vascular Surgery®: Dr. Porter

1998

The Year Book of CRITICAL CARE MEDICINE®

Editor-in-Chief

Joseph E. Parrillo, M.D.

James B. Herrick Professor of Medicine, Rush Medical College; Chief, Division of Cardiovascular Disease and Critical Care Medicine; Director, Section of Cardiology; Medical Director, Rush Heart Institute, Rush-Presbyterian-St. Luke's Medical Center, Chicago, Illinois

Associate Editors

Robert A. Balk, M.D.

Professor of Medicine, Rush Medical College; Director, Section of Pulmonary and Critical Care Medicine, Rush-Presbyterian-St. Luke's Medical Center, Chicago, Illinois

James E. Calvin, Jr., M.D.

Associate Professor of Medicine, Rush Medical College; Director, Coronary Care Unit, Rush-Presbyterian-St. Luke's Hospital, Chicago, Illinois

Cory M. Franklin, M.D.

Professor of Medicine, Finch University of Health Sciences/Chicago Medical School; Director, Medical Intensive Care Unit, Cook County Hospital, Chicago, Illinois

Barry A. Shapiro, M.D.

James E. Eckenhoff Professor, Northwestern University Medical School; Chair, Department of Anesthesiology, Northwestern Memorial Hospital, Chicago, Illinois

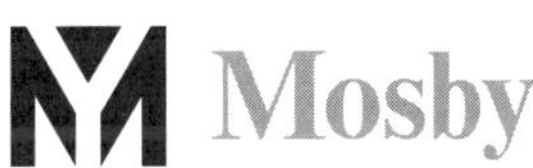

St. Louis Baltimore Boston Carlsbad Naples New York Philadelphia Portland London
Madrid Mexico City Singapore Sydney Tokyo Toronto Wiesbaden

Table of Contents

Journal of Clinical Investigation
Journal of Clinical Microbiology
Journal of Neurosurgery
Journal of Pediatric Surgery
Journal of Pediatrics
Journal of Perinatology
Journal of Pharmacology and Experimental Therapeutics
Journal of Surgical Research
Journal of Thoracic and Cardiovascular Surgery
Journal of Vascular Surgery
Journal of the American College of Cardiology
Journal of the American Geriatrics Society
Journal of the American Medical Association
Journal of the American Society of Nephrology
Lancet
Mayo Clinic Proceedings
Medical Journal of Australia
Neurology, Dialysis, Transplantation
Neuroradiology
Neurosurgery
New England Journal of Medicine
Pediatric Infectious Disease Journal
Pediatrics
Pharmacotherapy
Radiology
Southern Medical Journal
Stroke
Surgery
Surgical Neurology
Thorax
Thrombosis and Haemostatis
Transfusion
World Journal of Surgery

STANDARD ABBREVIATIONS

The following terms are abbreviated in this edition: acquired immunodeficiency syndrome (AIDS), cardiopulmonary resuscitation (CPR), central nervous system (CNS), cerebrospinal fluid (CSF), computed tomography (CT), deoxyribonucleic acid (DNA), electrocardiography (ECG), health maintenance organization (HMO), human immunodeficiency virus (HIV), intensive care unit (ICU), intramuscular (IM), intravenous (IV), magnetic resonance (MR) imaging (MRI), and ribonucleic acid (RNA).

NOTE

The YEAR BOOK OF CRITICAL CARE MEDICINE is a literature survey service providing abstracts of articles published in the professional literature. Every effort is made to ensure the accuracy of the information presented in these pages. Neither the editors nor the publisher of the YEAR BOOK OF CRITICAL CARE MEDICINE can be responsible for errors in the original materials. The editors' comments are their own opinions. Mention of specific products within this publication does not constitute endorsement.

To facilitate the use of the YEAR BOOK OF CRITICAL CARE MEDICINE as a reference tool, all illustrations and tables included in this publication are now identified as they appear in the original article. This change is meant to help the reader recognize that any illustration or table appearing in the YEAR BOOK OF CRITICAL CARE MEDICINE may be only one of many in the original article. For this reason, figure and table numbers will often appear to be out of sequence within the YEAR BOOK OF CRITICAL CARE MEDICINE.

1 Cardiopulmonary Resuscitation

Cardiovascular Function During the Postresuscitation Phase After Cardiac Arrest in Pigs: A Comparison of Epinephrine Versus Vasopressin
Prengel AW, Lindner KH, Keller A, et al (Univ of Ulm, Germany; Univ of Minnesota, Minneapolis)
Crit Care Med 24:2014–2019, 1996   1–1

Introduction.—In pigs undergoing cardiopulmonary resuscitation during cardiac arrest, administering vasopressin provides significantly greater blood flow to the vital organs when compared with epinephrine. However, it is unclear how vasopressin affects cardiovascular function after resuscitation. Vasopressin and epinephrine were compared for their effects on cardiovascular function after CPR.

Methods.—Cardiac arrest was induced in 16 anesthetized, mechanically ventilated pigs. The animals were randomized to receive either epinephrine 0.045 mg/kg or vasopressin 0.4 U/kg after 4 minutes. At intervals of up to 4 hours after successful CPR, the pigs underwent measurement of hemodynamic parameters, left ventricular contractility, and myocardial blood flow.

Results.—In the 15 minutes after spontaneous circulation was restored, mean aortic pressure was 64 mm Hg in the epinephrine group vs. 84 mm Hg in the vasopressin group. Systemic vascular resistance was 1,285 dyne·sec/cm^5 in the epinephrine group vs. 2,314 dyne·sec/cm^5 in the vasopressin group (Fig 1). Cardiac index was 140 vs. 99 mL/min/kg; myocardial contractility, calculated as dp/dt$_{max}$/P, was 52.8 vs. 36.3/sec; and left ventricular epicardial blood flow was 241 vs. 142 mL/min/100 g with epinephrine and vasopressin, respectively. However, none of these variables was significantly different between groups by 4 hours after CPR.

Conclusions.—In the early phase after successful CPR, systemic blood pressures are higher in pigs receiving vasopressin than in those receiving epinephrine. Vasopressin also has a reversible depressant effect on myocardial function. However, vasopressin does not appear to be associated with an irreversible or critical impairment of overall cardiovascular function in this situation.

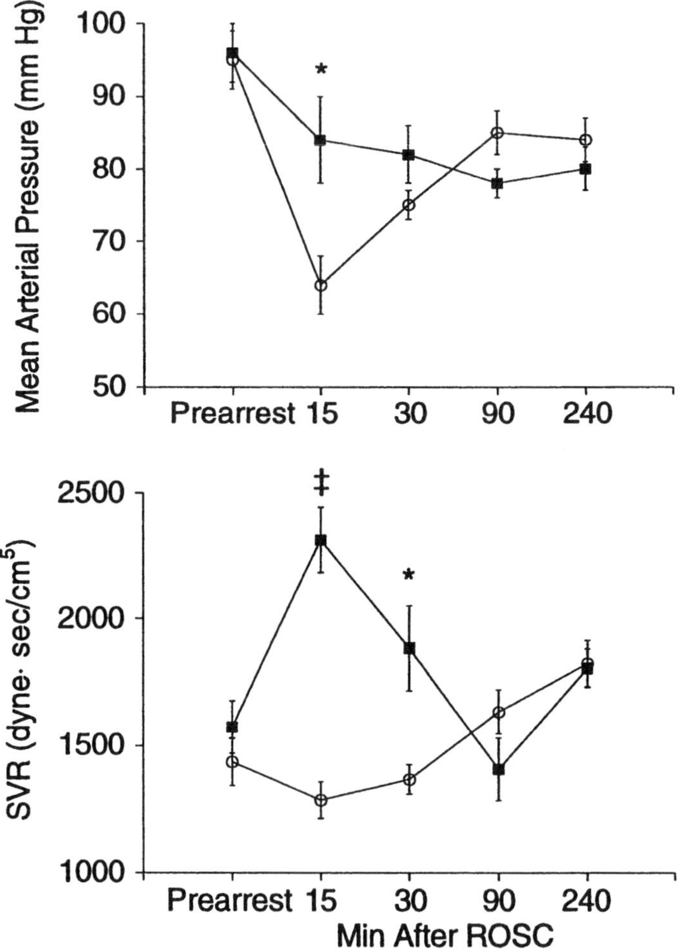

FIGURE 1.—Mean arterial pressure and systemic vascular resistance (SVR) before arrest and after cardiopulmonary resuscitation with 0.045 mg/kg of epinephrine and 0.4 U/kg of vasopressin. Mean arterial pressure is higher 15 minutes after restoration of spontaneous circulation (ROSC), and systemic vascular resistance is higher 15 and 30 minutes after restoration of spontaneous circulation, in animals treated with vasopressin (*squares*) vs. epinephrine (*circles*). Values are expressed as mean ± SEM. *$p < .05$; ‡$p < .001$. (Courtesy of Prengel AW, Lindner KH, Keller A, et al: Cardiovascular function during the postresuscitation phase after cardiac arrest in pigs: A comparison of epinephrine versus vasopressin. *Crit Care Med* 24:2014–2019, 1996.)

▶ Vasopressin primarily exerted a vasoconstrictor response in this excellent study. While vasopressin increased systemic vascular resistance and blood pressure, it also lowered cardiac index and coronary blood flow, making it less than ideal as a treatment in resuscitating cardiac arrest.

J.E. Calvin, Jr., M.D.

J.E. Parrillo, M.D.

Efficacy of Cardiopulmonary Resuscitation Using Intratracheal Insufflation

Brochard L, Boussignac G, Adnot S, et al (Hôpital Henri Mondor, Créteil, France)
Am J Respir Crit Care Med 154:1323–1329, 1996   1–2

Introduction.—Constant-flow ventilation at high flow rates of 1–3 L/min/kg, administered with an intraairway catheter has been shown to maintain gas exchange in the absence of respiratory movement in animal models. The ventilatory and hemodynamic effects of constant-flow insufflation (CFI) of air in the trachea during cardiopulmonary resuscitation (CPR) were assessed in anesthetized, paralyzed pigs.

Findings.—The ventilatory effect of CFI at 15 L/min producing a positive pressure of approximately 10 cm H_2O with concomitant chest compression was evaluated first. When 9 sedated, paralyzed pigs were disconnected from the ventilator, CFI alone could not significantly alter the reduction in partial pressure of arterial oxygen and the increase in partial pressure of arterial carbon dioxide that occurred during apnea. The combination of precordial compression and CFI was able to hold arterial blood gases over a 4-minute period at the same level achieved during mechanical ventilation. Next, ventricular fibrillation was provoked and CFI-CPR was compared in random order with standard CPR using conventional mechanical ventilation during 2 successive 4-minute periods. Ventilatory parameters were the same for both situations and hemodynamic parameters were similar or better when CFI-CPR was used, compared with standard CPR. There were significant differences between CPR and CFI-CPR for systolic aortic pressure and systolic and mean common carotid blood flows.

Conclusion.—During cardiac arrest in pigs, tracheal gas injection resulted in a 10 cm H_2O rise in airway pressure that was sufficient as the sole mode of ventilation. The hemodynamic benefits of this approach were superior to those of standard CPR. This method deserves further investigation as it may also be beneficial in humans.

▶ Constant-flow insufflation is well known to provide a constant positive airway pressure at the carina of approximately 10 cm H_2O. In concert with chest compressions that will result in intrathoracic pressure variations, CFI should provide a reasonable degree of lung ventilation. This pig study not only documents the fact that the above hypothesis is true, it also demonstrates that the constant airway pressure appears to cause less hemodynamic embarrassment during CPR than does traditional positive pressure ventilation. Importantly, this technique requires endotracheal intubation to assure a patent airway. As the authors conclude, CFI with CPR deserves further investigation.

B.A. Shapiro, M.D.

2   Cardiovascular

Acute Myocardial Infarction

Outcome of Acute Myocardial Infarction According to the Specialty of the Admitting Physician
Jollis JG, DeLong ER, Peterson ED, et al (Duke Univ, Durham, NC)
N Engl J Med 335:1880–1887, 1996   2–1

Background.—One strategy used by health care organizations to reduce the use of medical services and lower health care costs is to limit access to specialists. It is not known whether this practice affects the outcome of patients, especially those who are acutely ill. It has been suggested that patients with acute cardiac illnesses may have a poorer outcome when treated by a primary care physician, partially because family practitioners and internists may be less aware of life-saving drugs than cardiologists. The association between the outcome of patients with acute myocardial infarction and the type of physician who provides their care was investigated.

Methods.—The medical records were reviewed of 8,241 patients from 4 states receiving Medicare who were hospitalized for acute myocardial infarction during a 7-month period in 1992. Also analyzed were the insurance claims and survival data for all 220,535 patients receiving Medicare who were hospitalized for acute myocardial infarction during 1992. Data were analyzed according to the specialty of the admitting physician.

Results.—Patients admitted by cardiologists were more likely to have had prior myocardial infarction, coronary bypass surgery, anterior myocardial infarction, and to have lower blood pressure than other patients. After adjusting for patient and hospital characteristics, analysis showed that patients admitted by a cardiologist had a 12% lower risk of death within 12 months than patients admitted by a primary care physician. Cardiologists had the highest use rate of cardiac procedures, cardiac medications, and other medications associated with improved survival.

Discussion.—In treating elderly patients with acute myocardial infarction, cardiologists use more resources, but patients are more likely to have a better outcome than patients admitted by primary care physicians. Cardiologists were more likely to use thrombolytic agents, β-blockers, aspirin, nitrates, and heparin than other physicians. Shifting the care of were calculated for patients with AMI outside of a hospital and in patients with nonfatal, serious cardiac events, including shock, sustained ventricular tachycardia, ventricular fibrillation, and asystole.

Results.—Complete medical records were available for 2,708 patients. Of these, 2,542 had AMI outside of the hospital. These patients arrived at a hospital at a median of 81 minutes after symptom onset. The median time to treatment after arrival at the hospital was 85 minutes. Compared with other patients enrolled in the GUSTO-I trial in other countries, a significantly greater proportion of Canadian patients reached the hospital within 2 hours of symptom onset, but a significantly greater proportion of Canadian patients experienced in-hospital treatment delays of >1 hour. The number of nonfatal cardiac events in patients treated 4 to 6 hours after symptom onset was significantly higher than in patients treated within 2 hours.

Conclusion.—Canadian patients enrolled in GUSTO-I experienced significant in-hospital delays in thrombolytic therapy, compared with enrollees from other countries. These delays reduce the rate of short-term survival after AMI. Findings indicate that delays also increase the odds of nonfatal, serious cardiac events. All hospitals should routinely assess ways to decrease treatment delays in patients with AMI.

▶ This multicenter Canadian study focuses on an important question: Why are there continuing delays in treatment with thrombolytic therapy? The time to in-hospital treatment is higher than current U.S. figures. Some factors associated with delays in treatment included age, hypertension, high pulse rate, and anterior MI. Other important reasons for delay also include an initial nondiagnostic ECG and consideration of primary percutaneous transluminal coronary angioplasty.

J.E. Calvin, Jr., M.D.

J.E. Parrillo, M.D.

Patient-Specific Predictions of Outcomes in Myocardial Infarction for Real-Time Emergency Use: A Thrombolytic Predictive Instrument
Selker HP, Griffith JL, Beshansky JR, et al (New England Med Ctr, Boston; Tufts Univ, Boston; Boston Univ; et al)
Ann Intern Med 127:538–556, 1997   2–4

Introduction.—For reducing the most common cause of death in the United States, thrombolytic therapy for acute myocardial infarction has great potential. Treating appropriate candidates as early as possible is key for the benefits of this therapy to be evident. A real-time method is needed in the emergency clinical setting that identifies patients most likely to benefit from thrombolytic therapy to broadly maximize the benefits of thrombolytic therapy. To identify patients likely to benefit and to facilitate the earliest possible use of this therapy, a thrombolytic predictive instrument for real-time use in emergency medical service settings was developed.

Methods.—There were 3,483 patients of 4,911 patients with acute myocardial infarction and ST-segment elevation on the electrocardiogram who received thrombolytic therapy. Presenting clinical and electrocardiographic features were included in the input variables. Predictive models generated probabilities for acute 30-day mortality, 1-year mortality and cardiac arrest in patients treated and not treated with thrombolysis, thrombolysis-related intracranial hemorrhage, and a thrombolysis-related major bleeding episode requiring transfusion. The thrombolytic predictive instrument was constructed with these models.

Results.—For the patients in the Thrombolytic Predictive Instrument Database, the predictive models generated the following mean predictions: 1-year mortality rate, 10.9%; 30-day mortality rate, 7.1%; rate of thrombolysis-related intracranial hemorrhage, 0.6%; rate of cardiac arrest, 3.7%; rate of other thrombolysis-related major bleeding episodes, 5.0%. Between persons having and those not having the predicted outcome, they discriminated well. For the 5 outcomes, areas under the receiver-operating characteristic curve were between 0.77 and 0.84. There was excellent calibration between each instrument's predicted and observed rates.

Conclusion.—The predictions of the thrombolytic predictive instrument can be printed on the electrocardiogram report after the basic features of a clinical presentation are entered into a computerized electrocardiograph. In patients with acute myocardial infarction, earlier and more appropriate use of thrombolytic therapy may result from this decision aid.

▶ The models derived to predict poor outcome in this study were very straightforward and included for 1-year mortality rate, age, heart rate, anterior location of myocardial infarction, number of leads with Q waves, and right bundle-branch block. The predictors for cardiac arrest included time from onset, systolic blood pressure, age, size of infarct based on ECG, QT interval, and use of thrombolytic therapy. The area beneath each receiver-operating characteristic curve presented indicated that the models were reasonably robust. The predicted outcomes were similar to those of the national database on myocardial infarction.

What is new is the way the authors present these predictions to the treating physicians; they place the predictions on the ECG. The hope is that such information can speed up the decision-making process in the emergency room. More studies are necessary to assess the impact of having this information. One of the reasons for decision delay is the consideration of primary percutaneous transluminal coronary angioplasty. This should be incorporated into the predictive model.

J.E. Calvin, Jr., M.D.

J.E. Parrillo, M.D.

Effects of RheothRx on Mortality, Morbidity, Left Ventricular Function, and Infarct Size in Patients With Acute Myocardial Infarction

Yusuf S, for Collaborative Organization for RheothRx Evaluation (Hamilton Gen Hosp, Ont, Canada)
Circulation 96:192–201, 1997   2–5

Introduction.—Preliminary experimental and human data suggest that RheothRx may be effective in treating acute myocardial infarction (AMI). RheothRx is a formulation of poloxamer 188, which is a nonionic block copolymer surfactant with no known anticoagulant, thrombolytic, or antiplatelet properties or hypotensive effects. The effects of various doses of RheothRx were assessed in a randomized, placebo-controlled trial of 2,948 patients with AMI.

Methods.—Patients were randomized to either a control group or to receive RheothRx in varying doses: regimen A, 1-hour bolus only; regimen Y, additional 11-hour infusion with target serum concentration of 0.5 mg/mL; regimen B, additional 23-hour infusion at a low dose. Three higher doses, with 1-hour bolus plus low-dose infusion for 47 hours, 1-hour bolus plus high dose with target serum concentrations of 1.0 mg/mL for 24 hours, or 1-hour bolus plus high dose for 48 hours, were discontinued because of high rates of renal dysfunction (8.8%).

Results.—Compared with the control group, renal dysfunction was observed at lower doses for regimen A, Y, and B (1.0% vs. 3.1%, 2.7%, and 4.1%, respectively). There were no significant between-group differences in the composite outcome of death, cardiogenic shock, or repeated infarction at 35 days (12.7% control; 13.6% all RheothRx). Compared with the control group, patients in all RheothRx group had higher rates of sinus tachycardia (24.7% vs. 21.6%, $p = 0.02$), atrial flutter (3.0% vs. 1.3%, $p = 0.019$), atrial fibrillation (10.2% vs. 7.3%, $p = 0.082$), pericarditis (6.6% vs. 4.7%, $p = 0.055$), and clinical evidence (21.9% vs. 17.9%, $p = 0.005$) and radiologic evidence (15.3% vs. 12.3%, $p = 0.12$) of heart failure. These findings were correlated with a lower left ventricular ejection fraction in treated patients, but with little difference in infarct size.

Conclusion.—RheothRx did not significantly affect rates of mortality, repeated infarction, or cardiogenic shock. Its use had an adverse effect on renal function, left ventricular ejection fraction, and various clinical manifestations of left ventricular dysfunction or heart failure.

▶ There was a great deal of hope that poloxamer 188 would prove to be a useful adjuvant to thrombolytic therapy. Unfortunately, this study showed no benefit in a fairly convincing fashion. Because of the superior results of primary percutaneous transluminal coronary angioplasty for the treatment of AMI, we expect continuing research on novel agents that may improve results of thrombolytic therapy.

J.E. Calvin, Jr., M.D.

J.E. Parrillo, M.D.

Angiographic Findings and Outcome in Diabetic Patients Treated With Thrombolytic Therapy for Acute Myocardial Infarction: The GUSTO-I Experience
Lundergan CF, for the GUSTO-I Angiographic Investigators (George Washington Univ, Washington, DC)
J Am Coll Cardiol 28:1661–1669, 1996   2–6

Introduction.—For coronary artery disease, diabetes is a risk factor and is associated with increased mortality, which may be caused by decreased rates of successful early thrombolysis, a greater degree of diastolic left ventricular dysfunction, or increased adverse outcome after revascularization procedures. In diabetic and nondiabetic patients with an acute myocardial infarction, the clinical and angiographic determinants of outcome were assessed.

Methods.—In 2,431 diabetic and nondiabetic patients, patency rates and global and regional left ventricular function were determined. Thrombolytic therapy and angiographic data were analyzed. A comparison was also made in 30-day mortality differences.

Results.—Among the patients with diabetes, there was a significantly higher proportion of female and elderly patients who came to the hospital later, were more often hypertensive, had a higher number of previous myocardial infarctions and bypass surgery procedures, and had more congestive heart failure. In patients with diabetes, the 90-minute infarct-related artery patency rate was 40.3%, and for patients without diabetes, it was 37.6%. For patients with diabetes, the reocclusion rate was 9.2%, and for those without diabetes, it was 5.3%. In both groups of patients, the ejection fraction at 90 minutes after thrombolysis was similar, as was regional ventricular function. Less compensatory hyperkinesia in the non-infarct zone was seen in the diabetic patients (1.3 ± 0.2) than in nondiabetics (1.7 ± 0.1). At 5- to 7-day follow-up, no significant difference in ventricular function was seen. In diabetic patients, the 30-day mortality rate was 11.3% and in the nondiabetic patients, it was 5.9%. Diabetes remained an independent determinant of 30-day mortality after adjustment for clinical and angiographic variables.

Conclusion.—There was no difference between patients with and without diabetes after thrombolytic therapy in terms of early (90-minute) infarct-related artery patency or regional and global ventricular function, except for reduced compensatory hyperkinesia in the noninfarct zone among patients with diabetes. After correction for clinical and angiographic variables, diabetes remained an independent determinant of 30-day mortality.

▶ This study suggests that the poor outcome of diabetic patients is unrelated to early patency rates after thrombolytic therapy or regional and global left ventricular function. The reason for the increased mortality rate in diabetics remains unknown and needs further study.

J.E. Calvin, Jr., M.D.
J.E. Parrillo, M.D.

Cardiovascular Surgery

Long-term Outcome and Quality of Life of Patients Requiring Multidisciplinary Intensive Care Unit Admission After Cardiac Operations
Trouillet J-L, Scheimberg A, Vuagnat A, et al (Hôpital Bichat, Paris)
J Thorac Cardiovasc Surg 112:926–934, 1996   2–7

Introduction.—Up to 33% of patients who survive cardiac operations may have at least 1 adverse event, and this may require a long stay in an ICU. Complications include mediastinitis, respiratory failure, shock, hemodynamic instability, and multiorgan failure. Long-term mortality and quality of life were examined in surviving patients with organ failure or severe infection after cardiac operations.

Methods.—There were 116 patients who had cardiac operations and were transferred to a multidisciplinary ICU. Several clinical characteristics were recorded, including New York Heart Association functional class before cardiac surgery, duration of cardiopulmonary bypass, use of intra-aortic balloon pumping, number and type of organ dysfunctions, and

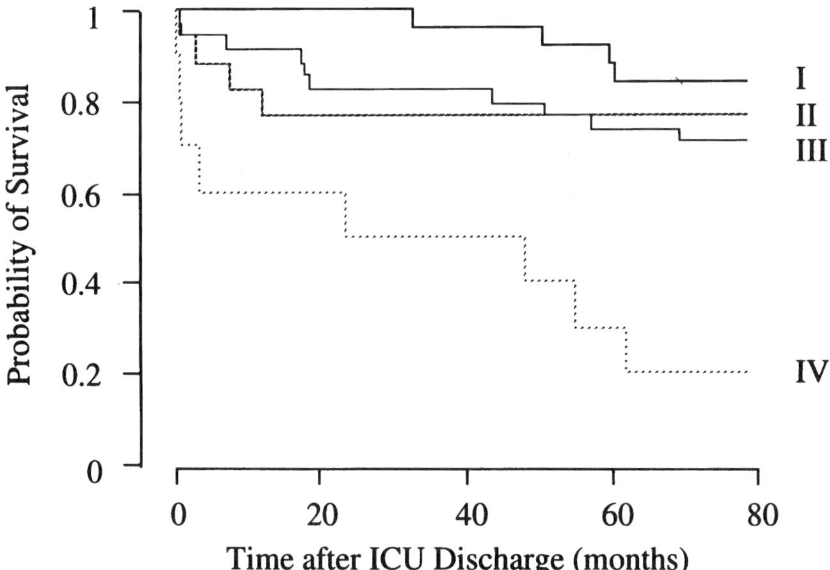

FIGURE 1.—Kaplan-Meier survival analysis of the 86 survivors grouped by preoperative New York Heart Association functional class. The *P* value of the overall log-rank test comparing the survival distribution of the 4 New York Heart Association classes is 0.002. (Courtesy of Trouillet J-L, Scheimberg A, Vuagnat A, et al: Long-term outcome and quality of life of patients requiring multidisciplinary intensive care unit admission after cardiac operations. *J Thorac Cardiovasc Surg* 112:926–934, 1996.)

severity of illness. The patients were classified as survivors or nonsurvivors (died in the ICU). During the last interview, morbidity, New York Heart Association class, and health status were recorded. The patients were also evaluated for quality of life in respect to 38 items.

Results.—The main causes of transfer were respiratory failure (88.8%) and hemodynamic instability (81.9%). In 23.3% of patients, infection was present at entry into the ICU. In the ICU, 27 patients died. Independent predictors of death in the ICU were presurgical New York Heart Association functional class, postoperative bacteremia before admission to the ICU, and severity of illness on ICU admission. Sixty-nine percent of the patients who were alive at transfer were still alive at an average follow-up of 81 months.

Conclusion.—The only long-term independent prognostic factor was preoperative New York Heart Association functional class (Fig 1). For more than 70% of the survivors, quality of life, as evaluated by the Nottingham Health Profile, was good. With the exception of age, quality of life was not influenced by any recorded variables.

▶ The good news is that quality of life was good in the majority of survivors. The bad news is that we cannot predict who the survivors are going to be. New York Heart Assocation class was the only predictor, but the mortality rate of class IV patients was 50% (literally a flip of a coin).

J.E. Calvin, Jr., M.D.

J.E. Parillo, M.D.

Arrhythmias

Management of Paroxysmal Atrioventricular Nodal Reentrant Tachycardia in the Critically Ill Surgical Patient

Kirton OC, Windsor J, Weddeburn R, et al (Univ of Miami, Fla; St Luke's Roosevelt Hosp Ctr, New York)
Crit Care Med 25:761–766, 1997   2–8

Introduction.—Atrioventricular nodal reentrant tachycardia is a clinically significant form of paroxysmal supraventricular tachycardia observed in critically ill surgical patients. The efficacy of a new treatment algorithm involving the sequential administration of various classes of antiarrhythmic agents until conversion to sinus rhythm was accomplished was evaluated in 27 critically ill patients from the ICU.

Methods.—All hemodynamically stable patients admitted to surgical and trauma ICUs with new-onset atrioventricular nodal reentrant tachycardia were prospectively evaluated over 11 months. Sixteen patients had trauma, with a median Injury Severity Score of 20; and 11 were general surgical patients, with a median Acute Physiology and Chronic Health Evaluation II score of 17. The algorithm drugs were given in rapid sequence through a central venous catheter, using successive doses of adenosine, verapamil, and esmolol until conversion to sinus rhythm.

Results.—The mean time from ICU admission to onset of atrioventricular nodal reentrant tachycardia was 4.5 days. Arrhythmia termination was accomplished in all patients within a mean of 13 minutes. Only 44% of initial episodes of atrioventricular nodal reentrant tachycardia were converted with administration of incremental sequential adenosine by itself. There were 38 relapses of paroxysmal supraventricular tachycardia in the ICU after initial conversion to sinus rhythm in 14 patients. Additional antiarrhythmic drugs were required for relapses. Adenosine was effective in 34% of relapses. In 7 of the 14 patients, relapses were multiple. Two patients were taking suppressive calcium channel or β-adrenergic receptor blockers when relapse occurred.

Conclusion.—A multiagent algorithm was able to effect initial conversion in patients with new-onset atrioventricular nodal reentrant tachycardia to sinus rhythm in surgical and trauma patients who were critically ill. Adenosine was marginally effective in this patient cohort. Suppressive therapy for arrhythmias during maximal cardiovascular stress is crucial, regardless of agents used for initial control.

▶ The diagnosis of atrioventricular nodal reentrant tachycardia was based on surface ECG and was not overread by a cardiologist. Because of adenosine's short half-life and the ongoing conditions of the critically ill that predispose to arrhythmia, it is not unexpected that the recurrence rate would be high and that longer acting agents would be necessary. Adenosine is still a useful agent to diagnose atrioventricular nodal reentrant tachycardia, in large part because of its short half-life and selective effects on the atrioventricular node. The algorithm used in this study is sensible.

J.E. Calvin, Jr., M.D.

J.E. Parrillo, M.D.

Intravenous Dofetilide, a Class III Antiarrhythmic Agent, for the Termination of Sustained Atrial Fibrillation or Flutter
Falk RH, for the Intravenous Dofetilide Investigators (Boston Med Ctr)
J Am Coll Cardiol 29:385–390, 1997   2–9

Background.—Dofetilide, a pure class III antiarrhythmic agent, selectively blocks the rapid component of the delayed rectifier current that causes action potential prolongation. Thus, it may be effective in the treatment of atrial fibrillation and flutter. The safety and efficacy of a single bolus of IV dofetilide in the termination of sustained atrial fibrillation or flutter were established.

Methods.—Seventy-five patients with sustained atrial fibrillation and 16 with flutter were enrolled in the double-blind, randomized, multicenter trial. Two doses of dofetilide, 4 and 8 µg/kg body weight, and placebo were compared.

Findings.—Arrhythmia was terminated in 31% of the patients given 8 µg/kg of dofetilide. This dose was significantly more effective than the lower dose or placebo. The conversion rate for patients with atrial flutter given dofetilide was 54%, compared with 14.5% among those with atrial fibrillation.

Conclusions.—The IV administration of dofetilide can convert sustained atrial fibrillation or flutter to sinus rhythm. Its efficacy is greater in patients with flutter, which contrasts with the poorer response observed with class I agents. This may be an important advance in the pharmacologic termination of atrial flutter.

▶ There is continuing interest in pharmacologic termination of atrial flutter and fibrillation. The results of this study show that dofetilide had greater efficacy with atrial flutter compared with atrial fibrillation. This difference was also noted with ibutilide, although ibutilide appeared to have greater efficacy overall. Proarrhythmic effects were observed in this study, including Torsades des Pointes in 3.2%. Dofetilide also increased QT intervals. Patients should be carefully monitored when using this drug. How it interacts with other antiarrhythmics that might also be used to maintain sinus rhythm is unknown.

J.E. Calvin, Jr., M.D.

J.E. Parrillo, M.D.

Miscellaneous

The Effect of Digoxin on Mortality and Morbidity in Patients With Heart Failure

Gorlin R, and the Digitalis Investigation Group (Mount Sinai Med Ctr, New York)

N Engl J Med 336:525–533, 1997   2–10

Background.—Digoxin is a common drug used to treat heart failure, but its long-term safety and efficacy are unclear. Recent studies have shown that discontinuing digoxin in patients with heart failure can worsen functional status, exercise capacity, and left ventricular ejection fraction. The effects of digoxin on hospitalization and mortality rates in patients with heart failure were assessed in a randomized, double-blind, placebo-controlled trial.

Methods.—Patients with heart failure and a left ventricular ejection fraction of 0.45 or less were treated with digoxin or placebo, plus angiotensin-converting enzyme inhibitors and diuretics. The median dose of digoxin was 0.25 mg/day. The average follow-up was 37 months. In a substudy of patients with a left ventricular ejection fraction of greater than 0.45, 492 patients were treated with digoxin and 496 were given placebo.

Results.—In the main study, the mortality rate was similar in both groups of patients. In patients treated with digoxin, there was a trend toward a lower risk of death from worsening heart failure. Also in patients treated with digoxin, the hospitalization rate was 6% less than in patients given placebo, and fewer patients were admitted for worsening heart

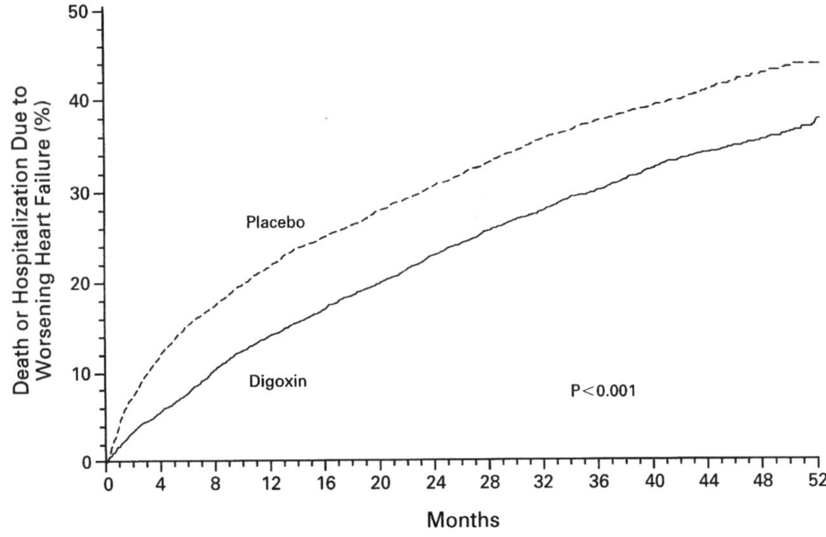

No. of Patients at Risk

Placebo	3403	2915	2674	2473	2328	2197	2071	1954	1659	1397	1111	859	546	250
Digoxin	3397	3120	2888	2696	2544	2392	2241	2115	1825	1521	1188	916	578	255

FIGURE 3.—Incidence of death or hospitalization caused by worsening heart failure in the digoxin and placebo groups. The number of patients at risk at each 4-month interval is shown below the figure. (Reprinted by permission of *The New England Journal of Medicine*, courtesy of Gorlin R, and the Digitalis Investigation Group: The effect of digoxin on mortality and morbidity in patients with heart failure. *N Engl J Med* 336:525–533, copyright 1997, Massachusetts Medical Society. All rights reserved.)

failure (Fig 3). In the substudy, the mortality and hospitalization rates from worsening heart failure were consistent with the rates in the main study.

Discussion.—In these patients, digoxin did not affect overall mortality rates in patients also receiving angiotensin-converting enzyme inhibitors and diuretics, but it lowered the death and hospitalization rates from worsening heart failure. In clinical practice, it is unlikely that digoxin would affect survival rates.

▶ Although all patients had ejection fractions of less than 45%, they were in sinus rhythm and approximately 65% were in class I or II heart failure. The trend toward fewer hospitalizations with digoxin is still an important finding for managing patients with milder heart failure. Current clinical practice guidelines recommend digoxin for heart failure classes II, III, and IV. These data support those recommendations.

J.E. Calvin, Jr., M.D.
J.E. Parrillo, M.D.

Significance of Magnesium in Congestive Heart Failure

Douban S, Brodsky MA, Whang DD, et al (Univ of California, Irvine; Christ Hosp, Cincinnati, Ohio; Univ of Hawaii, Honolulu)
Am Heart J 132:664–671, 1996   2–11

Background.—In patients with congestive heart failure, hypomagnesemia and hypokalemia may play a role in mortality and sudden death. Increased losses of these cations may occur as a result of the underlying disease. Decreased caloric intake and increased bowel edema are usually associated with treatment for heart failure. The clinical implications of magnesium in patients with congestive heart failure are reviewed.

Magnesium in Congestive Heart Failure.—There is debate over the significance of magnesium to cardiovascular stability. Uncertainty arises from the difficulty of accurate measurement and other associated factors. Similar to the situation with serum potassium, serum magnesium accounts for less than 1% of total body stores and does not reflect total-body magnesium concentration. Magnesium plays an important role in several different enzymatic reactions involved in cardiovascular hemodynamics and electrophysiologic functioning.

Magnesium deficiency is a common problem that can be linked to the risk factors and complications of heart failure. Changes in magnesium balance may occur with several of the treatments for heart failure, including digoxin, diuretics, and ACE inhibitors. Improvements in hemodynamics and reductions in arrhythmias have been reported with magnesium deficiency replacement, and with higher pharmacologic doses. Except for patients with kidney dysfunction, magnesium deficiency is rare.

Discussion.—On the biochemical and cellular levels, magnesium plays a key role in the maintenance of cardiovascular hemodynamics and electrophysiologic function. Total body magnesium is an important prognostic factor in patients with congestive heart failure. For these patients, ensuring an adequate magnesium level can reduce arrhythmias, digitalis toxicity, and hemodynamic abnormalities.

▶ This is a non-systematic review, which means that there has been no real attempt to quantify the evidence of the medical literature. The authors do provide some evidence that hypomagnesemia is common. Hypomagnesemia has important implications for heart function and requires surveillance and treatment. Some of the interesting effects of magnesium deficiency include some influences on the development of coronary artery disease and cardiomyopathy, an association with hypercholesterolemia, electrophysiological abnormalities including prolonged QT interval and Torsades des Pointes and inducing digitalis toxicity.

J.E. Calvin, Jr., M.D.

J.E. Parrillo, M.D.

ACE Inhibitors Unmask Incoordinate Diastolic Wall Motion in Restrictive Left Ventricular Disease

Henein MY, Amadi A, O'Sullivan C, et al (Royal Brompton Hosp, London)
Heart 76:326–331, 1996   2–12

Purpose.—For patients with left ventricular disease, treatment with angiotensin-converting enzyme (ACE) inhibitors can improve exercise tolerance and lengthen life. The variable nature of the ventricular function disturbance in these patients seems likely to have a major effect on the action of these drugs. The effects of ACE inhibitor treatment on left ventricular filling and wall motion in patients with heart failure were prospectively studied.

Methods.—The study included 30 outpatients with a clinical diagnosis of heart failure starting treatment with an ACE inhibitor. There were 27 men and 3 women, mean age 61 years. A group of controls of similar age were studied as well. Before and 3 weeks after the start of ACE inhibitor therapy, the patients underwent M-mode echocardiography and pulsed and continuous wave Doppler US to assess left ventricular systolic and diastolic function. The findings were analyzed to determine the effects of ACE inhibition on the abnormally functioning left ventricles.

Results.—The patients showed dilation of the left ventricular cavity both at end systole and end diastole, along with reduced fractional shortening. They had a normal mean isovolumetric relaxation time (IVRT) and ratio of transmitral early (E) to late (A) filling velocity. However, 2 groups could be identified based on a value of 1.0 on the normal frequency plot of the E/A ratio: group A, 20 patients with an E/A ratio greater than 1.0, and group B, 10 patients with an E/A ratio less than 1.0. Patients in group A had a shortened IVRT and transmitral E wave deceleration time, consistent with restrictive left ventricular physiology. They had coordinate left ventricular wall motion during IVRT, with increased left ventricular end-diastolic pressure on the apexcardiogram. Patients in group B had a lengthened E wave deceleration time, incoordinate relaxation, and a normal apexcardiogram.

After the start of ACE inhibitor treatment, patients in group A showed a decrease in the left ventricular dimensions at end diastole and end systole, but no change in fractional shortening. Total excursion of the long axis increased in this group, as did the peak rate of shortening. They also had increased IVRT accompanied by highly incoordinate wall motion, minor axis lengthening, and long axis shortening. A wave amplitude and velocity were increased, while transmitral E wave velocity was decreased. In group B, ACE inhibition caused no change in any of the left ventricular minor and long axis or transmitral Doppler variables measured.

Conclusions.—In patients with heart failure, the baseline hemodynamic characteristics determine the response to ACE inhibitor therapy. Patients with restrictive left ventricular physiology show a reduction in cavity size and a prolongation of IVRT, consistent with decreased left atrial pressure. These changes are accompanied by delayed and incoordinate ventricular relaxation, which reduces early diastolic left ventricular filling velocity considerably. For patients with restrictive left ventricular disease and a clinical diagnosis of heart failure, ACE inhibitor treatment may uncover major diastolic abnormalities.

▶ This study highlights the complexity of the pathophysiology of heart failure. These investigators demonstrate hidden abnormalities of diastolic function in heart failure patients who appear to have primarily systolic failure. Because these abnormalities were induced by ACE inhibition, there is an implied need for combination therapy to ameliorate the abnormal diastolic function. Whether echocardiography is better than clinical response—and what combinations of medical therapy are best—is still unanswered.

J.E. Calvin, Jr., M.D.

J.E. Parrillo, M.D.

Hemofiltration in a Cardiac Intensive Care Unit: Time for a Rational Approach
Tsang GMK, Khan I, Clayton D, et al (Walsgrave Hosp, Coventry, UK)
ASAIO J 42:M710–M713, 1996   2–13

Purpose.—Because of the high mortality, morbidity, and cost of renal replacement therapy for acute renal failure after cardiac surgery, it would be useful to have prognostic factors for use in decision making. Such prognostic factors were sought in an analysis of 48 consecutive patients requiring continuous hemofiltration (CHF) for acute renal failure after cardiac surgery.

Patients.—The patients—34 men and 14 women, mean age 65 years— were operated on over a 2-year period. The cardiac operations performed included 26 coronary artery bypass grafts, 8 aortic valve replacements, 3 aortic/mitral valve replacements, 2 postinfarction ventricular septal defect repairs, and 1 thoracoabdominal aneurysmectomy. Sixty-nine percent of patients had oliguria and fluid overload as their indication for hemofiltration, 56% had uremia, 33% had acidosis, and 13% had hyperkalemia. In-hospital mortality was 52%, plus another 21% mortality within 9 months after discharge. This left 13 survivors, 46% of whom were in New York Heart Association class III or IV. Factors affecting patient outcome were analyzed.

Findings.—Mean ICU stay per patient was 15 days, with a mean hospital stay of 25 days. Survivors and nonsurvivors were similar in age, preoperative renal function, ejection fraction, duration of cardiopulmonary bypass, and urine output before CHF. None of 7 patients with a cardiac index less than 1.7 L/m^2 and an adrenalin requirement more than 30 µg/min survived.

Conclusions.—Patients who develop acute renal failure requiring CHF after cardiac surgery have poor short- and long-term outcomes, this study finds. Because of its expense, a rational basis for the use of CHF in these patients should be established, particularly if persistent low cardiac output is present. The findings may be useful in selecting potential prognostic factors for detailed, prospective analysis.

▶ This retrospective review of 48 patients suggest a poorer outcome in patients who require continuous hemofiltration after cardiac operations and a relatively poor quality of life for survivors. The finding that there were no survivors when the cardiac index was less than 1.7 L/m/m² or catecholamine requirements were more than 30 µg/min does help give us some guidance as to when this technique should, probably, be withheld. However, the patient sample is small. More information, perhaps through a large clinical database like Project IMPACT, would be of some help.

J.E. Calvin, Jr., M.D.

J.E. Parrillo, M.D.

Detecting Acute Thoracic Aortic Dissection in the Emergency Department: Time Constraints and Choice of the Optimal Diagnostic Test
Sarasin FP, Louis-Simonet M, Gaspoz J-M, et al (Univ of Geneva)
Ann Emerg Med 28:278–288, 1996   2–14

Background.—The longer it goes undiagnosed and untreated, the higher the early mortality of acute dissection of the thoracic aorta. Many different factors affect the choice of diagnostic procedures for patients with suspected aortic dissection. In the emergency setting, the impact of delays related to the availability of tests must be considered in terms of the tests' diagnostic accuracy. Decision analysis was used to compare various techniques for the emergency assessment of suspected aortic dissection.

Methods.—Data for the analysis—including the risks of performing 1 or 2 sequential tests, test accuracy, the risks and benefits of treatment, and the mortality of untreated dissection—were obtained from published studies. The decision analysis model considered patients presenting to the emergency department with chest pain and possible acute dissection of the thoracic aorta. The risks and benefits of the following tests were assessed, alone or in combination: CT, MR, transesophageal echocardiography (TEE), and transthoracic echocardiography (TTE). The effects of delayed testing on the choice of procedure were assessed as well. Thirty-day survival was the main study outcome.

Results.—The clinical probability of aortic dissection did not have to be high for the benefits of testing to outweigh the risks. The threshold probability was only 2% for MRI and 9% for TTE, the most and least reliable procedures, respectively. For patients with less than a 15% probability of dissection, all tests except TTE were adequate to exclude dissection. The results were little affected by delayed testing. For patients with higher probabilities of dissection, a better approach was to do another diagnostic test after the first was negative. At a probability of 15%, the preferred approach was CT followed by aortography; at a probability of 35%, MRI followed by aortography was preferred.

Long delays affected test selection only for patients with a high likelihood of dissection—50% or higher. In this situation, a CT scan performed within 2 hours or a TEE study performed within 6 hours after presentation in the emergency department provided a better survival than an MRI scan performed within 9 hours. In this situation, the benefits of performing a second test after the first test was negative exceeded the risks only if the delay to testing was no longer than 10 hours.

Conclusions.—All patients with suspected aortic dissection—even if the index of suspicion is very low—should undergo diagnostic testing. If the clinical probability of dissection is moderate to high, a second test is indicated if the results of the first are negative. For patients with a high probability of dissection, it is best to order the most readily available test, even if it is less accurate.

▶ This study used a clinical decision methodology to determine the best strategies for evaluating aortic dissection, based on a current review of the literature reporting sensitivity and specificities for a variety of imaging techniques. The most reliable test is thought to be MRI, and the least reliable, transthoracic echocardiography. Using a classical clinical decision-making approach, the authors determined that patients with high clinical likelihood of aortic dissection would require 2 negative diagnostic tests before reliably excluding the diagnosis. The threshold probability for ordering a second test depends on the clinical circumstances and the predictive value of the individual test. The authors also determined that excessive delays could influence survival rates. The major limitations of this study appears to be the assessment of pretest probability based on clinical grounds. There are no clinical rules provided, so the clinical probability of aortic dissection discussed in the paper is not clinically meaningful. Therefore, clinicians still have to rely on their clinical judgment. The take-home message of this paper would appear to be: when your suspicion is high, get a diagnostic test quickly and do not accept a single negative test.

J.E. Calvin, Jr., M.D.

J.E. Parrillo, M.D.

Capacitive Function of the Heart: Influence of Acute Changes in Heart Volume on Mean Right Atrial Pressure
Sheriff DD, Luo Z (St Elizabeth's Med Ctr, Boston)
Am J Physiol 272:H553–H558, 1997   2–15

Objective.—There have been several studies of the ways in which central volume—i.e., the blood volume contained in the central veins, heart, and pulmonary vessels—is affected by various stresses. In terms of central venous pressure, net transfer of a given volume of blood into or out of the cardiac chambers should have the same effect as transfer of the same blood volume into or out of the peripheral organs. Experiments were conducted in pigs to see if reducing the volume of blood in the heart can increase right atrial pressure.

Methods.—Rapid atrial pacing was induced in anesthetized pigs to reduce the time-averaged blood volume contained in the heart. Cardiac output in this state was equalized to that in the resting state, about 2.35 L/min; this was done by balancing the frequency of cardiac contractions against stroke volume to prevent changes in cardiac output from changing central blood volume and pressure. Drugs were used to reduce autonomic reflex mechanisms. The hypothesis tested was that the blood volume distending the central veins determines the mean right atrial pressure and that atrial contractions are the main factor determining the variation in atrial pressure around its central value.

Results.—The change from sinus rhythm to rapid atrial pacing—from 89 to 165 bpm—had little effect on mean arterial pressure. At the start of rapid pacing in 4 of 5 pigs, mean right atrial pressure increased sharply, from 2.8 to 3.5 mm Hg. This appeared to result from a reduction in cardiac blood volume and the resulting increase in central venous volume. The fifth animal had reduced cardiac output as a result of tachycardia. This caused a greater increase in mean right atrial pressure than that caused by a bradycardia-induced reduction in cardiac output.

Conclusions.—As heart rate increases, the heart may play a key role in maintaining or increasing its own filling pressure. Cardiac blood volume seems to be reduced by tachycardia but increased by bradycardia. In ventricular tachycardia and other pathologic conditions, changes in the capacitive function of the heart may play a key role in governing mean atrial pressure.

▶ This animal study concludes that the heart plays an important role in maintaining and raising its own filling pressure when the heart rate rises. I agree with the authors that the most plausible explanation was reciprocal expansion of central venous volume because of the heart's inability to adequately fill. It is likely that the direction of change in right atrial pressure seen with rapid pacing is different than what occurs with physiological exercise when diastolic volumes are known to be well preserved. What is unanswered by this study is what the capacitive function of the splanchnic circulation would be over time under states of rapid increases in the heart rate. It is likely that, over time, the rising right atrial pressure induced by heart rate increases would dissipate.

J.E. Calvin, Jr., M.D.

J.E. Parrillo, M.D.

A Technique to Remove Knotted Pulmonary Artery Catheters

Tan C, Bristow PJ, Segal P, et al (Liverpool Hosp, Sydney, NSW)
Anaesth Intens Care 25:160–162, 1997

2–16

Objective.—There is ongoing debate over the indications for pulmonary artery (PA) catheterization, and the treatment information provided. In addition to catheter-related infection and pulmonary infarction, catheter knotting may occur as a complication. A case of PA catheter knotting is reported, including a technique to remove the knotted catheter.

Case.—Man, 75, was undergoing insertion of a 7.5F, 5-lumen PA catheter through a right subclavian line in preparation for laparotomy. The catheter could not be advanced into the pulmonary outflow tract. A knot in the catheter was unrecognized on chest radiograph. After surgery, it proved impossible to remove the catheter through its introducing sheath. A left internal jugular PA catheter was then successfully placed, after which the knot in the other PA catheter was recognized.

The next day, attempts were made to remove the knotted catheter. A guidewire was placed into the superior vena cava, and passed through the loop in the knot of the PA catheter. A 5F angioplasty balloon catheter was then placed over the guidewire so that the knot was located in the middle part of the balloon. Further traction was placed on the PA to tighten the knot around the balloon. The balloon was then inflated, opening up the knot. This permitted the catheter to be withdrawn further, moving the knot toward the distal tip of the PA catheter. After the procedure was repeated 5 times, the knot was eliminated and the catheter removed.

Conclusions.—A technique for removal of a knotted PA catheter is presented. The method is safer than previously proposed techniques, particularly in patients with coagulopathy. Avoiding multiple attempts at flotation and using the right internal jugular or left subclavian insertion site will help to reduce the risk of catheter knotting.

▶ Another use of a balloon catheter. This time it is to retrieve another balloon catheter. This was a very novel and innovative approach to help solve a problem that, fortunately, is rare.

J.E. Calvin, Jr., M.D.
J.E. Parrillo, M.D.

Very Poor Prognosis in Cases With Extravasation of the Contrast Medium During Angiography

Yasui T, Kishi H, Komiyama M, et al (Osaka City Gen Hosp, Japan)
Surg Neurol 45:560–565, 1996   2–19

Objective.—Patients with rebleeding of a ruptured intracranial aneurysm during the acute stage are believed to have a very poor prognosis. However, the authors' experience suggests that outcomes are still worse for patients with rupture and extravasation of contrast medium during angiography. They compared the outcomes of patients with extravasation vs. those with rerupture under circumstances other than angiography, including factors contributing to the worse outcomes of the former group.

Methods.—A 10-year review identified 641 cases of ruptured intracranial aneurysm. Thirty-six of these patients had rebleeding before surgery could be performed, a rate of 5.6%. Of these, 13 had rebleeding during angiography and 23 under other circumstances. The outcomes of the 2 groups were compared.

Results.—In 80% of patients, rebleeding occurred within 6 hours of the initial rupture. Just 1 of 13 patients with extravasation achieved, according to the Glasgow Outcome Scale, SD—the rest died. In the group with rebleeding under other circumstances, 8 were in GR or MD, 2 were in SD, and 13 died. Patients with extravasation showed a greater deterioration in clinical grade after rebleeding.

Conclusions.—In patients with ruptured intracranial aneurysm, rebleeding during angiography commonly occurs in the acute stage. The prognosis is very bad for patients with extravasation. This review suggests that angiography should be delayed for at least 3–6 hours after the initial rupture.

▶ The authors of this study recommend delaying angiography 3–6 hours if extravasation is found on head CT. This study really doesn't answer the question of when is the best time interval for angiography. Clinical judgment, based on the patient's clinical status and CT findings, is still paramount, but certainly some caution is key.

J.E. Calvin, Jr., M.D.

J.E. Parrillo, M.D.

Effects of Motion on the Performance of Pulse Oximeters in Volunteers

Barker SJ, Shah NK (Univ of Arizona, Tucson; Univ of California, Irvine)
Anesthesiology 85:774–781, 1996   2–20

Introduction.—Pulse oximetry is a standard of care in the operating room and recovery room. The dropout rates in the recovery room are significantly greater than those in the operating room; motion artifact is a common cause of data dropout and false alarms in the awake patient. The accuracy and dropout rates of 3 current pulse oximeters were evaluated during standardized motion in 10 healthy volunteers.

Methods.—The 3 pulse oximeters were Nellcor N-200, Nellcor N-3000, and Masimo SET (prototype). The test hand was strapped to a mechanical motion table and sensors were placed on the second, third, and fourth digits. The ipsilateral hand acted as a stationary control and was monitored with the same pulse oximeters and an arterial cannula. The inspired oxygen concentration was varied by face mask to produce an arterial oxygen saturation rate from 100% to 75%. When pulse oximetry was both constant and changing, the oximeter sensors were attached before and during motion. A continuous digital record was kept of oximeter errors and dropout rates during each experiment.

Results.—If the oximeter was working before motion began, the percentages of time when the instrument displayed a pulse oximetry value within 7% of control were 76% in N-200, 87% in N-3000, and 99% in Masimo. When the oximeter sensor was attached after the beginning of motion, the values were 68% for N-200, 47% for N-3000, and 97% for Masimo. When the alarm threshold was selected as pulse oximetry less than 90%, the positive predictive values were 73% for N-200, 81% for N-3000, and 100% for Masimo.

Conclusions.—Oximeter function was significantly affected by mechanical motions, especially when the sensors were connected during motion. The Masimo unit was superior to the N-200 and N-3000 oximeters during all test conditions, perhaps because the Masimo uses a new paradigm for oximeter signal processing. This may be a significant advance in low signal-to-noise performance.

▶ Motion artifact in pulse oximetry is a problem that we all have learned to live with in the ICU. This well-designed volunteer study is enlightening regarding the sophisticated computer algorithms that improve the rejection of motion artifact. Technology that can minimize motion artifact without increasing equipment cost would be welcome. As the authors suggest, the clinical value of these devices must now be tested in the operating room and ICU.

B.A. Shapiro, M.D.

Accuracy of Pulse Oximetry in Patients With Low Systemic Vascular Resistance
Secker C, Spiers P (Leicester Gen Hosp NHS Trust, England)
Anaesthesia 52:127–130, 1997   2–21

Introduction.—High skin blood flow may cause inaccurate readings from a pulse oximeter in normal volunteers. Abnormal readings can also occur clinically when skin flow is increased, particularly in septic shock, but also with regional or conduction anesthesia or reperfusion after ischemic injury. Pulse oximetry was compared in a population of patients with low systemic vascular resistance and a population with normal or unaffected. Plasma epinephrine and cortisol levels were also unaffected. The warm infusion produced no changes in any measured parameter.

Conclusions.—Mild hypothermia induced by isolated core cooling is associated with an adrenergic response characterized by peripheral sympathetic nervous system activation with no significant adrenocortical or adrenomedullary response. Core cooling produces a shivering-induced increase in metabolic rate, norepinephrine-mediated peripheral vasoconstriction, and increased arterial blood pressure.

▶ This study demonstrates the difference in the physiologic responses between external cooling and core cooling without external cooling. It suggests a potential adrenergic mechanism to explain hypothermia-induced cardiovascular complications. The authors showed that core cooling, in the absence of external cooling, increased peripheral sympathetic nervous system activity by four- to sevenfold without any effect on adrenomedullary or adrenocortical activity. However, because this study involved healthy young individuals, it remains to be seen whether similar changes also happen in elderly patients with other medical problems.

J. Samuel, M.D.

Panic Disorder in Emergency Department Chest Pain Patients: Prevalence, Comorbidity, Suicidal Ideation, and Physician Recognition
Fleet RP, Dupuis G, Marchand A, et al (Université du Québec, Montréal; Univ of Missouri, Columbia)
Am J Med 101:371–380, 1996   2–24

Background.—Psychological factors have long been suspected as a cause of noncardiac chest pain. Recent studies have shown that about 30% of patients with noncardiac chest pain have panic disorder (PD). The current study determined the prevalence of PD in patients with chest pain in one emergency department (ED), psychological distress and recent suicide ideation in patients with and without PD, psychiatric co-morbidity, and physician recognition of PD.

Methods and Findings.—A total of 441 consecutive patients with a chief complaint of chest pain were included in the prospective study. About one fourth met the *DSM-III-R* criteria for PD. Patients with PD had significantly higher panic-agoraphobia, anxiety, depression, and pain scores than patients without PD. Of the patients with PD, 25% had thought about killing themselves in the week preceding their ED visit, compared with 5% of patients without PD. This difference continued to be significant, even after adjustment for coexisting major depression. Of the patients with PD, 57% also met criteria for 1 or more current AXIS I disorders. Although 44% of the patients with PD had a documented history of coronary artery disease, 80% had atypical or nonanginal chest pain. Seventy-five percent were discharged with a diagnosis of "noncardiac pain." Of the patients with PD, 98% were unrecognized by attending cardiologists in the ED.

Conclusions.—Panic disorder is a very distressing condition found to be prevalent among patients with chest pain who visit the ED. The physicians in this study rarely recognized PD. Such lack of recognition may result in the mismanagement of a significant group of distressed patients who may or may not have coronary artery disease.

▶ The authors studied over 400 emergency department patients with chest pain to determine the prevalence of pain associated with panic disorder. Over 25% of the patients met *Diagnostic and Statistical Manual of Mental Disorders* criteria for panic disorder. These patients displayed a higher psychological score for agoraphobia, anxiety, depression, and pain when compared with nonpanic disorder patients. At least one fourth of the patients had recent suicidal ideation, even when controlled for coexisting major depression. Interestingly, many of the panic disorder patients also had a prior documented history of coronary artery disease and, although 75% of them were discharged with noncardiac pain, patients were identified with both organic disease and panic disorder.

The major point in the study is that psychological factors causing cardiac-like pain are not routinely recognized by emergency room physicians and cardiologists, even though earlier recognition facilitates treatment of these patients. Although the authors suggest that early recognition might reduce medical costs, the high proportion of patients with both psychological and organic disease makes a thorough workup of chest pain in these patients imperative. It is not clear whether cost-savings would ensue, especially since the patients surveyed in the study were ambulatory patients who presented themselves to the emergency department and may not be representative of patients who are brought to the hospital by ambulance. Nonetheless, it is important for emergency room physicians and cardiologists to understand the significant impact of psychological disorders on patients with cardiac-like and cardiac chest pain.

R.V. Rege, M.D.

Multivessel Palmaz-Schatz Stenting: Early Results and One-Year Outcome
Laham RJ, Ho KKL, Baim DS, et al (Harvard Med School, Boston; Beth Israel Hosp, Boston)
J Am Coll Cardiol 30:180–185, 1997   2–25

Introduction.—Percutaneous transluminal coronary angioplasty (PTCA) is commonly used in patients with single-vessel coronary artery disease. Its use has been extended to selected patients with multivessel coronary disease. Palmaz-Schatz stenting is associated with a higher success rate and a lower restenosis rate, compared with conventional PTCA. The short-term results of Palmaz-Schatz stenting in patients with multivessel disease were assessed in 103 patients who underwent placement of 273 stents in 212 vessels.

Correlation of Angiographic Morphology and Clinical Presentation in Unstable Angina

Dangas G, Mehran R, Wallenstein S, et al (Mount Sinai Med Ctr, New York)
J Am Coll Cardiol 29:519–525, 1997   2–27

Introduction.—New markers of myocardial injury and necrosis have been developed and are being evaluated in clinical trials, but there is no technology to confirm the diagnosis and severity of unstable angina. Angiographic findings of intracoronary thrombus and complex lesions were directly correlated with the severity of clinical presentation in 284 patients with unstable angina.

Methods.—Cardiac catheterizations were prospectively conducted in 284 patients with unstable angina. A blinded angiographer interpreted all angiograms. Two hundred patients had culprit lesions that were quantitatively analyzed and classified as simple or complex (complex architecture, intracoronary thrombus (ICT), or total occlusion). Flow was measured according to the Thrombolysis in Myocardial Infarction (TIMI) classification. Braunwald classes III, C, and c were sequentially compared with classes <III, <C, and <c, respectively.

Results.—There were significant associations between class III and complex lesions and decreased TIMI flow. Class C angina was significantly associated with complex lesions, ICT, and decreased TIMI flow. Class c angina was significantly correlated with ICT. The degree of stenosis by quantitative angiography was not correlated with any special Braunwald class.

Conclusion.—Complex lesions were independently correlated with clinical severity of unstable angina syndrome. Recent rest pain and refractory or postinfarction unstable angina or both were strongly correlated with the general category of complex lesions, especially with angiographically detected ICT and reduced TIMI flow.

▶ Several groups have now studied the utility of a risk stratification scheme in unstable angina originally proposed by Braunwald. This study is consistent with others that have correlated morphologic features on coronary angiography with clinical presentation. Recent rest pain, refractory pain, and postinfarction angina are all associated with worse outcome and a higher grade of complexity in lesion morphology.

J.E. Calvin, Jr., M.D.

J.E. Parrillo, M.D.

Penetrating Cardiac Injuries
Karmy-Jones R, van Wijngaarden MH, Talwar MK, et al (Henry Ford Hosp, Detroit; Univ of Alberta Hosps, Edmonton, Canada)
Injury 28:57–61, 1997   2–28

Objective.—United States recommendations for dealing with penetrating cardiac injuries are evaluated with respect to the Canadian experience.

Methods.—Between April 1, 1992 and December 31, 1994, a total of 1,054 patients with an Injury Severity Score (ISS) of 12 were admitted to an urban tertiary-care trauma center. Ambulance, emergency department, operating room, hospital records, and autopsy reports were reviewed. Probability of survival (POS) was determined.

Results.—There were 8 patients with blunt myocardial injuries and 8 (7 men) with penetrating injuries. The 8 penetrating injuries were stab wounds; 7 occurred at home, 2 involved alcohol, 4 were assaults, and 3 were self-inflicted. Five patients died, and 3 of 5 with detectable vital signs survived. Six had thoracotomy performed in the emergency department, and 4 of these died. The medical examiner's records showed an additional 76 patients with penetrating chest injuries, 67 of whom were dead at the scene. A literature review revealed that 35% of penetrating wounds involved the right ventricle and 25% the left ventricle. All patients with penetrating thoracic and upper abdominal wounds may have associated cardiac injuries. Unstable patients should be operated on as soon as possible, and a median sternotomy should be performed for anterior penetrating injuries. Pericardiocentesis can reduce mortality when a thoracotomy is performed in the emergency department. Patients with blunt injury, no detectable vital signs, no pupillary responses, and extrathoracic injuries do not survive. Thoracotomy can be beneficial in other patients. Prehospital intubation, fast transport, isolated penetrating injuries, signs of life, single cardiac chamber injury, penetrating injury, stab wounds, and tamponade are associated with survival.

Conclusions.—Three patients survived cardiac stab wounds without neurologic sequelae. All 3 had tamponade. Emergency department thoracotomy should be performed in patients that have a probability of survival.

▶ The incidence of penetrating cardiac injuries in Canada is low and most frequently related to stab wounds. Interestingly, the outcome was reasonable. Outcome is likely related to rapid surgical therapy in the operating room. The authors recommend median sternotomy in anterior penetrating injuries and thoracotomy in posterolateral injuries.

J.E. Calvin, Jr., M.D.

J.E. Parrillo, M.D.

3 Shock

Hypovolemic

Safe Hemoglobin or Hematocrit Levels in Surgical Patients
Lundsgaard-Hansen P (Univ of Berne, Switzerland)
World J Surg 20:1182–1188, 1996   3–1

Objective.—Red blood cells (RBCs) are transfused for their ability to carry oxygen from the lungs to the systemic microcirculation. Clinically, RBC transfusion is "triggered" by accepted "critical levels" of hemoglobin and hematocrit: 10 g/dL and 30%, respectively. It has recently been suggested that these triggers might be set lower to reduce the number of transfusions. The literature on safe hemoglobin and hematocrit levels was reviewed, with a focus on the perioperative period.

Discussion.—In nonseptic states, RBC transfusion can increase oxygen consumption. The response to RBC transfusion in acute sepsis is less predictable; however, if there are signs of a potentially fatal oxygen deficit, the attempt to raise oxygen delivery is warranted. For critically ill patients, anything that increases the cardiac index to supranormal values improves the chances of survival. This may include raising hemoglobin to about 11 g/dL and hematocrit to 33%. Reports as to the general tolerance of anemia vary significantly; critical levels have ranged from 4 or 5 to 11 g/dL for hemoglobin and from 12% or 15% to 33% for hematocrit. All of these estimates are affected by the behavior of certain "non-hemoglobin variables" affecting venous oxygen tensions. Critically ill patients commonly have abnormalities of these non-hemoglobin variables, making them more dependent on high hemoglobin or hematocrit levels to protect against oxygen deficit. This suggests that there is no generally valid transfusion trigger; the critical hemoglobin or hematocrit level must be individualized to the patient. Silent myocardial ischemia appears to play a central role in anemia tolerance. Unless this entity has been excluded, patients older than 40 years should not be subjected to a hemoglobin of less than 10 g/dL or a hematocrit of less than 30%.

Summary.—The use of "critical" hemoglobin and hematocrit values as "triggers" for blood transfusion has been questioned. The literature suggests that the most appropriate trigger will vary by patient and clinical condition. Although the traditional hemoglobin trigger of 10 g/dL has often been dismissed as unsupported, it may still be appropriate for the assessment of individual cases.

▶ Strategies for increasing tissue oxygen delivery have been advocated as a method of increasing survival in critically ill patients. This study reviewed published data on the use of red blood cell transfusions as a means of increasing tissue oxygen delivery. The conclusion drawn from this review is that a target hemoglobin of 11 gm/dL appears to result in the "best outcome" for the nonseptic critically ill adult patient. The potential for silent myocardial ischemia is the rationale that typically drives the use of red blood cell transfusions. The same reported benefit has not been demonstrated in the septic population.

On closer consideration, the whole topic of defining the "optimum" tissue oxygen delivery strategy is confusing and controversial. Unless the oxygen consumption is measured with indirect calorimetry and other variables—including the clinical diagnosis and severity of the illness—are strictly controlled, it is difficult to make any definite conclusions from the literature. It does appear that the earlier claims of oxygen supply dependence do not seem to be operational in most clinical circumstances. In addition, a recent, large, multicenter trial failed to demonstrate that there was a survival benefit associated with therapeutic strategies to increase tissue oxygen delivery.[1]

In regard, specifically, to the use of blood product transfusions, there appears to be a strong movement away from the early and frequent use blood products, unless there is a definite need to rapidly control bleeding or correct a severe anemia in an unstable patient. The definition of a "safe" level of hemoglobin in the acutely ill is a moving target at the present time, and I am not sure that anyone can identify the exact level at this time.

R.A. Balk, M.D.

Reference

1. Gattinoni L, Brazzi L, Pelosi P, et al: A trial of goal-oriented hemodynamic therapy in critically ill patients. *N Engl J Med* 333:1025–1032, 1995.

Central and Regional Hemodynamics During Acute Hypovolemia and Volume Substitution in Volunteers
Riddez L, Hahn RG, Brismar B, et al (Huddinge Univ, Sweden; St Görans Hosp, Stockholm; Univ Hosp, Uppsala, Sweden)
Crit Care Med 25:635–640, 1997   3–2

Objective.—Whereas it is agreed that volume replacement is an important treatment for blood loss of 10% to 20%, there is little information about the blood flow and metabolism in the kidney and liver during "preshock" bleeding. The central and regional hemodynamics and oxygen consumption were measured in healthy volunteers exposed to a 900-mL venesection. The effectiveness of crystalloid and colloid volume substitution in restoring normal circulation was compared in this prospective, randomized, laboratory investigation.

Methods.—Catheters were inserted into the cubital vein, brachial, artery, pulmonary artery, thoracic aorta, right hepatic vein, and left renal artery in 18 fasting male volunteers, aged 21–35 years. Systemic arterial pressure, pulmonary artery pressure, total and central blood volume, extravascular lung water, and liver and renal flow rates were measured, respiratory and blood gases were analyzed, and plasma catecholamine concentrations were determined.

Results.—Withdrawal of 900 mL of blood reduced arterial blood pressure slightly, but decreased cardiac output by 16%, stroke volume by 19%, pulmonary arterial pressures by 25%, central blood volume by 10%, and extravascular water by 10%. Vascular resistance increased in the lung by 32% and in the systemic vascular bed by 18%. Blood flow to the kidneys and liver decreased by 20%, whereas arterial-venous oxygen consumption increased slightly. Norepinephrine increases paralleled increases in peripheral vascular resistance. Epinephrine increases occurred in all volunteers. Oxygen uptake and carbon dioxide elimination in the lungs decreased, whereas other blood-gas and acid-base measures were unchanged. Infusion of 900 mL of 5% albumin restored total blood volume, cardiac output, stroke volume, and systemic vascular resistance significantly more effectively than Ringer's acetate solution. Volume substitution restored liver but not renal blood flow, and returned arterial-venous oxygen content minute volume, oxygen uptake, and carbon dioxide elimination to baseline levels. Heart rate and most central pressures were elevated above baseline values, and blood volume, central blood volume, and pulmonary resistance measures were restored by 1,800 mL of Ringer's acetate.

Conclusions.—Withdrawal of 900 mL of blood reduces cardiac, liver, and renal output. A 5% albumin solution (900 mL) is more effective than Ringer's acetate (900 mL) in restoring blood volume. Infusion of Ringer's acetate in a 1:1 rather than 2:1 ratio of blood lost is more effective at restoring hemodynamic parameters.

▶ This carefully performed study in human volunteers sought to determine the effects of hypovolemia on central and regional blood flows, and on oxygen uptake, and the effects of volume replacement. This study along with previous studies suggest that albumin is more effective than Ringer's at restoring cardiac index to normal. Replacement with Ringer's requires a volume between 100% and 200% of estimated blood loss. This implies that volume replacement with crystalloid is more effective than was previously thought.

J.E. Calvin, Jr., M.D.
J.E. Parrillo, M.D.

Initial Evaluation of Diaspirin Cross-linked Hemoglobin (DCLHb) as a Vasopressor in Critically Ill Patients

Reah G, Bodenham AR, Mallick A, et al (Gen Infirmary at Leeds, England; Baxter Healthcare Corp, Round Lake, Ill)
Crit Care Med 25:1480–1488, 1997

3–3

Introduction.—Experimental studies have shown diaspirin cross-linked hemoglobin (DCLHb)—a highly purified hemoglobin solution extracted from outdated volunteer-donated human erythrocytes—to be an effective blood substitute during resuscitation for hemorrhagic shock. Its vasopressor effect has been accompanied by indirect evidence of improved tissue perfusion, and DCLHb also appears to be a nitric oxide scavenger and a modulator of adrenoreceptor sensitivity. These favorable preliminary results led to an evaluation of the benefits of DCLHb in critically ill patients in shock.

Methods.—The prospective, observational study enrolled 14 patients hospitalized in an ICU with clinical signs of shock. Each had a low systemic vascular resistance index (SVRI) and/or was receiving increasing doses of vasopressor to maintain adequate mean arterial pressure (MAP). All patients had secondary organ dysfunction. Treatment with DCLHb (10 g/dL) consisted of a maximum of five 100-mL boluses administered over 15 minutes and 60 to 90 minutes apart. Reduction in the dose of norep-

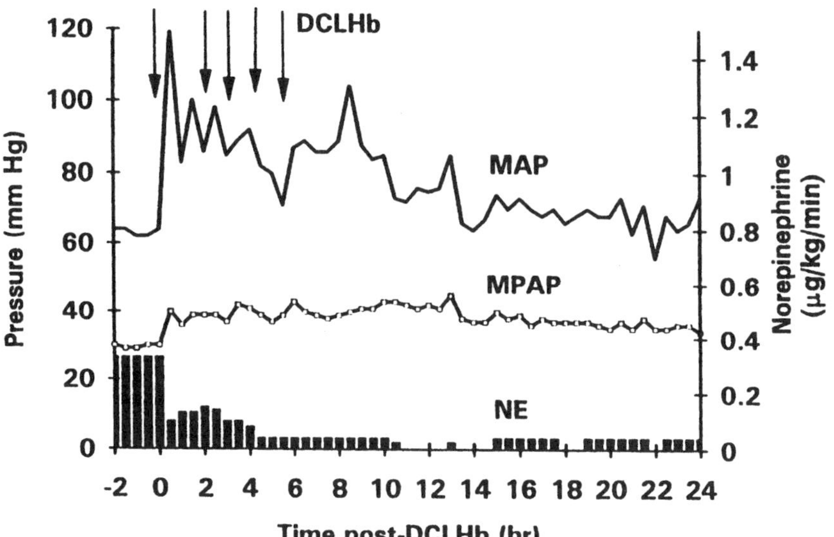

FIGURE 1.—Hemodynamic effects of diaspirin cross-linked hemoglobin (*DCLHb*) over a 24-hour period post infusion in 1 patient. The patient received a total of 5 boluses (500 mL) of DCLHb. *Arrows* indicate each infusion. *Abbreviations: MAP,* mean arterial pressure; *MPAP,* mean pulmonary arterial pressure; *NE,* norepinephrine requirements. (Courtesy of Reah G, Bodenham AR, Mallick A, et al: Initial evaluation of diaspirin cross-linked hemoglobin (DCLHb) as a vasopressor in critically ill patients. *Crit Care Med* 25:1480–1488, 1997.)

inephrine was the main end point in assessing the efficacy of DCLHb as a vasopressor.

Results.—All 14 patients had an immediate vasopressor response within 5 minutes of receiving the initial bolus of DCLHb, an effect that lasted for 72 hours. Norepinephrine requirements were reduced, and cardiac index was significantly decreased at several time points. Throughout the 72-hour period, no significant changes were observed in MAP, heart rate, pulmonary arterial occlusion pressure, SVRI, central venous pressure, or urine output (Fig 1). The pulmonary vascular resistance index increased at 7.5 hours despite nonsignificant increases in mean pulmonary arterial pressure. Total plasma bilirubin levels increased significantly during DCLHb treatment but returned to baseline values within 5 days.

Conclusions.—The vasopressor effect of DCLHb was confirmed in this group of critically ill patients who required vasopressor therapy to maintain MAP. Patients responded within minutes of receiving the infusion, and norepinephrine requirements were reduced with each bolus infusion. The magnitude of response declined, however, with each subsequent bolus.

▶ This is a prospective, observational study only. A control group is really necessary. This novel agent is a highly purified hemoglobin solution modified to optimize the oxygen dissociation curve. The authors speculate on the mechanism of the pressor effect, including enhanced adrenergic responsiveness and attenuation of nitric oxide effects. However, in this study, pressor response was really measured by decreasing epinephrine requirements. It is possible that the cardiac index decreased and systemic vascular resistance increased as a result of the increase in oxygen-carrying capacity.

J.E. Calvin, Jr., M.D.

J.E. Parrillo, M.D.

Septic

The Effects of Ibuprofen on the Physiology and Survival of Patients With Sepsis

Bernard GR, for the Ibuprofen in Sepsis Study Group (Vanderbilt Univ, Nashville, Tenn; et al)
N Engl J Med 336:912–918, 1997   3–4

Background.—Sepsis is associated with significant morbidity and a mortality rate of 30% to 50%. The effect of the inflammatory response and infection on morbidity and mortality is unknown. The production of arachidonic acid metabolites by cyclooxygenase increases in patients with sepsis, but the pathophysiologic role of prostaglandins has not been determined. Studies of animal models of sepsis have shown that treatment with nonsteroidal antiinflammatory drugs decreases physiologic abnormalities and improves survival.

Methods.—In a randomized, double-blind, placebo-controlled trial, intravenous ibuprofen 10 mg/kg (maximum, 800 mg) or placebo was administered every 6 hours to 455 patients with sepsis.

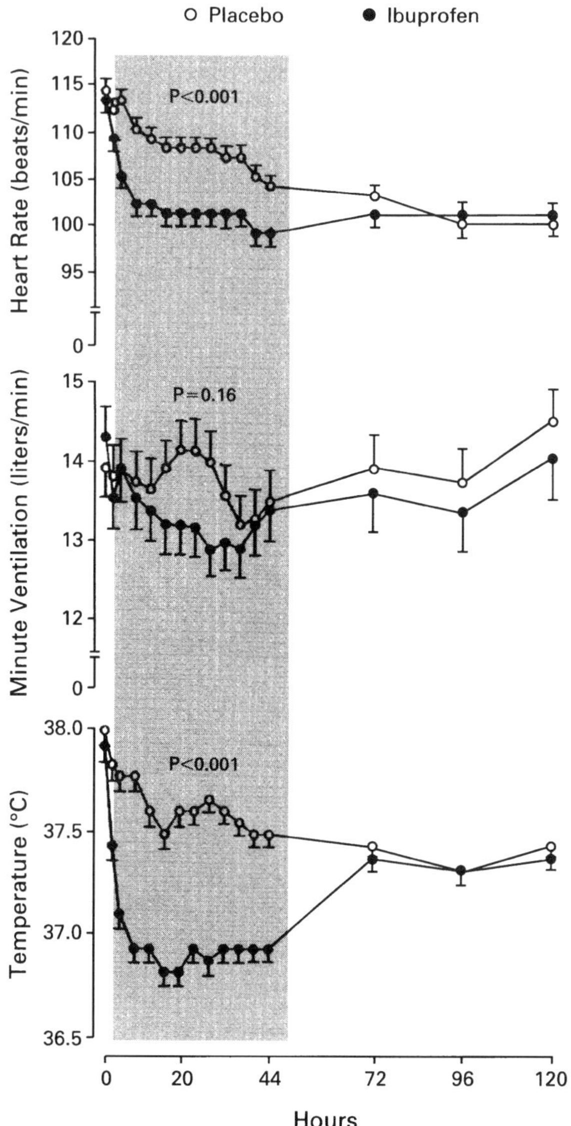

FIGURE 1.—Mean (± SE) temperature, heart rate, and minute ventilation in the study patients. The *shaded area* indicates the duration of administration of the study drug. Data on temperature and heart rate are for the entire study population; data on minute ventilation are for intubated patients only (175 patients in the ibuprofen group and 176 patients in the placebo group). *P* values are for the comparison between the groups with respect to the values measured during administration of the study drug. (Reprinted by permission of *The New England Journal of Medicine*, courtesy of Bernard GR, for the Ibuprofen in Sepsis Study Group: The effects of ibuprofen on the physiology and survival of patients with sepsis. *N Engl J Med* 336:912–918, copyright 1997, Massacheusetts Medical Society. All rights reserved.)

Results.—In patients given ibuprofen, temperature, heart rate, oxygen consumption, lactic acidosis, and urinary levels of prostaglandin and thromboxane decreased significantly (Fig 1). These decreases were not seen in patients given placebo. Treatment with ibuprofen was not associated with increased rate of renal dysfunction, gastrointestinal bleeding, or other adverse effects. Ibuprofen did not lower the incidence or length of shock or acute respiratory distress syndrome, and did not significantly improve survival at 30 days; mortality was 37% in patients given ibuprofen and 40% in patients given placebo.

Discussion.—These results indicate that treatment with ibuprofen in patients with sepsis is safe and can significantly reduce the synthesis of prostaglandin and thromboxane. Ibuprofen did not improve survival or rate of organ failure in these patients. Though patients were given ibuprofen very early, this study did not address the effects of ibuprofen given even earlier or as prophylaxis.

▶ The long-awaited final results of the multicenter trial of ibuprofen in the treatment of patients with severe sepsis and septic shock has now been published. Despite the impressive array of beneficial results in a number of experimental animal models of sepsis, the use of ibuprofen in humans with well-defined sepsis has proven to be useless in regard to the two major endpoints, shock prevention and survival. The use of ibuprofen was associated with a reduction in fever, tachycardia, oxygen consumption, and lactic acidosis. In addition, there was a beneficial blockade on the products of cyclooxygenase metabolism of arachidonic acid, thromboxane and prostacyclin. Again, the scientific community has been misled by an agent which appeared to be extremely promising in the well-controlled environment of the experimental laboratory. Once the intervention is introduced into the extremely variable world of the prospective, randomized, placebo-controlled, double-blind, clinical trial almost anything can happen. Lately, in the field of sepsis, "anything" does not seem to include a positive effect on survival from the use of well-intentioned interventions.

R.A. Balk, M.D.

---

p55 Tumor Necrosis Factor Receptor Fusion Protein in the Treatment of Patients With Severe Sepsis and Septic Shock: A Randomized Controlled Multicenter Trial
Abraham E, for the Ro 45–2081 Study Group (Univ of Colorado, Denver)
JAMA 277:1531–1538, 1997   3–5

Background.—Because tumor necrosis factor-α is implicated in systemic manifestations of severe sepsis and septic shock, the p55 tumor necrosis factor receptor fusion protein (p55-IgG) was evaluated for safety and efficacy in the treatment of severe sepsis or septic shock.

Methods.—A randomized, prospective, multicenter, double-blind, placebo-controlled clinical trial enrolled 498 patients with signs of severe sepsis or septic shock. Interventions, assigned randomly, were placebo or a single infusion of p55-IgG, 0.083, 0.042, or 0.008 mg/kg, all with standard aggressive medical and surgical care. Clinical condition and laboratory values were monitored at baseline (before treatment) and throughout the 28-day protocol. The primary efficacy variable was 28-day mortality from all causes.

Results.—Interim analysis showed no benefit for the 0.008 mg/kg dose of p55-IgG, which was discontinued. A total of 444 patients from the 3 remaining arms of the study were available for the final analysis on day 28. Of those, 197 (44%) were in refractory septic shock at enrollment; the remaining 247 were in the severe sepsis group (including early septic shock). There was a nonsignificant trend toward reduced 28-day mortality from all causes among all patients treated with p55-IgG (5% reduction vs. placebo for 0.042 mg/kg and 15% reduction vs. placebo for 0.083 mg/kg; $P = 0.30$), primarily as a result of decreased mortality among patients with severe sepsis. There was no survival increase among patients with refractory shock. Overall 28-day mortalities among patients with severe sepsis were 23% for the 0.83 mg/kg group, 37% for the 0.042 mg/kg group, and 36% for the placebo group. Reduction in mortality among patients treated for severe sepsis with the 0.083 mg/kg p55-IgG was 36% ($P = 0.07$), greater among patients with baseline hypotension (48%) than among those without (24%). Significantly improved outcome—which included a decrease in mortality from that expected and decreased interleukin-6—was demonstrated in the 0.82 mg/kg group of patients with severe sepsis ($P = 0.01$). Serious adverse events were reported in 65% of patients in the placebo group and 56% in the treatment groups. No hypersensitivity was reported.

Discussion.—Treatment of severe sepsis or early septic shock, but not refractory septic shock, was apparently enhanced by the infusion of 0.083 mg/kg p55-IgG. A large confirmatory clinical trial is underway.

▶ The search for the magical compound that would improve the outcome of patients with severe sepsis and septic shock has again turned toward the inhibition of circulating tumor necrosis factor. This attempt involved the use of p55-IgG to neutralize the proinflammatory cytokine, tumor necrosis factor. This phase 2 dose-defining trial was well designed and involved a prospective, multicenter, double-blind, placebo-controlled approach in patients with well defined severe sepsis and septic shock. Nearly 500 patients were enrolled in the trial and mortality was assessed after 28 days of study.

As with the multitude of past sepsis trials, there was no significant benefit of the inhibitory compound with respect to survival; however, a population was identified for future trials to assess whether this compound has any benefit or role in the management of septic patients. The vast number of negative trials conducted to date is a cause for concern. Perhaps we are asking too much of these various novel therapies, or perhaps we should direct our questions toward a more specific target population.

R.A. Balk, M.D.

Treatment of Severe Systemic Inflammatory Response Syndrome and Sepsis With a Novel Bradykinin Antagonist, Deltibant (CP-0127): Results of a Randomized, Double-blind, Placebo-controlled Trial

Fein AM, for the CP-0127 SIRS and Sepsis Study Group (Winthrop-Univ, Mineola, NY; et al)

JAMA 277:482–487, 1997

3–6

Background.—Despite our best efforts to date, about 1 of every 2 patients with sepsis syndrome and septic shock dies. Drug treatments have been aimed at influencing the systemic inflammatory response syndrome (SIRS), particularly the kinin peptide mediators of this process. Because deltibant blocks the bradykinin receptor B_2 subclass, these investigators examined its role in treating patients with SIRS presumed to be caused by sepsis.

Methods.—Eventually, 504 patients from 47 centers were studied for 28 days. All enrollees had SIRS and either hypotension or evidence of organ system dysfunction in 2 different systems plus suspected infection. Patients were randomized into a placebo group (n = 126) or groups receiving deltibant doses of 0.3 (n = 124), 1.0 (n = 129), or 3.0 (n = 125) µg/kg/min. Placebo (lactated Ringer's solution) or deltibant infusion was started within 12 hours of enrollment in the study and continued for 72 hours.

Findings.—Risk-adjusted survival did not differ statistically in any of the 3 treatment groups, nor was the median time to death significantly longer in any group. In the 112 patients with pure gram-negative infection, after adjusting for severity and assuming a linear dose–response, the largest deltibant dose reduced 28-day mortality significantly compared with placebo (from 50% to 22.2%). Serious adverse effects did not differ significantly among any of the groups.

Conclusions.—Despite its pharmacologic actions, deltibant had little affect on treating SIRS caused by sepsis. The only significant effect of deltibant was seen with the largest dose (3 µg/kg/min) in patients with pure gram-negative sepsis. Further studies of the use of deltibant in this specific situation seem warranted.

▶ The search for the "magic bullet" or the key to improved survival in patients with severe sepsis or SIRS has consumed the efforts of a multitude of investigators and pharmaceutical corporations. There have been refinements in the design and implementation of the phase II and phase III clinical trials along the way, but at this time there has not been a "winning compound or intervention." This is a well-designed prospective, multicentered, randomized, placebo-controlled, double-blind, dose-ranging trial to evaluate the use of a competitive bradykinin antagonist in the treatment of patients with severe sepsis or severe SIRS. As with other trials to discover the elusive "magic bullet" this trial also was unsuccessful. There were suggestions that in a subpopulation of patients with sepsis and SIRS, those with gram-negative infections, there could be a survival benefit. Thus, the success of the trial was in demonstrating safety of the test article and defining the hypothesis for subsequent trials. The sad end to the story is that the subsequent trial, although unpublished as yet, was also *negative.* "Another one bites the dust."

R.A. Balk, M.D.

Effects of Pentoxifylline on Hemodynamics and Oxygenation in Septic and Nonseptic Patients

Bacher A, Mayer N, Klimscha W, et al (Univ of Vienna)
Crit Care Med 25:795–800, 1997   3–7

Introduction.—The main goals in the treatment of sepsis are to achieve a stable hemodynamic and respiratory condition by fluid resuscitation, administration of drugs acting on the circulatory system, and mechanical ventilation. Some of the focus has been directed to the pharmacologic modulation of the immune system and the microcirculation. Pentoxifylline has been shown to reduce the production of free oxygen radicals by neutrophils, and results in marked improvements in tissue oxygenation and microcirculatory blood flow. Few studies have been conducted on the effects of pentoxifylline on hemodynamic function in patients, particularly with inflammatory/infectious diseases. In septic and nonseptic critically ill patients, the effects of pentoxifylline on hemodynamics and systemic oxygenation were evaluated.

Methods.—Nineteen critically ill patients were studied, 12 of whom had a systemic inflammatory response syndrome and were considered to be septic, whereas the other 7 were not septic. All patients were mechanically ventilated, pulmonary and radial artery catheters were inserted, and the dose of catecholamines was kept constant. During a period of 180 minutes at a rate of 100 mL/hr, 5 mg/kg of pentoxifylline was administered intravenously. Before the administration of pentoxifylline, after 2.5 mg/kg of pentoxifylline, after 5 mg/kg of pentoxifylline, and 60 minutes after the termination of pentoxifylline, hemodynamic variables, oxygen transport, oxygen uptake, and the oxygen extraction ratio were determined.

Results.—The mean pulmonary arterial pressure at baseline was significantly different in septic and nonseptic patients (31 ± 5 mm Hg and 26 ± 7 mm Hg, respectively). For septic patients, the pulmonary vascular resistance was 344 ± 121 dyne·sec/cm⁵·m², and for nonseptic patients, it was 233 ± 100 dyne·sec/cm⁵m². Significant increases in heart rate and cardiac index were seen in the septic group. There was a decrease in systemic vascular resistance index and pulmonary vascular resistance index. In the nonseptic group, there were no significant changes in hemodynamic variables. There was a significant increase in oxygen transport and oxygen uptake in both the septic and nonseptic patients, with no change in the oxygen extraction ratio.

Conclusions.—A significant improvement in hemodynamic performance results with the administration of pentoxifylline in septic patients in comparison with that seen in critically ill nonseptic patients. An increase in oxygen transport and oxygen uptake accompanies the better hemodynamic state, with an unchanged oxygen extraction ratio.

▶ The nonspecific phosphodiesterase inhibitor, pentoxifylline, may have a number of potential benefits in the management of septic patients. Included in the list of potential benefits are (1) decreased polymorphonuclear leukocyte (PMNL) production of free oxygen radicals; (2) decreased PMNL expression of cell surface adhesion molecules; (3) decreased endothelial cell release of thromboxane and increased production of prostacyclin, resulting in modulation of platelet aggregation; and (4) decreased tumor necrosis factor release from macrophages and T lymphocytes. This trial evaluated the use of pentoxifylline in 19 consecutive critically ill adult patients who were also receiving renal dose dopamine. The patients were classified according to whether they met the criteria for sepsis/systemic inflammatory response syndrome (SIRS). In the septic/SIRS patients, there was an improvement in hemodynamic function, primarily manifested as an increase in cardiac index and heart rate without changing the pulmonary capillary wedge pressure. Both groups demonstrated an increase in oxygen delivery and oxygen consumption without a change in the oxygen extraction ratio.

This interesting observation sets the stage for future prospective, randomized, placebo-controlled, double-blind trials to better assess the potential utility of pentoxifylline in the management of sepsis. When such a trial is conducted, it would be beneficial to serially measure cytokine levels in an attempt to elucidate the mechanism of benefit.

R.A. Balk, M.D.

Oxygen Transport Patterns in Patients With Sepsis Syndrome or Septic Shock: Influence of Treatment and Relationship to Outcome
Hayes MA, Timmins AC, Yau EHS, et al (St Bartholomew's and Homerton Hosps, London; Charing Cross Hosp, London)
Crit Care Med 25:926–936, 1997   3–8

Introduction.—Numerous studies of critically ill patients report improved survival rates for those with early increases in cardiac index and higher levels of oxygen delivery and oxygen consumption. Despite this relationship, there is controversy over the value of treatment aimed at improving oxygen transport patterns. A retrospective study of patients with sepsis syndrome or septic shock, managed according to 2 different treatment regimens, sought to characterize the hemodynamic and oxygen transport patterns of survivors and nonsurvivors.

Methods.—Seventy-eight patients with sepsis syndrome or septic shock were drawn retrospectively from a randomized trial of patients at risk of multiple organ failure. All patients received controlled oxygen therapy on admission to the ICU. If volume expansion to an optimal pulmonary artery occlusion pressure did not achieve therapeutic goals (cardiac index of

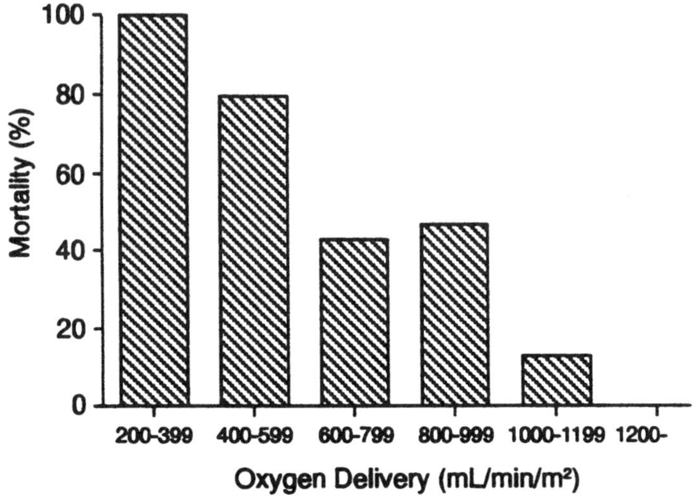

FIGURE 5.—Relationship between maximal oxygen delivery (at time of maximal resuscitation) and outcome. (Courtesy of Hayes MA, Timmins AC, Yau EHS, et al: Oxygen transport patterns in patients with sepsis syndrome or septic shock: Influence of treatment and relationship to outcome. *Crit Care Med* 25:926–936, 1997.)

greater than 4.5 L/min/m^2, oxygen delivery of more than 600 mL/min/m^2, and oxygen consumption of greater than 170 mL/min/m^2), patients were randomized to treatment or control groups. The treatment group received dobutamine (5 to 200 µg/min) to increase cardiac index and oxygen delivery; controls were given dobutamine only if the cardiac index was less than 2.8 L/min/m^2. All patients received norepinephrine (0.05 to 10 µg/ kg/min) if required to maintain mean arterial pressure at 80 mm Hg. Measurements of hemodynamic, oxygen transport, and lactate values were obtained at frequent intervals.

Results.—In both the treatment and control groups, survivors significantly increased cardiac index and oxygen delivery in response to maximal resuscitation (Fig 5). They also had a significant increase in oxygen consumption, despite an associated decrease in oxygen extraction. Nonsurvivors from both groups had significant increases in cardiac index and oxygen delivery, but oxygen extraction decreased and oxygen consumption was unchanged. Compared with survivors, nonsurvivors had significantly lower maximum increases in oxygen delivery and oxygen consumption and exhibited persistently high lactate concentrations.

Conclusion.—Survivors and nonsurvivors of septic syndrome and septic shock had qualitatively similar hemodynamic and oxygen transport responses, whether allocated to dobutamine or control groups. But in both groups, survivors responded with greater increases in cardiac index, left ventricular stroke work index, and oxygen delivery, and their lactate concentrations were lower.

▶ The controversy surrounding the use of strategies to increase oxygen delivery and oxygen consumption in critically ill patients persists, despite recent large-scale multicenter trials and concerns about mathematical coupling.[1-3] This retrospective review of a subgroup of patients enrolled in a sepsis trial evaluated the use of dobutamine dosed to achieve therapeutic goals (cardiac index greater than 4.5 L/min/m², oxygen delivery greater than 600 mL/min/m², and oxygen consumption greater than 170 mL/min/m²) vs. standard therapy of sepsis syndrome and septic shock after adequate volume resuscitation. Serial hemodynamic, oxygen transport, and lactate measurements were performed.

The authors found that survivors of severe sepsis were able to increase their cardiac index, oxygen delivery, and oxygen consumption and had a decrease in the oxygen extraction and oxygen extraction ratio. In nonsurvivors, there was an increase in the cardiac index and in oxygen delivery, but there was a significant decrease in oxygen extraction and no change in oxygen consumption. Overall, the oxygen delivery and oxygen consumption were significantly lower in nonsurvivors, compared with survivors. The nonsurvivors also had persistently elevated whole-blood arterial lactate levels. The inability of nonsurvivors to increase their oxygen consumption and oxygen extraction in the setting of increased oxygen delivery may be a marker of poor cardiac reserve that then manifests as poor outcome.

It would be preferable to repeat this trial in a prospective fashion at multiple centers and to control the treatment protocols related to oxygen delivery strategies. In this trial, the oxygen consumption must be measured using indirect calorimetry. After such a trial is completed, perhaps we will then truly understand which path to take in the management of oxygen delivery in critically ill patients.

R.A. Balk, M.D.

References

1. Gattinoni L, Brazzi L, Pelosi P, et al: A trial of goal-oriented hemodynamic therapy in critically ill patients. *N Engl J Med* 333:1025–1032, 1995.
2. Phang PT, Cunningham KF, Ronco JJ, et al: Mathematical coupling explains dependence of oxygen consumption on oxygen delivery in ARDS. *Am J Resp Crit Care Med* 150:318–323, 1994.
3. Ronco JJ, Fenwick JC, Wiggs BR, et al: Oxygen consumption is independent of increases in oxygen delivery by dobutamine in septic patients who have normal or increased plasma lactate. *Am Rev Respir Dis* 147:25–31, 1993.

Whole Gut Washout for Severe Sepsis: Review of Technique and Preliminary Results

Alverdy J, Piano G (Univ of Chicago)
Surgery 121:89–94, 1997   3–9

Background.—Luminal intestinal flora may have a significant role in sepsis syndrome. Over time, positive pressure ventilation, antibiotic therapy, total parenteral nutrition, and vasoactive agents may compromise the microecology of the intestinal tract. In animal models, it has been shown that catabolic stress can disturb the luminal microbial flora and impair normal defense strategies that contain these mucosal pathogens. Animal models indicate that a gut-driven proinflammatory state may cause multiple organ failure, but human models have not supported this.

Methods.—The feasibility and safety of a whole gut washout procedure was studied in 5 critically ill patients with sepsis syndrome. High volume polyethylene glycol-3500 was administered to all patients. Body temperature, white blood cell count, and ventilatory indices were measured 24 hours before and after gut washout.

Results.—In the 5 patients, a significant decrease in febrile response occurred after whole gut washout. PaO_2, positive end-expiratory pressure, and peak airway pressure improved. Whole gut washout with polyethylene glycol was well tolerated in 4 of 5 patients.

Discussion.—These results show that whole gut washout can be safely performed in critically ill patients with sepsis. This treatment may help clarify the mechanism of systemic inflammation in the intestinal tract during severe catabolic stress. Larger studies are needed to test the efficacy of this treatment in critically ill patients.

▶ The authors present 5 cases of patients who had severe ongoing sepsis and who were treated with a high-volume polyethylene glycol-3500 whole gut washout procedure. Although anecdotal, the cases show the marked improvement of the patients. This was especially true in 2 patients who had very dramatic resolution of their septic symptoms. The premise behind whole gut washout is that removal of bacteria and stool from the gut eliminates a source of endotoxin and bacterial contamination to the vascular system. The results presented are limited to clinical responses, and there was no evidence presented that whole bowel washout decreased reflux of endotoxin or bacteria into the vascular system from the bowel. The results are interesting and provocative. It is shown that whole gut washout can be performed safely, but this needs to be studied in a larger number of patients. In addition, more study is needed to determine the mechanism by which whole gut washout improves the septic course of these patients.

R.V. Rege, M.D.

Cytokine Profile and Correlation to the APACHE III and MPM II Scores in Patients With Sepsis
Presterl E, Staudinger T, Petterman M, et al (Univ of Vienna)
Am J Respir Crit Care Med 156:825–832, 1997   3–10

Introduction.—In the care of critically ill patients, sepsis is a major problem. Mortality of patients with sepsis approximates 30% despite the availability of potent antibiotics and intensive supportive care. To assess the acute clinical condition of seriously ill patients with sepsis, several prognostic scoring systems have been used. During the course of sepsis in patients with proven infection, the roles of tumor necrosis factor-α, interleukin-6, tumor necrosis factor–soluble receptor, interleukin-12, and C-reactive protein levels were defined. The blood cytokine levels were correlated with the clinical condition found in other scoring systems to evaluate whether repeated measurement of blood cytokine levels may contribute to mortality risk estimation of clinical scoring systems.

Methods.—Determinations were made on days 1–7, 14, 21, and 28 of tumor necrosis factor-α, interleukin-6, tumor necrosis factor–soluble receptor, interleukin-12, and C-reactive protein levels, as well as the Acute Physiology and Chronic Health Evaluation III (APACHE III) scores, in 35 patients who had systemic inflammatory response syndrome of infectious origin. At the time of admission into the study, an assessment was also made of the Mortality Probability Models II (MPM II) sepsis score.

Results.—On day 1, the MPM II sepsis score correlated with interleukin-6 plasma levels. On days 2–7, the APACHE III scores correlated with plasma levels of tumor necrosis factor–soluble receptor. On days 3–7, the APACHE III scores correlated with plasma levels of interleukin 6, and on days 4–7, the APACHE III scores correlated with plasma levels of C-reactive protein. Between survivors and nonsurvivors and between patients with and without shock, the MPM II sepsis score, the APACHE III score, and interleukin-6, C-reactive protein, and tumor necrosis factor–soluble receptor levels were significantly different.

Conclusions.—Only in the survivor group was there a significant decrease of the APACHE III scores, and interleukin-6 and C-reactive protein levels over the study period. The risk of estimation of mortality could not be found with the dynamics of tumor necrosis factor-α or interleukin-12 plasma levels.

▶ This study correlated plasma cytokines with 2 prognostic scoring systems. The authors found that MPM II and the APACHE III scores correlated with plasma levels of interleukin-6 (IL-6), tumor necrosis factor–soluble receptor (TNF-sR), and C-reactive protein (CRP). However, the correlations were different depending on what day the samples were obtained. Whether plasma IL-6 and/or CRP will improve the prognostic scoring systems has yet to be determined and would require "real-time" assay to be of any clinical value. The technology for providing real-time cytokine analysis exists, but industry is hesitant to spend the money required to bring the equipment on line until there is proven clinical usefulness of having real-time cytokine analysis.

L.C. Casey, M.D., Ph.D.

Epidemiology of Sepsis Syndrome in 8 Academic Medical Centers

Sands KE, for the Academic Medical Center Consortium Sepsis Project Working Group (Harvard Med School, Boston, et al)
JAMA 278:234–240, 1997

Background.—Sepsis syndrome, in which organ perfusion is altered as a systemic response to infection, is a major cause of death among hospitalized patients. However, little is known about its epidemiology on a hospital-wide basis; this information would have important implications for research. The epidemiology of sepsis syndrome was examined in a prospective, multicenter study.

Methods.—The study used data from 8 academic tertiary care centers. At each center, sepsis monitoring was performed in a weighted random sample of ICU patients, non-ICU patients who had blood cultures drawn, and all patients receiving a novel therapeutic agent or dying in the emergency department or ICU. The diagnosis of sepsis syndrome was made by the presence of a positive blood culture or the combination of fever, tachypnea, tachycardia, clinically suspected infection, and any 1 of 7 confirmatory criteria. On the basis of the number of cases observed, the observation period, and the sampling fraction, total cases expected annually were estimated.

Results.—In the total of 12,759 patients monitored, there were 1,342 documented episodes of sepsis syndrome. The data suggested a hospital-wide incidence of 20 cases per 100 admissions, or 2.8 cases per 1,000 patient-days. The various centers varied by as much as 3 times in unadjusted attack rate of sepsis syndrome; however, the variation from expected was not significant after adjustment for differences in organ transplant population. Of extrapolated cases, 59% were in ICU patients, 11% in non-ICU patients with positive blood cultures, and 30% in non-ICU patients with negative blood cultures. One fourth of patients with sepsis syndrome were in septic shock at the time of onset. Twenty-eight percent had confirmed bloodstream infection, most often with Gram-positive organisms. One-month mortality was 34% and 5-month mortality, 45%.

Conclusions.—Sepsis syndrome is a common condition in academic hospitals, depending on the patient population. Many cases occur in non-ICU patients. This information will help guide the planning and treatment of sepsis syndrome in hospitals, particularly as expensive new treatment agents become available.

▶ The participating members of the Academic Medical Centers Consortium are to be congratulated for this report, which attempted to assess the incidence and epidemiology of sepsis both in and out of the ICU environment. Such a report should add greatly to our understanding of this elusive process we term sepsis and could validate or refute the new definitions that were posed by the SCCM/ACCP Consensus Conference.[1] Unfortunately, the study group modified the definitions put forth by the Consensus Conference for this trial and proposed new criteria for the definition of sepsis syndrome.

The new definition is a modification of the original sepsis syndrome definition proposed by Bone and colleagues.[2] The findings of the consortium are interesting and reflect changes over the past decades. The mortality rate of severe sepsis and septic shock continues to be in the 30% to 40% range and approximately 25% of these patients met the septic shock definition at the time of identification. Only 28% of this population had positive blood cultures and it now appears that the Gram-positive organisms have become the most frequent identifiable cause of severe sepsis and septic shock. Another interesting observation was the increase in mortality rate up to 45% at 5 months that was seen in these patients over time. This highlights both the significance of the septic insult and the major contribution of the patient's underlying health status.

R.A. Balk, M.D.

References

1. American College of Chest Physicians–Society of Critical Care Medicine Consensus Conference: Definitions for sepsis and organ failure and guidelines for the use of innovative therapies in sepsis. *Crit Care Med* 20:864–875, 1992.
2. Bone RC, Fisher C Jr, Clemmer TP, et al: Sepsis syndrome: A valid clinical entity. *Crit Care Med* 17:389–393, 1989.

Magnitude and Duration of the Effect of Sepsis on Survival
Quartin AA, for the Department of Veterans Affairs Systemic Sepsis Cooperative Studies Group (Univ of Miami, Fla)
JAMA 277:1058–1063, 1997   3–12

Introduction.—Sepsis is viewed as a deadly acute disease, with most studies addressing outcomes of 30 days or fewer. In the long-term after an episode of sepsis, the risk of death appears to be higher than explained by comorbidity, suggesting that the sepsis has some prolonged effect beyond the episode itself. The magnitude and duration of the effect of an episode of sepsis on patient survival were analyzed.

Methods.—The study included 1,505 patients who had probable sepsis and were screened for inclusion in the Department of Veterans Affairs Cooperative Study of Corticosteroids in Systemic Sepsis during the 1980s. The controls were 91,830 nonpsychiatric patients who were free of infection and discharged from the same medical centers during the same approximate period. The 2 groups were compared for mortality during the 8 years after the index hospitalization. The comparison was based on a proportional hazards model constructed from the characteristics of the control group. The relative contributions of sepsis and underlying disease to mortality were assessed.

Results.—Throughout the 8-year follow-up period, the risk of death was higher for patients with sepsis than it was for the control group. One-year mortality from nonseptic causes among patients with sepsis, as predicted from the model, was 26%. This figure was similar for patients with uncomplicated or severe sepsis or septic shock. For the first 5 years after screening, the daily risk of death for patients with sepsis was greater than that predicted by the model. Thereafter, the risk was similar to that observed in patients with similar underlying disease but without sepsis. For the first year, the hazard rate associated with sepsis rose along with the severity of the septic episode. For patients in the septic group who survived for 30 days, the mean life span was reduced from a predicted 8.03 years to 4.08 years. Within the first 30 days after screening, the septic group had 452 more deaths than predicted. Within the first year among 30-day survivors, there were 192 more deaths. Among 1-year survivors, there were 51 more deaths within 5 years.

Conclusions.—Sepsis increases mortality risk not only within the first 30 days but also for up to 5 years after the septic episode. This is so, even with adjustment for comorbid conditions. The severity of sepsis influences the risk of death for the first year after the episode. Studies of treatment for sepsis should consider possible late benefits because some of these treatments may improve long-term survival without apparent immediate benefits.

▶ This interesting report used the extremely large Veterans Administration database of patients from the mid-1980s to determine the impact of an episode of severe sepsis on long-term prognosis. Although this study can be criticized for its methods and the fact that the study population was identified and treated 12 years ago, it nonetheless brings out a conclusion that many have suspected for some time. This conclusion centers on the finding that there was an increased 8-year mortality rate among the recovered patients who had septic shock, compared with a matched control group. This supports the hypothesis that there may be either a genetic or other immune system abnormality that may be responsible for the increased predilection to the septic process and may have a role in the subsequent increase in the 8-year mortality rate. The observed postsepsis survival rate was 50% of the nonseptic population, even with corrections for the underlying disease process. More investigations are warranted to further evaluate this observation and to uncover the process that may be responsible.

R.A. Balk, M.D.

Sepsis and Fat Metabolism
Samra JS, Summers LKM, Frayn KN (Radcliffe Infirmary, Oxford, England)
Br J Surg 83:1186–1196, 1996   3–13

Sepsis is a frequent complication of surgery and is associated with changes in lipid metabolism. Fats are the preferred fuels for oxidation in such patients, yet their fat mobilization exceeds fat oxidation. Improving fat oxidation could provide more energy for cellular repair mechanisms.

However, these changes in lipid metabolism have significantly different effects in the septic state. For example, the metabolism of nonesterified fatty acids (NEFAs) in a nonseptic state produces ketone bodies, but in sepsis, the increased NEFA levels actually produce fewer ketone bodies (presumably because of esterification in the liver). Furthermore, the increase of very-low-density lipoprotein levels, leading to hypertriglyceridemia, is thought to play a protective role in the septic patient. These changes must be kept in mind when considering exogenous lipid therapy.

The administration of exogenous lipids can help meet the increased metabolic fuel demands of these patients. However, they also can increase NEFA levels even more, and they can exacerbate the hypertriglyceridemia. Thus, they should constitute no more than 30% to 60% of the nonprotein energy intake in patients with sepsis. Because fatty acids help regulate the immune response, it can be altered by changing the composition of the different fatty acids being delivered. For example, the administration of n-3 fatty acids has been shown to shorten the hospital stay in these patients.

Parenteral or enteral routes can be used to deliver the exogenous lipids, although the parenteral route is associated with a greater likelihood of gross lipemia. Thus, in all patients receiving exogenous lipids, but particularly in those receiving lipids by the parenteral route, lipid tolerance should be monitored closely.

▶ Nutrition has been emphasized as an increasingly important aspect of the management of critical illness. The role of lipids has received a lot of attention as a vital component of the fuel for metabolic functions, as well as a possible beneficial effect on body defense mechanisms. This article reviews the complex alterations in lipid metabolism and their relationship to the inflammatory mediators that are activated in the setting of sepsis. The specific role of lipid emulsions as a fuel source and as a modifier of the host–immune response are reviewed, but much is unanswered at this time and deserving of further research efforts.

R.A. Balk, M.D.

Nitric Oxide (NO) Production Correlates With Renal Insufficiency and Multiple Organ Dysfunction Syndrome in Severe Sepsis

Groeneveld PHP, Kwappenberg KMC, Langermans JAM, et al (Univ Hosp Leiden, The Netherlands; British Biotechnology Limited, Cowley, Oxford, England)
Intensive Care Med 22:1197–1202, 1996   3–14

Background.—Mortality from septic shock in patients with overwhelming infection from gram-negative or gram-positive microorganisms is from 20% to 60%. The hemodynamic abnormalities are characterized by peripheral vasodilatation with lowered sensitivity to catecholamines. It has been shown that peripheral vasodilatation in septic shock is related to production of nitric oxide by vascular endothelial cells. It is unclear if

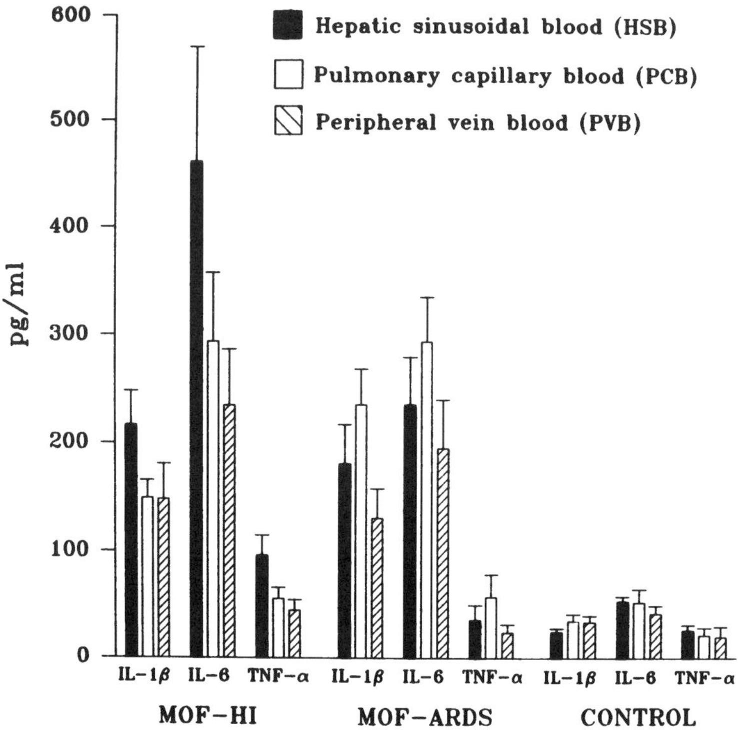

FIGURE 1.—Mean ± SE serum levels of IL-1β, IL-6, and TNF-α from the three different sites of blood sampling in the MOF groups and the control group in the study of regional concentrations. (Courtesy of Douzinas EE, Tsidemiadou PD, Pitardis MT, et al: The regional production of cytokines and lactate in sepsis-related multiple organ failure. *Am J Respir Crit Care Med* 155:53–59, 1997. Official Journal of the American Thoracic Society. Copyright 1997 American Lung Association.)

organ failure (MOF). Sepsis and MOF are also associated with overproduction of lactate, which may be a marker of tissue hypoxia. Organ-specific patterns of cytokine and lactate concentrations were assessed in patients with MOF.

Methods.—The study included 10 patients with MOF and hepatic involvement (MOF-HI), 8 patients with MOF and adult respiratory distress syndrome (MOF-ARDS), and 5 control patients with head injury. In each patient, blood was obtained from the hepatic vein, pulmonary capillaries, and peripheral veins for measurement of interleukin (IL)-1β, IL-6, and TNF-α and lactate. In addition, arteriovenous pulmonary concentration gradients of these cytokines and lactate were studied in 10 patients.

Results.—For patients in the MOF-HI group, mean IL-1β level was 216 pg/mL in the hepatic sinusoidal blood, 149 in the pulmonary capillary blood, and 148 in the peripheral venous blood. Mean IL-6 levels were 461, 293, and 234, respectively. For patients in the MOF-ARDS group, IL-1β levels were 180 pg/mL in the hepatic sinusoidal blood, 235 in the pulmonary capillary blood, and 130 in the peripheral venous blood. Corresponding values for IL-6 were 235, 280, and 194, respectively. The pattern of differences in TNF-α levels was comparable (Fig 1).

Mean lactate levels were, for patients in the MOF-HI group, 3.1 mmol/L in the hepatic sinusoidal blood, 1.5 mmol/L in the pulmonary capillary blood, and 1.3 mmol/L in the peripheral venous blood; and in the MOF-ARDS group, 1.1, 1.8, and 1.0 mmol/L, respectively. For the liver and lungs, the 2 MOF groups differed significantly in the levels of all substances measured. The study of transpulmonary gradients found lower cytokine and lactate levels in arterial blood than in mixed venous blood for patients in the MOF-HI group, but the opposite pattern in MOF-ARDS patients.

Conclusions.—For patients with MOF, cytokine excretion continues to occur mainly from the organs involved in sepsis-related organ failure, even when peripheral venous blood levels are normal. Regional lactate production occurs on a similar basis, particularly in the hepatic veins of MOF patients with hepatic involvement. For patients with liver failure, the pulmonary alveolar capillary bed seems to play a major role in lactate metabolism.

▶ This study measured cytokines and lactate production across the lungs and across the liver in patients with either acute lung injury or acute liver injury. They found that whether an organ metabolizes or releases cytokines and lactate depends on the severity of organ injury. For instance, if the lungs are not injured but the liver is, the lungs take up cytokines and metabolize lactate. On the other hand, if the lungs are injured, the lungs produce both lactate and cytokines. While this is interesting information, it has little practical use for the practicing clinician.

L.C. Casey, M.D., Ph.D.

HSP Induction Inhibits iNOS mRNA Expression and Attenuates Hypotension in Endotoxin-challenged Rats

Hauster GJ, Dayao EK, Wasserloos K, et al (Georgetown Univ, Washington, DC; Univ of Pittsburgh, Pa; Children's Hosp Med Ctr, Cincinnati, Ohio)
Am J Physiol 271:H2529–H2535, 1996   3–17

Introduction.—A highly conserved stress response, the heat shock response, attenuates inflammatory gene expression and confers cytoprotection under nonthermal and thermal stimuli. Different heat shock proteins (hsp) are expressed, depending on the stimulus and the cell type. Survival rates have been improved after endotoxin challenge in rats with lipopolysaccharide when the animals had prior induction of hsp 70 by external heating or by the administration of sodium arsenate. Induction of nitric oxide synthase, release of nitric oxide, and suppression of vascular reactivity mediate endotoxin-induced hypotension. The effect of hsp induction in vivo on the following effects was studied: inducible nitric oxide synthase messenger RNA (mRNA) expression in vivo; hypotension in vivo, and suppression of contraction of mesenteric vessels to norepinephrine ex vivo.

Methods.—Heat shock protein–inducer sodium arsenite (6 mg/kg IV) or saline as control was used to treat rats. Saline control or 10 mg/kg of *Escherichia coli* lipopolysaccharide O127:B8 IV was used to challenge the rats 17 hours later.

Results.—Attenuation of lipopolysaccharide-induced hypotension in vivo, reversal of the lipopolysaccharide-induced hyporesponsiveness to norepinephrine ex vivo in isolated mesenteric arteries, inhibition of lipo-polysaccharide-mediated inducible nitric oxide synthase mRNA induction, and expression of hsp 70 mRNA and of hsp 70 and heme oxygenase-1 proteins were the results of arsenite pretreatment.

Conclusion.—By blocking lipopolysaccharide-induced inducible nitric oxide synthase expression, induction of hsp expression protects rats from lipopolysaccharide. This leads to inhibition of the overproduction of nitric oxide and reverses lipopolysaccharide-induced hypotension and lipopoly-saccharide-induced vasoplegia. Although it is still not known how suppression of inducible nitric oxide synthase by hsp occurs, there is an alteration in gene expression characterized by transient inhibition of transcription and translation of various genes, with priority given to substantial expression of hsp.

▶ The induction of heat shock proteins (hsp) is a highly conserved response (from bacteria to humans) which causes cytoprotection to both thermal as well as non-thermal stimuli. The induction of hsp also attenuates inflammatory gene expression. This article reports that the induction of hsp inhibits nitric oxide expression which has been linked to endotoxin-induced hypotension in rats. This article has no direct clinical application at the present time, but it makes you wonder whether we should stop using Tylenol to control fevers. Maybe fever is beneficial and provides a cytoprotective response.

L.C. Casey, M.D., Ph.D.

Left Ventricular Systolic and Diastolic Function in Septic Shock
Poelaert J, Declerck C, Vogelaers D, et al (Univ Hosp, Gent, Belgium; Free Univ, Amsterdam)
Intensive Care Med 23:553–560, 1997   3–18

Objective.—The mechanism responsible for myocardial depression resulting from septic shock has not been explained. Left ventricular (LV) diastolic filling characteristics in persistently vasopressor-dependent patients with septic shock were assessed using transesophageal 2-dimensional color and Doppler echocardiography (TEE).

Methods.—Transesophageal echocardiography was performed at a midpapillary short axis view of the LV to measure end-systolic and end-diastolic areas; at the level of the mitral valve to measure early (E) and late

(A) filling parameters; and at the level of the right upper pulmonary vein to measure systolic (S) and diastolic (D) filling characteristics in 31 patients with septic shock who were in circulatory failure for more than 48 hours and required ventilatory support. Patients were 23 men and 8 women, with a mean age of 53 years. Hemodynamic variables were monitored using the pulmonary artery. All parameters were described as maximal flow velocity, time velocity integral, and flow time.

Results.—There were 25 evaluable patients. Transesophageal echocardiography identified 3 types of patients based on analysis of the transmitral and pulmonary vein flow characteristics: E/A greater than 1 and S/D greater than 1; E/A greater than 1 and S/D less than 1 in patients with normal LV contractility; E/A less than 1 and S/D less than 1 in patients with global LV dysfunction. Group 3 patients were significantly older than patients in the other 2 groups and showed diastolic dysfunction and ventricular systolic dysfunction.

Conclusions.—Three patterns of septic shock were demonstrated, ranging from normal LV contractility through diastolic dysfunction, to global LV dysfunction. Additional studies are needed to investigate LV diastolic dysfunction in these patients.

▶ This study extends our knowledge about the cardiovascular abnormalities in septic shock by identifying a group of patients in septic shock with predominant diastolic dysfunction. It is unclear from the design of the study whether the abnormalities might have predated the episode of septic shock or whether the abnormalities were reversible. If the abnormalities had disappeared once the sepsis had resolved, the argument would have been more convincing.

J.E. Calvin, Jr., M.D.

J.E. Parrillo, M.D.

Cytokines, Nitrite/Nitrate, Soluble Tumor Necrosis Factor Receptors, and Procalcitonin Concentrations: Comparisons in Patients With Septic Shock, Cardiogenic Shock, and Bacterial Pneumonia
de Werra I, Jaccard C, Corradin SB, et al (Centre Hospitalier Universitaire Vaudois-Lausanne, Switzerland; Inst of Biochemistry, Basel, Switzerland; Institut Gustave Roussy, Villejuif, France)
Crit Care Med 25:607–613, 1997   3–19

Introduction.—Proinflammatory cytokines are thought to play a key pathogenetic role in septic shock. The role of nitric oxide in septic shock is unclear. Procalcitonin is a newly recognized marker of sepsis, of unknown metabolic action. Plasma levels of tumor necrosis factor (TNF)-α, interleukin (IL)-6, soluble TNF receptors, nitrite/nitrate, and procalcitonin were measured in patients with septic shock, cardiogenic shock, and bacterial pneumonia without shock.

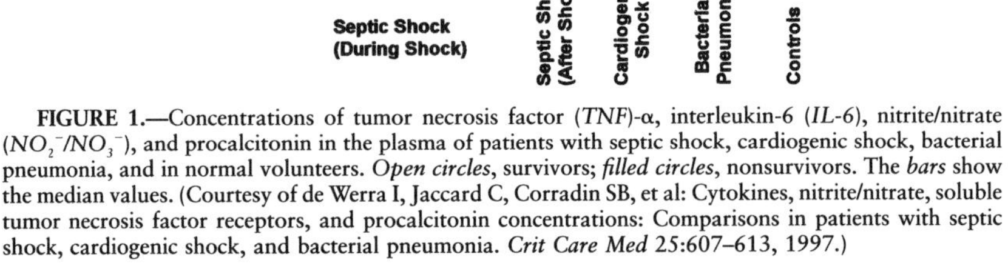

FIGURE 1.—Concentrations of tumor necrosis factor (*TNF*)-α, interleukin-6 (*IL-6*), nitrite/nitrate (NO_2^-/NO_3^-), and procalcitonin in the plasma of patients with septic shock, cardiogenic shock, bacterial pneumonia, and in normal volunteers. *Open circles*, survivors; *filled circles*, nonsurvivors. The *bars* show the median values. (Courtesy of de Werra I, Jaccard C, Corradin SB, et al: Cytokines, nitrite/nitrate, soluble tumor necrosis factor receptors, and procalcitonin concentrations: Comparisons in patients with septic shock, cardiogenic shock, and bacterial pneumonia. *Crit Care Med* 25:607–613, 1997.)

Methods.—All mediators were measured in 15 patients with septic shock, during both the shock and recovery phases; 7 patients with cardiogenic shock during the recovery phase; and 7 patients with severe bacterial pneumonia. The values were compared with those of normal volunteers. The mediators' predictive value in identifying patients with septic shock was assessed.

Results.—Plasma concentrations of TNF-α were 53–131 pg/mL in patients with septic shock, peaking during the acute phase; 32 pg/mL in bacterial pneumonia; and nonelevated in cardiogenic shock. Acute septic shock was associated with the highest concentrations of IL-6, 85–385 pg/mL. Interleukin-6 concentrations were elevated to 78 pg/mL in patients with cardiogenic shock, but were normal in patients with bacterial pneumonia. All 3 patient groups had elevated levels of soluble TNF receptors, particularly those with septic shock. Patients with septic shock had nitrite/nitrate levels of 72–140 mmol; these levels were less than 40 mmol in all other groups. The only group with a significant elevation in procalcitonin concentration were the patients with septic shock, with levels of 72–135 ng/mL. Plasma nitrite/nitrate and procalcitonin concentrations were the best predictors of septic shock (Fig 1).

Conclusions.—Inflammation, not shock, is the cause of increased proinflammatory cytokine levels, these findings suggest. Measuring nitrite/nitrate and procalcitonin concentrations may be useful tests for identifying patients with septic shock. Infection and shock appear to play complementary roles in the stimulation of circulating proinflammatory cytokines.

▶ The authors undertook a trial to define the markers of inflammation that would be indicative of septic shock in contrast to other inflammatory or shock states. The 4 groups of patients (septic shock, cardiogenic shock, bacterial pneumonia, and normal controls) underwent serial sampling to assess plasma levels of TNF, IL-6, soluble TNF receptors, nitrite/nitrate, procalcitonin, and creatinine concentrations. Unfortunately, the number of patients studied was small, and there was a large amount of overlap in the individual patient values demonstrating the expected contribution of the inflammatory response. The authors did find that the plasma concentrations of nitrite/nitrate and procalcitonin were the highest in the group of patients with septic shock and that these levels decreased as the patient's septic shock improved. This observation may help direct future attempts to better identify patients with septic shock and may even have prognostic capability. We must await a larger, prospective study to substantiate the potential diagnostic and prognostic abilities of plasma nitrite/nitrate and procalcitonin concentrations.

R.A. Balk, M.D.

Soluble E-Selectin Levels in Sepsis and Critical Illness: Correlation With Infection and Hemodynamic Dysfunction

Cummings CJ, Sessler CN, Beall LD, et al (Virginia Commonwealth Univ, Richmond; Otsuka American Pharmaceutical Inc, Rockville, Md)
Am J Respir Crit Care Med 156:431–437, 1997   3–20

Background.—Like other members of the selectin family, E-selectin is an early mediator of endothelial-leukocyte adhesion in inflammatory states. Soluble E-selectin is found in the supernatant of cytokine-activated endothelial cells, and serum E-selectin levels are increased in patients with various inflammatory conditions. E-selectin serum levels were studied for their relationship to systemic inflammation, infection, hemodynamic compromise, organ dysfunction, and outcome in critically ill patients.

Methods.—The study included 119 critically ill patients in a medical ICU. The initial sample consisted of 24 patients with severe sepsis. Subsequently, 95 consecutive HIV-negative patients were studied, including 43 who met the criteria for sepsis. Levels of soluble E-selectin were measured by a specific enzyme-linked immunosorbent assay.

Findings.—The log transformed mean E-selectin level was 5.28 ng/mL in the critically ill patients, compared to 1 ng/mL in normal controls. Mean E-selectin level was 15.39 ng/mL in 43 patients with culture-positive sepsis, compared to 4.87 ng/mL in 24 patients with culture-negative sepsis, 2.33 ng/mL in 44 patients with noninfectious systemic inflammatory re-

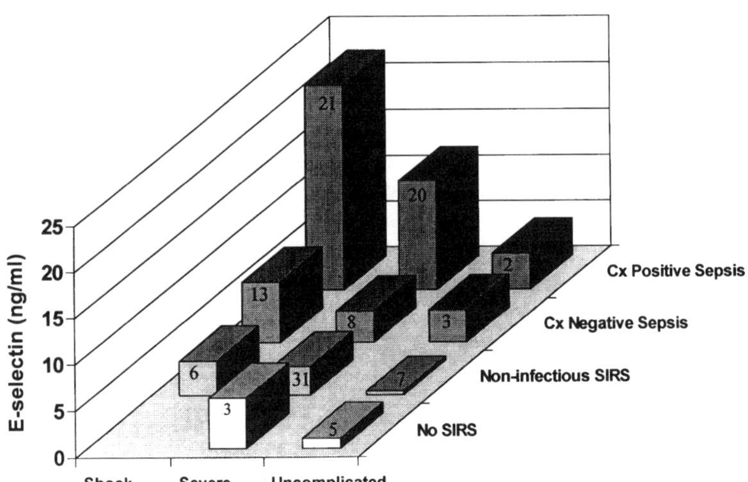

FIGURE 4.—Log-transformed mean E-selectin levels are displayed for subgroups categorized by hemodynamic severity (uncomplicated, severe, shock) and inflammation/infection (no SIRS, noninfectious SIRS, culture-negative sepsis, and culture-positive sepsis). The number of patients in each group is displayed on the corresponding column. *Abbreviation: SIRS,* systemic inflammatory response syndrome. (Courtesy of Cummings CJ, Sessler CN, Beall LD, et al: Soluble E-selectin levels in sepsis and critical illness: Correlation with infection and hemodynamic dysfunction. *Am J Respir Crit Care Med* 156:431–437, 1997. Official Journal of the American Thoracic Society. Copyright 1997 American Lung Association.)

sponse syndrome (SIRS), and 1.97 ng/mL in 8 patients without SIRS (Fig 4). There was a strong relationship between E-selectin level and degree of hemodynamic compromise. Microbiological and hemodynamic status were independently related to E-selectin level. The patients' E-selectin levels on the first ICU day were significantly correlated with peak organ failure score during ICU hospitalization. Mean E-selectin level was 10.61 ng/mL for patients who died vs. 4.35 ng/mL for those who lived.

Conclusions.—Patients with culture-positive sepsis have high serum levels of soluble E-selectin than other critically ill patients. The reason for this finding, and its clinical implications, remain to be determined. First-day E-selectin levels are strongly related to hemodynamic compromise, less so to organ dysfunction and survival.

▶ In this trial of critically ill patients with sepsis and SIRS. the use of E-selectin or endothelial leukocyte adhesion molecule-1 (ELAM-1) was found to be a marker of both culture-positive sepsis and shock. The elevation of ELAM-1 in shock states was irrespective of the presence of positive cultures. This finding may have future applicability in the identification of septic patients for inclusion in a septic trial if the findings are reproducible and the methodology can be utilized in "real time," preferably within a short diagnostic window. Another interesting observation that warrants further study was the correlation of initial ELAM-1 level with the subsequent development of organ system dysfunction. The ability to prognosticate future morbidity and mortality based on an initial circulating factor may have tremendous clinical implications both for treatment and triage decisions, providing this observation can be substantiated in subsequent prospective, multicenter trials.

R.A. Balk, M.D.

Interleukin-10 Prevents Early Cytokine Release in Severe Intraabdominal Infection and Sepsis
Rongione AJ, Kusske AM, Ashley SW, et al (Univ of California, Los Angeles; Sepulveda VA Med Ctrs, Los Angeles)
J Surg Res 70:107–112, 1997   3–21

Introduction.—Despite advances in critical care therapy and improved antibiotic regimens, sepsis and multiorgan system failure remain common surgical problems. The release of cytokines is a proposed common denominator of the sepsis syndrome, and both proinflammatory and anti-inflammatory cytokines may be critical factors in the pathogenesis of multiorgan system failure. Production of cytokines has been shown to be inhibited by interleukin-10, and its relevance in sepsis models has recently emerged. In a murine model of cecal ligation and puncture, it was determined whether interleukin-10 would decrease serum cytokine elevation.

Methods.—There were 4 groups of 14 mice: 1 group had laparotomy alone with intraperitoneal saline injection (sham group); 1 group had

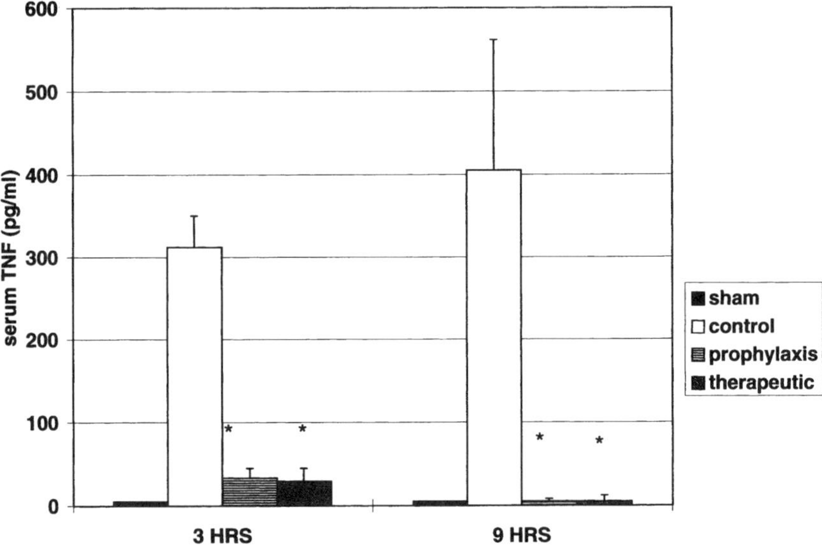

FIGURE 1.—Serum tumor necrosis factor-α (*TNF*)-α profile. Results are expressed as mean ± SEM. The expected rise in (*TNF*)-α was significantly attenuated by the prophylactic and therapeutic administration of interleukin-10 (*asterisk* indicates $P < 0.001$ vs. cecal ligation and puncture alone). There were no detectable serum cytokine levels in those that underwent sham operation. (Courtesy of Rongione AJ, Kusske AM, Ashley SW, et al: Interleukin-10 prevents early cytokine release in severe intraabdominal infection and sepsis. *J Surg Res* 70:107–112, 1997.)

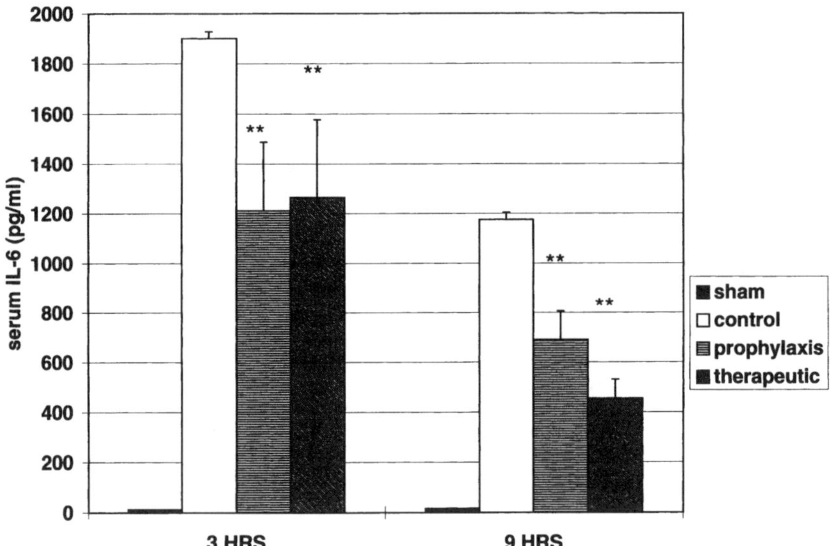

FIGURE 2.—Serum interleukin-6 (*IL-6*) profile. Results are expressed as mean ± SEM. The expected rise in IL-6 was significantly attenuated by the prophylactic and therapeutic administration of IL-10 (*asterisk* indicates $P < 0.05$ vs. cecal ligation and puncture alone). There were no detectable serum cytokine levels in those that underwent sham operation. (Courtesy of Rongione AJ, Kusske AM, Ashley SW, et al: Interleukin-10 prevents early cytokine release in severe intraabdominal infection and sepsis. *J Surg Res* 70:107–112, 1997.)

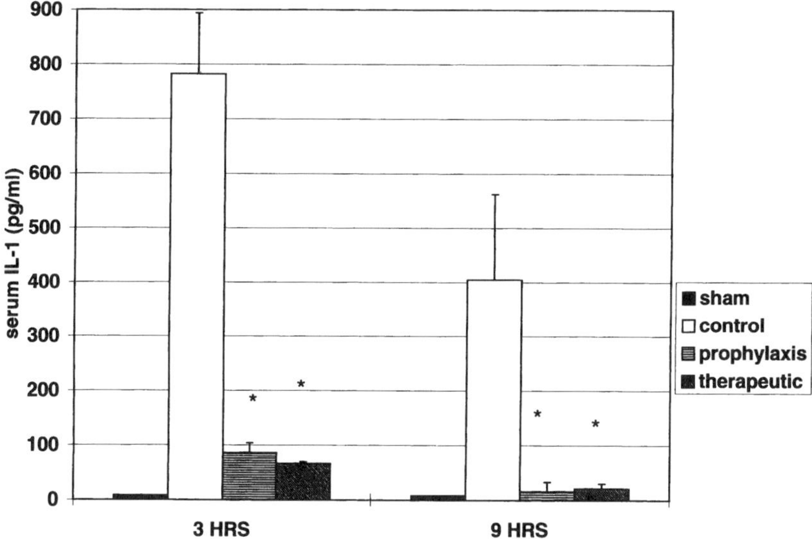

FIGURE 3.—Serum interleukin-1β (*IL-1*) profile. Results are expressed as mean ± SEM. The expected rise in IL-1β was significantly attenuated by the prophylactic and therapeutic administration of IL-10. (*asterisk* indicates $P < 0.001$ vs. cecal ligation and puncture alone). There were no detectable serum cytokine levels in those that underwent sham operation. (Courtesy of Rongione AJ, Kusske AM, Ashley SW, et al: Interleukin-10 prevents early cytokine release in severe intraabdominal infection and sepsis. *J Surg Res* 70:107–112, 1997.)

laparotomy and cecal ligation and puncture with intraperitoneal saline injection (control group); 1 group had laparotomy and cecal ligation and puncture with 10,000 U of interleukin-10 administered intraperitoneally 1 hour before cecal ligation and puncture and every 3 hours thereafter (prophylactic group); and 1 group had laparotomy and cecal ligation and puncture with 10,000 U of interleukin-10 administered intraperitoneally 1 hour after cecal ligation and puncture and every 3 hours thereafter (therapeutic group). At 3 and 9 hours after cecal ligation and puncture, the mice were killed. Enzyme-linked immunosorbent assay was used to determine serum tumor necrosis factor-α, interleukin-1β, and interleukin-6 levels.

Results.—In the control group, cecal ligation and puncture produced a significant rise in serum tumor necrosis factor, interleukin-6, and interleukin-1 (Figs 1–3). This early rise in serum cytokines was significantly attenuated with prophylactic or therapeutic administration of interleukin-10.

Conclusions.—An early systemic rise in macrophage-derived cytokines is produced by cecal ligation and puncture. This early release of macrophage-derived systemic mediators is inhibited by the administration of interleukin-10 before or after the onset of cecal ligation and puncture. In the therapeutic management of intra-abdominal infection and sepsis, interleukin-10 has potential clinical benefits.

▶ The anti-inflammatory cytokine, interleukin-10 (IL-10), is capable of suppressing the proinflammatory response by inhibiting the release of proinflammatory mediators from monocytes, macrophages, and T-helper cells. This trial evaluated cecal ligation and perforation as a "septic-like injury" in mice who were administered placebo or IL-10 intraperitoneally. The IL-10 was given 1 hour before the injury in one group and one hour after the injury in another. The use of IL-10 was associated with a significant decrease in serum tumor necrosis factor, IL-6, and IL-1 levels. The authors concluded that the use of this anti-inflammatory compound has potential clinical and therapeutic implications. This needs to be evaluated in a multicentered, prospective, randomized, placebo-controlled trial. Until we have the results from such a study, we must relegate this study to an interesting observation and use caution concerning the potential to suppress a potentially valuable and necessary inflammatory response in the war against infection.

R.A. Balk, M.D.

A Comparison of the Adrenocortical Response During Septic Shock and After Complete Recovery
Briegel J, Schelling G, Haller M, et al (Ludwig-Maximilians-Universität München, Germany)
Intensive Care Med 22:894–899, 1996   3–22

Introduction.—Serum cortisol concentrations are usually elevated in patients with septic shock when compared with those in unstressed, healthy individuals. The secretory reserve of cortisol may be reduced during septic shock and corticotropin-induced steroidogenesis has been shown to decrease with sepsis. It is still unclear whether an impairment of the adrenal reserve affects patients with septic shock. The adrenocortical response to corticotropin during septic shock and after recovery was demonstrated by using each patient as his or her own control.

Methods.—Twenty patients who survived septic shock with high-output circulatory failure with a cardiac index greater than 4L/min per m² were studied. Using the Acute Physiology and Chronic Health Evaluation (APACHE) II scoring system, severity of illness during septic shock and after recovery was graded. There were 17 patients (12 survivors and 5 nonsurvivors) who received stress doses of hydrocortisone after a corticotropin stimulation test was completed. A short corticotropin stimulation test was performed after fluid resuscitation, titration of vasopressors, and institution of life-supportive therapy.

Results.—There were no differences in the basal cortisol levels (18.8 μg/dL) recorded during septic shock and after recovery (18.9 μg/dL). During septic shock, the response to corticotropin was significantly attenuated when compared with the response after recovery (7.7 vs. 14.7

µg/dL). As indicated by a reduction in the APACHE II scores, patients' stress response was less after recovery.

Conclusions.—In patients with septic shock and high-output circulatory failure, adrenocortical response to corticotropin is attenuated when compared with the response in the less stressful condition after recovery. Effects of circulating mediators from the systemic inflammatory response may explain the attenuated adrenocortical responsiveness.

▶ This study prospectively evaluated patients with well-defined, high-output septic shock for their response to the short corticotropin stimulation test. Thirty-three patients were identified for the trial, but 13 died and were not available for repeat testing during the recovery period. In the 20 survivors, baseline and postrecovery cortisol response was similar, both at baseline and after stimulation with corticotropin. The increase in cortisol from baseline was greater during the recovery phase vs. during the period of septic shock. The implication of this apparent attenuation in cortisol response is uncertain at this time. Confounding these data are the fact that 17 of the 33 patients had received corticosteroid treatment as part of their therapeutic management of septic shock. The postrecovery corticotropin stimulation test was delayed until at least 24 hours after the last dose of corticosteroids.

Further study is needed to determine what is the significance, if any, of this observation. All the patients did manifest a normal corticotropin response despite the apparent decrease relative to the subsequent recovery period.

R.A. Balk, M.D.

Gastric Intramucosal pH and Blood Lactate in Severe Sepsis

Joynt GM, Lipman J, Gomersall CD, et al (Chinese Univ of Hong Kong, Sha Tin; Univ of the Witwatersrand, Soweto, South Africa)
Anaesthesia 52:726–732, 1997   3–23

Introduction.—In critically ill patients, an indication of the state of blood flow to the vital organs is given by routine measurement and assessment of blood pressure, heart rate, urine output, and peripheral perfusion. The balance of oxygen supply, demand and consumption at a tissue level, however, is not reflected by any of these measures. Tissue oxygen balance may be better reflected with gastric intramucosal pH and serum lactate levels. As predictors of outcome, gastric intramucosal pH and serum lactate were compared.

Methods.—During 5 days in a group of patients with newly diagnosed severe sepsis, the effect of conventional resuscitation on gastric intramucosal pH and serum lactate levels was prospectively investigated. Measurements were taken of the lactate concentration and gastric intramucosal pH at baseline, when resuscitation end points were met, every 8 hours for 48 hours, and every day for 5 days.

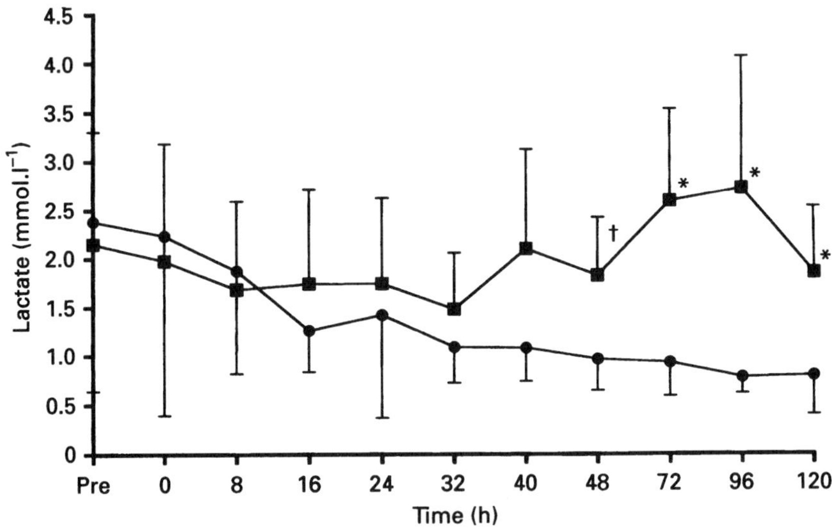

FIGURE 2.—Mean blood lactate concentration in survivors (*black circle*) and nonsurvivors (*black square*) during the study. *Error bars* indicate standard deviation. Significant differences between groups are indicated by *asterisks* ($P < 0.05$) and *dagger* ($P < 0.01$). (Courtesy of Joynt GM, Lipman J, Gomersall CD, et al: Gastric intramucosal pH and blood lactate in severe sepsis. *Anaesthesia* 52:726–732. Copyright 1997, by permission of WB Saunders Company Limited, London.)

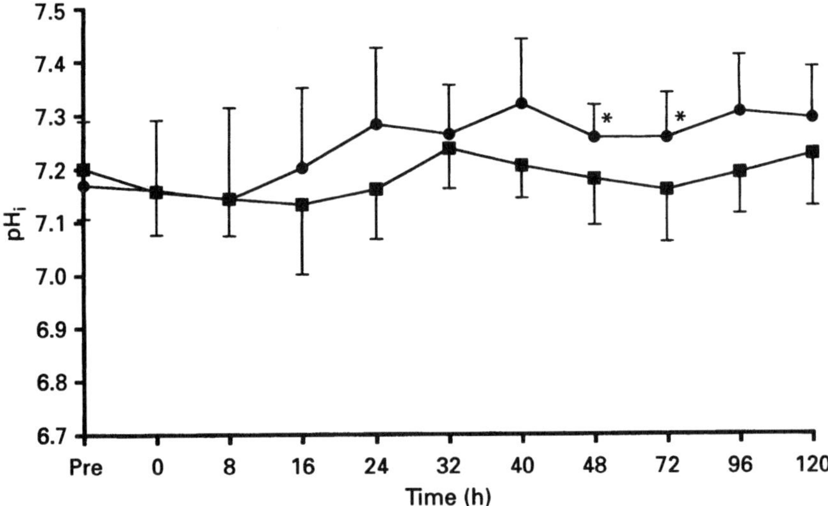

FIGURE 1.—Mean gastric intramucosal pH (pH_i) in survivors (*black circle*) and nonsurvivors (*black square*) during the study. *Error bars* indicate standard deviation. *Asterisks* indicate significant difference between groups: $P < 0.05$. (Courtesy of Joynt GM, Lipman J, Gomersall CD, et al: Gastric intramucosal pH and blood lactate in severe sepsis. *Anaesthesia* 52:726–732. Copyright 1997, by permission of WB Saunders Company Limited, London.)

Results.—At the time of diagnosis of severe sepsis, 16 of 18 patients had a low gastric intramucosal pH with a mean of 7.17. Serum lactate levels or gastric intramucosal pH could not distinguish between nonshocked or shocked patients. Over time, survivors were distinguished from nonsurvivors by serum lactate levels (Fig 2). Over time, survivors were not distinguished from nonsurvivors by gastric intramucosal pH (Fig 1). In survivors, serum lactate levels were lower at 48 hours and gastric intramucosal pH was higher. Lactate is a better predictor of survival, according to receiver operating characteristic curves.

Conclusions.—To guide resuscitation in patients who are severely ill and who have gastric intramucosal acidosis, gastric intramucosal pH should not be used because of its inability to distinguish survivors from nonsurvivors until 48 hours.

▶ The search for markers of survival in sepsis continues. Scoring systems,[1] cytokine levels,[2] and physiologic indicators such as oxygen consumption,[1] lactate levels,[3] and gastric mucosal pH (pH_i)[4] have all been reported to predict survival, although none of them is accurate enough for individual patient decision making. In recent years, there has been the recognition that changes in these measurements over time are more predictive than absolute values on admission. While methodologically more difficult to prove, this observation seems intuitively logical. This study contributes to this generally held belief.

Serum lactate levels were studied over 5 days in a homogeneous group of patients with newly diagnosed sepsis. Initial lactate levels were similar in both survivors and nonsurvivors. Over time, the lactate levels improved, while they remained abnormal in nonsurvivors. The lactate levels on day 2 through 5 were significantly higher in nonsurvivors than in survivors. These elevated levels were similar to those present on admission. Receiver operator curves demonstrate the value of lactate as a predictor of survival. Although statistically significant, it is not possible to use unchanging lactate levels 48 hours, 72 hours, or even 5 days after admission to withdraw or limit therapy based on a reduced probability of survival.

Changes in pH_i are even less predictive than lactate levels. There was a statistically significant improvement in the markedly reduced pH_i seen on admission, but the magnitude is quite modest in this study. Previous reports using pH_i as an indicator of survival have used a more heterogeneous patient population. In patients with sepsis, it appears that mucosal perfusion is reduced on presentation and remains reduced despite volume resuscitation. Technical factors such as probe placement and variation in pH_i measurements contribute to the problems with routine use of pH_i. Routine measurement of pH_i to aid in predicting survival cannot be recommended at the present time.

M.R. Silver, M.D.

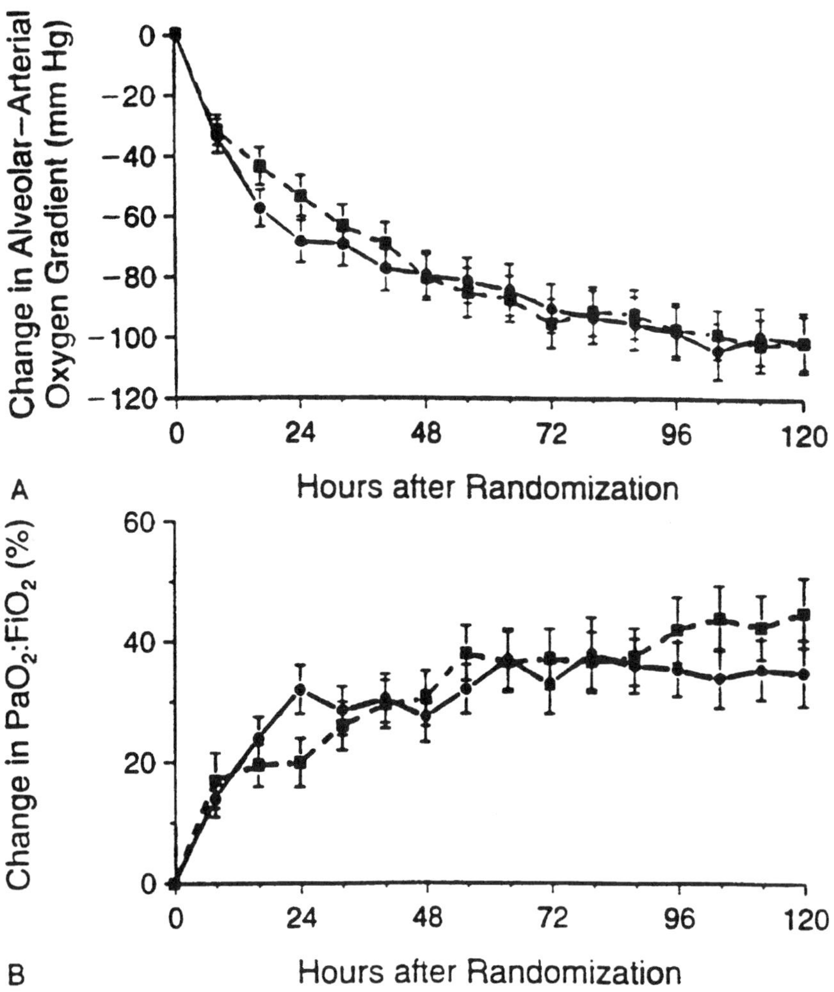

FIGURE 1.—Mean (±SD) changes in indexes of oxygenation in the surfactant and placebo groups. **Panel A** shows the decreases (indicated by negative numbers) in the alveolar-arterial oxygen gradient during the administration of placebo or surfactant. There were no significant differences between the two groups. **Panel B** shows the percent change in the ratio of PaO_2 to FiO_2 from base line. The surfactant group and the placebo group had similar changes during the 5-day treatment period. (Courtesy of Anzueto A, for the Exosurf Acute Respiratory Distress Syndrome Sepsis Study Group: Aerosolized surfactant in adults with sepsis-induced acute respiratory distress syndrome. *N Engl J Med* 334:1417–1421, 1996. Reprinted by permission of *The New England Journal of Medicine.* Copyright 1996, Massachusetts Medical Society. All rights reserved.)

ble-blind trial evaluated the use of surfactant versus saline aerosol in the treatment of well-defined, septic-induced ARDS. In the 725 patients randomized between the 2 treatment groups, no significant differences were found in 30-day survival, length of stay in the ICU, duration of mechanical

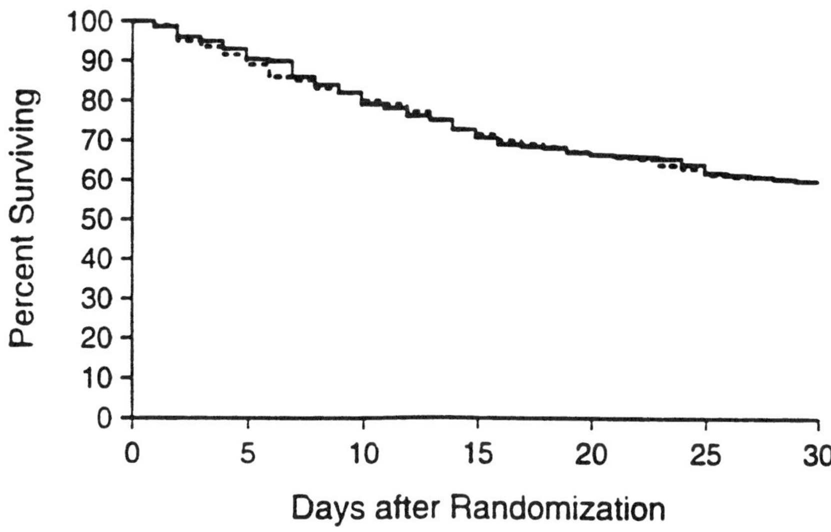

FIGURE 2.—Kaplan-Meier survival curves, showing the percentage of patients surviving in the placebo group (*solid line*) and surfactant group (*dashed line*). (Courtesy of Anzueto A, for the Exosurf Acute Respiratory Distress Syndrome Sepsis Study Group: Aerosolized Surfactant in Adults With Sepsis-induced Acute Respiratory Distress Syndrome. *N Engl J Med* 334:1417–1421, 1996. Reprinted by permission of *The New England Journal of Medicine.* Copyright 1996, Massachusetts Medical Society. All rights reserved.)

ventilatory support, or physiologic function. One of the major observations from this negative study was the 60% survival rate found in both patient groups over the 30 days. This survival rate in a large cohort of well-defined patients supports the contention that the outcome of patients with acute lung injury seems to be improving, in comparison to past reports. Unfortunately, a 40% mortality rate is still too high, and we must continue the search to identify the optimum treatment or support strategy to improve the survival of patients with ARDS.

R.A. Balk, M.D.

Influence of Prone Position on the Extent and Distribution of Lung Injury in a High Tidal Volume Oleic Acid Model of Acute Respiratory Distress Syndrome

Broccard AF, Shapiro RS, Schmitz LL, et al (Univ of Minnesota, St Paul; Hennepin County Med Ctr, Minneapolis, Minn)
Crit Care Med 25:16–27, 1997   4–2

Introduction.—Ventilator-induced lung injury may be more intense or extensive in the lower lung zones. An experiment was devised to determine the influence of position on the extent and distribution of lung injury in an oleic acid canine model of acute respiratory distress syndrome, using mechanical ventilation with high tidal volumes and positive end-expiratory pressure (PEEP).

Methods.—Twelve adult dogs were anesthetized, then injected with oleic acid. Ninety minutes after lung injury was induced with oleic acid, the animals were randomized to be ventilated for 4 hours in either the prone or supine position while using the identical ventilatory pattern (fraction of inspired oxygen [FIO_2] 0.6, PEEP 10 cm H_2O or greater, and a tidal volume that generated a peak transpulmonary pressure of 35 cm H_2O when implemented in the supine position). The tidal volumes, FIO_2, and PEEP were kept constant and the pulmonary artery occlusion pressure was held between 4 and 6 mm Hg, regardless of the dogs' position. At protocol completion, the animals were sacrificed and the lungs excised for gravimetric determination (wet/dry weight ratio) and histologic score. Changes over time in the static pressure-volume curve of the lungs (taken in the supine position) were assessed.

Results.—Both groups were similar in hemodynamic and respiratory variables and lung static-volume curves at baseline. At completion of the experiment, the lung gravimetric data in the 2 groups were similar, indicating a similar extent of edema. Histologic abnormalities were significantly less in the prone than in the supine group. There were marked differences in the extent and severity in the dependent regions of the lungs. There was significant improvement in static lung compliance in the prone, but not the supine, group.

Conclusion.—In an animal model of oleic acid–induced lung injury, dogs ventilated with high tidal volume and PEEP underwent less extensive histologic change in the prone position than in the supine position. The distribution of histologic abnormalities is altered in the prone position.

▶ Most clinicians intuitively believe that turning a critically ill patient to the prone position is personnel demanding and risky; therefore, they believe that it is not practical unless it is the only remaining alternative to invasive techniques for improving oxygenation. This article describes and discusses an animal experiment that lends some credence to the concept that the prone position may minimize lung injury in acute respiratory distress syndrome. I hope this stimulates further research into the role the prone position may play in limiting lung injury.

B.A. Shapiro, M.D.

Variability of Indices of Hypoxemia in Adult Respiratory Distress Syndrome

Gowda MS, Klocke RA (State Univ of New York, Buffalo)
Crit Care Med 25:41–45, 1997   4–3

Background.—Severe hypoxemia is a key component of adult respiratory distress syndrome (ARDS). Several different indices have been proposed to describe the altered arterial oxygenation of ARDS, all similar and all varying with alterations in inspired oxygen concentration. Hypoxemia in ARDS is usually interpreted as a complication of shunting, yet about

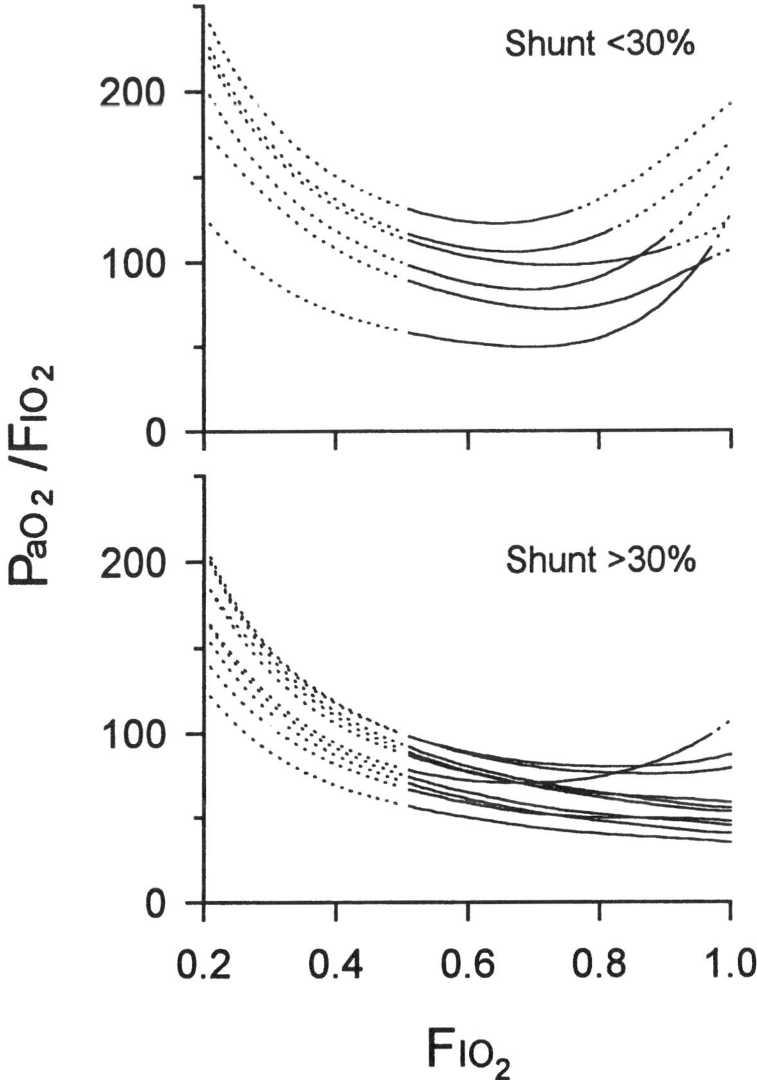

FIGURE 1.—Relationship between PaO_2/FIO_2 and FIO_2 for patients with less than 30% true shunt (**top**) and patients with more than 30% shunt (**bottom**). Ratios of PaO_2/FIO_2, characterized by FIO_2 values of 0.5 or greater and PaO_2 values of ≤100 (≤13.3 kPa), are shown by the *solid lines*. Ratios of PaO_2/FIO_2 outside these limits are indicated by the *dotted lines*. (Courtesy of Gowda MS, Klocke RA: Variability of indices of hypoxemia in adult respiratory distress syndrome. *Crit Care Med* 25(1):41–45, 1997.)

half of patients with ARDS have significant ventilation/perfusion abnormalities. This study, using published data and a computer model, analyzed the value of indices of hypoxemia in assessing patients with ARDS.

Methods.—The investigators collection published ventilation/perfusion distributions measured by the multiple inert gas elimination technique.

They then constructed a computer model of gas exchange, based on a 50-compartment model of ventilation/perfusion inhomogeneity plus true shunt and dead space. In the computer model, fraction of inspired oxygen (FIO_2) was varied from 0.21 to 1.0. Hypoxemia indices were calculated as a function of inspired oxygen concentration, including partial pressure of arterial oxygen (PaO_2)/FIO_2, arterial/alveolar ratio (PaO_2/alveolar partial pressure of oxygen (PO_2), alveolar-arterial PO_2 difference ($P[A-a]O_2$), respiratory index ($P[A-a]O_2$/PaO_2), and venous admixture.

Results.—For patients with moderate shunts of less than 30%, the PaO_2/FIO_2 ratio varied substantially with changing FIO_2. At either end of the range of FIO_2, PaO_2/FIO_2 was significantly greater than at intermediate FIO_2 values. For patients with larger shunts, PaO_2/FIO_2ratios were greater at low FIO_2 values, but relatively stable at FIO_2 values greater than 0.5 (Fig 1). The PaO_2/FIO_2 ratio was always relatively stable at FIO_2 values of 0.5 or greater and PaO_2 values of 100 mm Hg or less. Other PO_2-based indices had less stability, as FIO_2 was varied. When true shunting was the cause of hypoxemia, venous admixture was stable at all FIO_2 values. In about half of patients, significant hypoxemia resulted from mismatching between ventilation and blood flow. These patients had important changes in venous admixture with changes in FIO_2, in proportion to the fraction of cardiac output perfusing gas exchange units with ventilation/perfusion ratios of less than 0.1.

Conclusion.—Changes in FIO_2 affect indices of hypoxemia in ARDS. The index that is most stable at FIO_2 values of 0.5 or greater and PaO_2 values of 100 mm Hg or less is the PaO_2/FIO_2 ratio; it provides a useful estimate of gas-exchange abnormalities under the usual clinical conditions. In patients with significant ventilation/perfusion abnormalities, venous admixture does not provide a good reflection of the efficiency of pulmonary oxygen exchange, even if calculated from measured arterial and venous oxygen content values.

▶ The PaO_2/FIO_2 ratio is easy to calculate and has been incorporated into the operational definition for acute lung injury and ARDS, as proposed by the American European Consensus Conference.[1] This study evaluated the consistency of this oxygenation index over a wide range of FIO_2s, shunts, and hemoglobin levels. The authors concluded that the value was reasonably constant when used in the setting of an FIO_2 greater than 50%. Because most patients with ARDS are managed with ventilatory support strategies that usually involve an FIO_2 greater than 40%, this ratio should have utility, both as a means of comparing oxygenation status from 1 time point or intervention to another and as a standard with which we can identify patients with oxygenation abnormalities, as required by the proposed definition of acute lung injury and ARDS.

R.A. Balk, M.D.

Reference

1. Bernard GR, Artigas A, Brigham K, et al: The American-European Consensus Conference on ARDS: Definitions, mechanisms, relevant outcomes, and clinical trial coordination. *Am J Respir Crit Care Med* 149:818–824, 1994.

Inhaled Prostacyclin (PGI$_2$) Versus Inhaled Nitric Oxide in Adult Respiratory Distress Syndrome

Zwissler B, Kemming G, Habler O, et al (Ludwig-Maximilians-Universität München, Germany)
Am J Respir Crit Care Med 154:1671–1677, 1996   4–4

Introduction.—In patients with severe adult respiratory distress syndrome (ARDS), it can be very difficult to ensure a viable partial pressure of arterial oxygen (PaO$_2$). One way to increase PaO$_2$ in patients with acute lung injury is through inhalation of nitric oxide (NO) or prostacyclin (PGI$_2$), which induces selective pulmonary vasodilation and improves the ventilation-perfusion ratio in ventilated areas of the lung. This dose-response study evaluated the therapeutic efficacy of NO and PGI$_2$ in patients with ARDS.

Methods.—The study included 8 patients with ARDS; lung injury scores were 3.5 to 3.25 and Acute Physiology and Chronic Health Evaluation II scores were 20 to 27. All patients were treated with PGI$_2$ in doses of 1, 10, and 25 ng/kg/min and with NO at concentrations of 1, 4, and 8 ppm. Cardiorespiratory measurements were made at baseline, after each drug concentration was given, and after each drug was withdrawn.

Results.—Pulmonary artery pressure decreased significantly and selectively with PGI$_2$, from 35.1 mm Hg at baseline to 33.1 mm Hg at 1 ng/kg/min, 31.1 mm Hg at 10 ng/kg/min, and 29.6 mm Hg at 25 ng/kg/min. With inhaled NO, pulmonary artery pressure (PAP) was unchanged at 1 ppm, decreased from 34.5 mm Hg to 32.1 mm Hg at 4 ppm, and to 31.8 mm Hg at 8 ppm. Treatment with PGI$_2$ improved the PaO$_2$/FIO$_2$ ratio from 105 mm Hg to 125 mm Hg at 10 ng/kg/min and 131 mm Hg at 25 ng/kg/min, with no effect at the 1 ng/kg/min dose. With NO, PaO$_2$ improved significantly, and intrapulmonary shunt was reduced at all doses tested.

Conclusion.—In patients with severe ARDS, inhaled PGI$_2$ and NO can both induce selective pulmonary vasodilation, thus increasing PaO$_2$. The optimal 10 ng/kg/min dose of PGI$_2$ improves gas exchange while lowering PAP to an extent similar to that achieved with inhaled NO. The clinical significance of the changes produced may be questioned; however, these agents may be useful for patients in whom routine measures cannot produce a viable PaO$_2$, or who have acute right heart limitation.

▶ Delivery of vasodilators through the inhalation route has been shown to produce a beneficial effect upon oxygenation parameters and a reduction in the PAP and pulmonary vascular resistance. This small study of 8 patients with ARDS demonstrated that inhaled PGI_2 was as effective as inhaled nitric oxide when effective doses were administered. Both are naturally occurring vasodilators and appear to be safe and without systemic side effects when administered by the inhalation route.

Whether either of these agents will earn a role in the management of patients with acute lung injury remains to be seen. To date, there have been mixed results from trials of inhaled nitric oxide in patients with acute lung injury and ARDS. It seems that patients with septic shock with ARDS do not respond to the same degree as nonseptic patients with ARDS.

A recently completed multicenter trial of inhaled nitric oxide in 177 patients with ARDS failed to demonstrate an improvement in survival.[1] Future trials may better define the role of vasodilator therapy in acute lung injury. In my opinion, inhaled vasodilator therapy falls into the category of supportive or adjunctive therapy. Many people view ARDS as a systemic injury of endothelial cells, with the pulmonary system the initial clinical manifestation. Thus, an intervention that only targets the airways may ignore the real focus of the problem.

R.A. Balk, M.D.

Reference

1. Dellinger RP: Inhaled nitric oxide in ARDS: Preliminary Results of a Multicenter Clinical Trial (Abstract). *Crit Care Med* 24:A29, 1996.

Serum Ferritin as a Predictor of the Acute Respiratory Distress Syndrome

Connelly KG, Moss M, Parsons PE, et al (Univ of Colorado, Denver; Denver Gen Hosp; Natl Jewish Ctr for Immunology and Respiratory Medicine, Denver)

Am J Respir Crit Care Med 155:21–25, 1997   4–5

Background.—Patients with major trauma or sepsis are at risk for acute respiratory distress syndrome (ARDS), although it cannot be predicted which patients will actually develop it. The development of treatments to prevent ARDS or to minimize its severity makes an important goal of the identification of patients likely to develop this syndrome. Proinflammatory cytokines are involved in ARDS and increase ferritin synthesis. Oxidative stress in patients at risk for ARDS may free iron from ferritin, accelerating toxic hydroxyl radical formation. Therefore, serum ferritin levels were analyzed as a predictor of ARDS.

Patients.—Seventy-five patients at risk for ARDS and eight patients who had already developed the syndrome were studied. Serum ferritin levels were measured by radioimmunoassay and compared to levels in control subjects.

Results.—Serum ferritin levels were higher in patients with and at risk for ARDS than in control subjects. Levels were also higher in patients at risk who developed ARDS than in those who did not (Fig 1). In women,

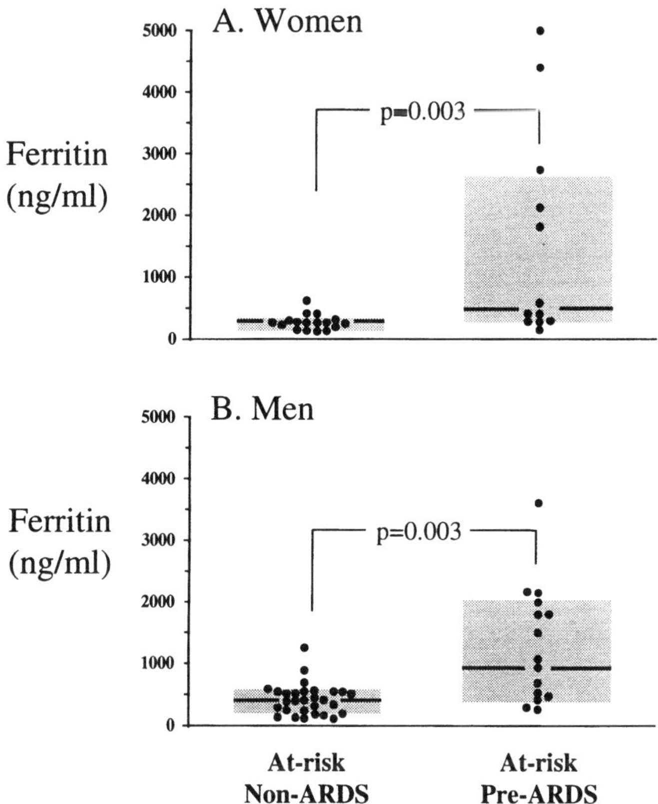

FIGURE 1.—Serum ferritin levels in: A, at-risk, non-ARDS women (n = 17; median: 265 ng/mL; 25% to 75% quartile range: 182 to 310 ng/mL) vs. at-risk, pre-ARDS women (n = 12; median: 490 ng/mL; 25% to 75% quartile range: 288 to 2,600 ng/mL); B, at-risk, non-ARDS men (n = 31; median: 420 ng/mL; 25% to 75% quartile range: 225 to 550 ng/mL) vs. at-risk, pre-ARDS men (n = 15; median: 925 ng/mL; 25% to 75% quartile range: 410 to 2,000 ng/mL). *Bar lines,* median values; *shaded boxes,* 25% to 75% quartiles. (Courtesy of Connelly KG, Moss M, Parsons PE, et al: Serum ferritin as a predictor of the acute respiratory distress syndrome. *Am J Respir Crit Care Med* 155:21–25, 1997. Official Journal of the American Thoracic Society. Copyright 1997, American Lung Association.)

a serum ferritin value greater than 270 ng/mL had 83% sensitivity, 71% specificity, 67% positive predictive value, and 86% negative predictive value in predicting acute respiratory distress syndrome (Table 3). In men, a serum ferritin value greater than 680 ng/mL had 60% sensitivity, 90% specificity, 75% positive predictive value, and 82% negative predictive value in predicting acute respiratory distress syndrome. There was no correlation between serum ferritin and C-reactive protein levels. Serum ferritin values were similar in medical and surgical patients at risk, and could not be accounted for by liver disease.

Discussion.—Determining serum ferritin levels in patients at risk for ARDS may help to identify those who will develop it and improve treat-

TABLE 3.—ARDS-Predictive Values of Serum Ferritin Levels in At-Risk Patients

Test	> 270 ng/ml in Females (n = 29)		> 680 ng/ml in Males (n = 46)	
	Percentage	95% CI	Percentage	95% CI
Sensitivity	83%	(62–100%)	60%	(35–84%)
Specificity	71%	(49–93%)	90%	(70–100%)
Positive predictive value	67%	(43–91%)	75%	(50–100%)
Negative predictive value	86%	(68–100%)	82%	(68–92%)
Accuracy	76%	(68–100%)	80%	(68–92%)

(Courtesy of Connelly KG, Moss M, Parsons PE, et al: Serum ferritin as a predictor of the acute respiratory distress syndrome. *Am J Respir Crit Care Med* 155:21–25, 1997. Official Journal of the American Thoracic Society. Copyright 1997. American Lung Association.)

ment. Elevated serum ferritin may regulate the role of iron in oxidative responses that contribute to ARDS.

▶ The ability to predict, with a relatively high degree of certainty, which patients with a defined risk for developing acute lung injury or ARDS will actually go on to develop these disorders would greatly improve our understanding of and therapeutic strategies for these processes. Many studies have attempted to identify circulating "factors" or expired gases that would predict the development of ARDS in an at-risk population. To date, none have been able to firmly establish their utility. Obviously, if we were able to identify with a reasonable degree of certainty which patients would go on to develop this dreaded complication, we would be able to target these patients for trials of prophylactic agents or initiate support strategies at an earlier point in time. We would likely enhance our understanding of the pathophysiologic processes at work in the production of this injury.

This study is a preliminary observation and needs to be confirmed by a randomized, multicentered, prospective trial. Strict definitions of the at risk population and the specific endpoints (including ARDS) need to be used in this trial. In addition, critically ill control patients and patients with preexisting pulmonary processes and systemic inflammatory conditions need to be included in the study populations to make sense of the results and to make them applicable to the clinical arena. Until we have this additional data and insight, this observation must be regarded as interesting, but not substantiated.

R.A. Balk, M.D.

Circulating IL-1ra and IL-10 Levels Are Increased but Do Not Predict the Development of Acute Respiratory Distress Syndrome in At-Risk Patients

Parsons PE, Moss M, Vannice JL, et al (Denver Gen Hosp; Univ of Colorado, Denver; Emory Univ, Atlanta, Ga; et al)
Am J Respir Crit Care Med 155:1469–1473, 1997   4–6

Introduction.—The development of acute lung injury may be impacted by cytokines in beneficial or detrimental ways. The pathogenesis of acute respiratory distress syndrome (ARDS) may be affected by interleukin (IL)-1, IL-8, and tumor necrosis factor. Potential modulators of the inflammatory process that leads to the development of acute lung injury are IL-1ra, IL-10, and IL-4. There has also been an increase in IL-10 in septic patients. It was hypothesized that IL-1ra, IL-10, and IL-4 are important modulators of the inflammatory cascade and may lead to the development of ARDS.

Methods.—In 77 patients who were identified as being at risk for the development of ARDS, serial levels of IL-1ra and IL-10 were measured. The patients had sepsis, pancreatitis, hypertransfusion, abdominal trauma, chest trauma, and multiple fractures.

Results.—In the patients, initial IL-1ra levels were significantly higher (7.82 ng/mL) than in the controls (0.24 ng/mL); however, the development of ARDS could not be predicted. In the patients who died, initial IL-1ra levels were higher (31.95 ng/mL) than in those who survived (6.61 ng/mL). Patients also had higher levels of IL-10 (155 ng/mL) than did the normal controls (0 ng/mL). The development of ARDS could not be predicted by IL-10 either. In patients who died, IL-10 levels were significantly higher than in the survivors None of the patients had IL-4 detected in the plasma samples.

Conclusion.—In patients at risk for ARDS who die, modulators of inflammation are increased; however, the syndrome cannot be predicted by measuring the levels of certain interleukins.

▶ Interleukin-10 and IL-1ra plasma levels do not predict the development of ARDS. Patient plasma levels were no different among those patients at risk for ARDS in whom ARDS did or did not subsequently develop. Plasma levels of IL-10 and IL-1ra were higher in patients who died, but there was no absolute level that could be used to predict mortality.

Clinical trials of IL-1ra infusion in septic patients have already failed, and there is interest in trying IL-10 infusions. This article points out that patients who die already have elevated levels of these cytokines. Who is designing these clinical trials? What are they thinking—that maybe the levels aren't high enough? More basic research is required to clarify the role of cytokines in the pathogenesis of sepsis and multisystem organ failure.

L.C. Casey, M.D., Ph.D.

Nutritional Status, ICU Duration and ICU Mortality in Lung Transplant Recipients

Plöchl W, Pezawas L, Artemiou O, et al (Univ of Vienna)
Intensive Care Med 22:1179–1185, 1996   4–7

Background.—Malnutrition is relatively common among patients with end-stage lung disease. Poor nutritional status is believed to increase the risk of postoperative complications in surgical patients, resulting in longer ICU stays. However some degree of malnutrition may benefit patients with end-stage lung disease by decreasing requirements for ventilation. The effects of nutritional status on early postoperative recovery in patients receiving lung transplants (LTX) has yet to be well described. The relationship of malnutrition of LTX patients with duration of stay and mortality in the ICU was explored in this retrospective study.

Methods.—Records were reviewed for 51 patients who had undergone LTX at a single hospital between 1992 and 1994. Data regarding diagnosis, surgical intervention, duration of ICU stay, ICU mortality, and body mass index (BMI) were collected. Body mass index was calculated by dividing body weight by height squared for each patient. Patients for whom the BMI was greater than the 25th percentile were regarded as adequately nourished. Those for whom the BMI was less than the 25th percentile or less than the 5th percentile were considered malnourished or severely malnourished, respectively.

Results.—The median duration of the ICU stay was 5 days, ranging from 2 to 123 days, for all patients. Median ICU stays were significantly shorter for patients with obstructive lung disease (4 days) than they were for those with either pulmonary hypertension (10 days) or restrictive lung disease (7 days). Patients receiving double-lung transplants spent a median of 10 days in the ICU, significantly longer than the 4-day median for those receiving single-lung transplants. The overall duration of ICU stays and ICU mortality did not vary significantly among patients, based on nutritional status. However, ICU mortality was significantly elevated in patients who had BMIs below the 25th percentile and who spent more than 5 days in the ICU.

Conclusions.—The underlying diagnosis and type of transplantation procedure are significant predictors of postoperative ICU stay duration. Malnutrition enhances the likelihood of ICU mortality after the fifth postoperative day. Interventions that maintain or improve nutritional status before LTX should be applied consistently. Further evaluation of postoperative nutritional enhancement strategies is necessary.

▶ Survival and causes of mortality after lung transplant in this study are consistent with other reports.[1, 2] In this study, patients with COPD undergoing single-lung transplant have the shortest ICU stay, whereas patients undergoing double-lung transplant with problems such as restrictive lung disease or pulmonary hypertension have longer ICU stays. Of the 9 mortalities observed, 6 were from infection, 2 were from severe reperfusion injury, and 1 was from a bronchial anastomosis dehiscence. Independent predictors of prolonged ICU stay included the type of transplant procedure and the underlying diagnosis. Predictors for ICU mortality were the development of severe reperfusion injury and a BMI of less than 25%.

Despite these findings, the role of nutritional status is not clear in this population. Patients were grouped into the following 3 categories: (1) severely malnourished with a BMI of less than 5%; (2) malnourished with a BMI of 5% to 25%, and (3) a BMI of more than 25%. Overall mortality was not affected by the patient's nutritional status. In a posthoc analysis, nutritional status affected patients who required an ICU stay of more than 5 days, with all 10 patients with a BMI of more than 25% surviving, whereas 6 of 9 patients with a BMI of less than 25% died. Interestingly, the patients with severe malnutrition did not have any greater hospital mortality than patients with moderate malnutrition (3 of 14 vs. 4 of 18). It is too early to tell whether the use of anabolic hormones, such as human recombinant growth hormone,[3] will have an impact on overall patient survival.

M.R. Silver, M.D.

References

1. Davis RD, Trulock EP, Manley J, et al: Differences in early results after single-lung transplantation. *Ann Thorac Surg* 58:1327–1335, 1994.
2. Chaparro C, Maurer JR, Chamberlain D, et al: Causes of death in lung transplant recipients. *J Heart Lung Transplant* 13:758–766, 1994.
3. Van den Berghe G, Zegher F, Van-haecke J, et al: Growth hormone as a rescue treatment after heart-lung or double-lung transplantation. *Endocrinol Metab* 1:187–190, 1994.

Higher Concentrations of Matrix Metalloproteinases in Bronchoalveolar Lavage Fluid of Patients With Adult Respiratory Distress Syndrome
Torii K, Iida K-I, Miyazaki Y, et al (Univ of Nagoya, Japan; Tosei Gen Hosp, Seto, Japan)
Am J Respir Crit Care Med 155:43–46, 1997   4–8

Introduction.—Characterized by high microvascular permeability, low-pressure edema, refractory hypoxemia, and respiratory failure, adult respiratory distress syndrome (ARDS) is a form of acute lung injury. The development of ARDS has been linked to the destruction of the basement membrane, of which a complex of type IV collagens occupies a substantial portion. Through the collagenolytic actions, type IV collagenolytic matrix metalloproteinases are known to degrade membrane structures. In the development of ARDS, the possible role of type IV collagenolytic matrix metalloproteinases and the respective specific tissue inhibitors of these metalloproteinases were investigated.

Methods.—Using newly developed, sensitive 1-step sandwich enzyme immunoassay methods, the concentrations of the enzymes were determined in the bronchoalveolar lavage fluid from 17 patients with ARDS. To analyze the number of the cellular component, bronchoalveolar lavage was obtained from the 17 patients and 8 healthy volunteers serving as controls. As markers of basement membrane disruption, concentrations of the 7S portion of type IV collagen and laminin in the bronchoalveolar lavage fluid were measured.

Results.—The concentration of metalloproteinase-2 was significantly higher in the patients with ARDS (66.7 ± 57.0 ng/mL) than in the controls (less than 7.0 ng.mL). The concentration of metalloproteinase-2 was also significantly higher in the patients with ARDS (118.0 ± 309.3 ng/mL) than in the controls (9.0 ± 9.5 ng/mL). The specific inhibitor of metalloproteinase-9 was higher in the patients with ARDS (161.0 ± 145.0 ng/mL) than in the controls (less than 50 ng/mL). The concentrations of 7S collagen and laminin correlated with those of metalloproteinase-2 in the patients with ARDS. The concentration of 7S collagen and the number of neutrophils also correlated with metalloproteinase-9 in the distress patients with ARDS.

Conclusion.—In the pathogenesis of ARDS, there is a role played by the increased concentration of collagenolytic metalloproteinases.

▶ Adult respiratory distress syndrome is defined by the presence of increased capillary permeability, causing noncardiogenic pulmonary edema. However, the mechanism(s) by which the increased capillary permeability occurs is unknown. This article sheds new light on 1 potential mechanism (i.e., that the release of matrix metalloproteinases by neutrophils may cause degradation of type IV collagen). Type IV collagen is basement membrane collagen, so it is easy to visualize how degradation of type IV collagen would cause membrane permeability. If specific inhibitors of matrix metalloproteinases were available, it might be possible to inhibit further membrane injury and, thus, limit the amount of lung injury. This line of work has potential, but it is not yet ready for clinical trials.

L.C. Casey, M.D., Ph.D.

Changes in Oxygenation and Compliance as Related to Body Position in Acute Lung Injury
Bittner E, Chendrasekhar A, Pillai S, et al (West Virginia Univ, Morgantown)
Am Surg 62:1038–1041, 1996   4–9

Introduction.—Acute lung injury (ALI) is thought to be part of the pathophysiologic spectrum associated with adult respiratory distress syndrome (ARDS). A change in body positioning—specifically, changing to the prone position—is known to improve ventilation-perfusion matching in patients with ARDS. However, the effects of body positioning during mechanical ventilation in patients with ALI are unclear. The effects of body position on lung function in ALI were studied.

Methods.—The prospective study included 16 patients with ALI who were receiving mechanical ventilation. All patients had a partial pressure

TABLE 1.—Compliance and Oxygenation Data at Various Body Positions

Position	Supine	30° Elevation	45° Elevation
Static compliance (cc/cm H_2O)	36.1 ± 1.6	23.8 ± 1.6*	24.0 ± 1.6*
Dynamic compliance (cc/cm H_2O)	34.0 ± 1.6	17.1 ± 1.6*	17.9 ± 1.6*
PaO_2 (mm Hg)	101.8 ± 7.3	101.7 ± 7.3†	97.9 ± 7.3†
PaO_2/FIO_2 ratio	221.3 ± 13.9	221.1 ± 13.9†	212.8 ± 13.9†

Note: Values are mean ± standard error of the mean.
*$P = 0.001$.
†P is nonsignificant, as compared with supine values.
Abbreviations: PaO_2, partial pressure of arterial oxygen; *FIO_2,* fraction of inspired oxygen.
(Courtesy of Bittner E, Chendrasekhar A, Pillai S, et al: Changes in oxygenation and compliance as related to body position in acute lung injury. *Am Surg* 62:1038–1041, 1996.)

of oxygen/fraction of inspired oxygen ratio of less than 300, with no clinical signs of congestive heart failure. Each patient was studied in the supine position, with the head elevated 30 degrees and with the head elevated 45 degrees. The patients were allowed to equilibrate in each position before measurements were made, including static pulmonary compliance and partial pressure of oxygen from arterial blood gas sampling. The study hypothesis was that changing from the supine to the upright position would not improve oxygenation or compliance.

Results.—Dynamic and static compliance were both significantly worse with the patients in the upright position. Oxygenation was unaffected, as were minute volume and carbon dioxide level (Tables 1 to 3).

Conclusion.—For mechanically ventilated patients with ALI, shifting from the supine to the upright position worsens compliance and does not

TABLE 2.—Individual Oxygenation and Static and Dynamic Compliance Data

Patient No.	Supine			30° Elevation			45° Elevation		
	C-S	C-D	PaO_2	C-S	C-D	PaO_2	C-S	C-D	PaO_2
1	52	50	101	26	20	85	27	23	87
2	19	15	135	22	18	153	22	16	167
3	40	36	80	22	16	80	30	25	75
4	50	45	88	28	21	100	27	22	79
5	42	38	80	22	16	70	37	31	65
6	42	39	152	18	12	146	18	12	112
7	30	27	113	18	12	118	22	12	110
8	32	30	98	32	24	90	27	15	103
9	38	36	114	38	30	114	21	20	89
10	40	38	165	20	12	146	21	15	159
11	29	28	106	20	14	123	17	14	100
12	39	38	78	20	14	80	23	17	86
13	35	35	87	25	20	96	24	16	105
14	37	35	58	20	12	59	22	15	56
15	27	26	84	20	12	87	27	21	86
16	30	28	90	29	20	80	19	12	87

Abbreviations: C-S, static compliance (cc/cm H_2O); *C-D,* dynamic compliance (cc/cm H_2) PaO_2, partial pressure of arterial oxygen (in arterial blood gas sample in mm Hg).
(Courtesy of Bittner E, Chendrasekhar A, Pillai S, et al: Changes in oxygenation and compliance as related to body position in acute lung injury. *Am Surg* 62:1038–1041, 1996.)

TABLE 3.—Ventilator Settings for Each Patient

Patient No.	Ventilator Mode	FIO$_2$	PEEP
1	SIMV	0.5	8
2	SIMV	0.5	10
3	SIMV	0.5	8
4	SIMV	0.45	12
5	SIMV	0.5	12
6	SIMV	0.55	14
7	SIMV	0.35	12
8	SIMV	0.4	12
9	SIMV	0.5	10
10	SIMV	0.6	8
11	SIMV	0.5	5
12	SIMV	0.45	11
13	SIMV	0.5	8
14	SIMV	0.3	8
15	SIMV	0.3	10
16	SIMV	0.45	10

Abbreviation: SIMV, Synchronized intermittent mandatory ventilation.
(Courtesy of Bittner E, Chendrasekhar A, Pillai S, et al: Changes in oxygenation and compliance as related to body position in acute lung injury. *Am Surg* 62:1038–1041, 1996.)

improve oxygenation. The authors call for more study to determine the effects of body position in patients receiving positive pressure ventilation with various pathophysiologic states.

▶ The authors proved their hypothesis that, in patients with ALI, there is no improvement in oxygenation or lung compliance when body position is changed from supine to upright. I was not aware that this particular issue was being challenged, but now we have the study that would end such a debate.

B.A. Shapiro, M.D.

Effect of Acute Respiratory Acidosis on the Limits of Oxygen Extraction During Hemorrhage

Ward ME (McGill Univ, Montreal)
Anesthesiology 85:817–822, 1996   4–10

Introduction.—The adverse effects of hypercapnia may be overstated. The attempt to achieve normocapnia in patients with severely diseased lungs can actually aggravate lung injury. Both bulk flow and the efficiency of oxygen extraction determine the ability to sustain tissue oxygenation. Increased sympathetic activity maintains bulk blood flow throughout hypercapnia. The effect of hypercapnia on cells' capacity to adapt to decreases in oxygen availability by increasing oxygen extraction was examined.

Methods.—Three groups of paralyzed, mechanically ventilated dogs were anesthetized using α-chloralose. Normocapnia, moderate hypercapnia, or severe hypercapnia were achieved by regulating the concentration of carbon dioxide in the inhaled gas mixture. Stepwise hemorrhage was used to destabilize each dog's blood pressure. Oxygen delivery, oxygen consumption, and oxygen extraction ratios were assessed at each stage of the hemorrhage protocol.

Results.—The oxygen delivery rate and the oxygen extraction ratio were 7.8 mL·kg^{-1}·min^{-1} and 0.72, respectively, in normocapnic dogs at the point of onset of delivery dependence of oxygen consumption. These parameters were not affected by moderate hypercapnia. In dogs with severe hypercapnia, the critical value for oxygen delivery was 12.5 mL·kg^{-1}·min^{-1}, and the critical value for the extraction ratio, was 0.54. These values were significantly different from those found in normocapnic dogs.

Conclusions.—These findings identify a previously unrecognized threat to tissue oxygenation. It is important that adequate oxygen delivery is maintained when using mechanical ventilatory strategies that allow respiratory acidosis to develop.

▶ This dog study shows that acute hypercapnia is not a significant detriment to oxygen delivery or extraction at the critical point where oxygen consumption becomes dependent on oxygen delivery. I interpret this data to be reassuring; permissive hypercapnia should not threaten tissue oxygenation, as long as cardiac output remains at normal levels or greater.

B.A. Shapiro, M.D.

Relative Production of Tumour Necrosis Factor α and Interleukin 10 in Adult Respiratory Distress Syndrome

Armstrong L, Millar AB (Univ of Bristol, UK)
Thorax 52:442–446, 1997

4–11

Objective.—Adult respiratory distress syndrome (ARDS) is characterized by an extreme inflammatory response, possibly to sepsis, involving the proinflammatory mediator tumor necrosis factor α (TNF-α) and its inhibitor, interleukin 10 (IL-10). To determine if the relative production of TNF-α and IL-10 proteins might be altered in ARDS, levels were measured in the plasma, broncheolar lavage (BAL) fluid, and alveolar macrophage culture supernatant of ARDS patients or patients at risk of ARDS.

Methods.—Within 24 hours of arrival in the intensive therapy unit, BAL fluid and venous blood were obtained from 6 patients with bowel perforation, 8 with multiple trauma, and 12 with sepsis. Ten patients had ARDS. Macrophages were isolated from BAL and cultured. IL-10 and TNF-α levels were measured using a double sandwich enzyme linked immunoabsorbent assay.

Results.—There was a tendency for TNF-α levels to be increased in the BAL fluid of ARDS patients compared with levels in at-risk patients (Fig 1). Findings in macrophages were similar. IL-levels in plasma and in BAL fluid, but not in macrophages of ARDS patients, were significantly

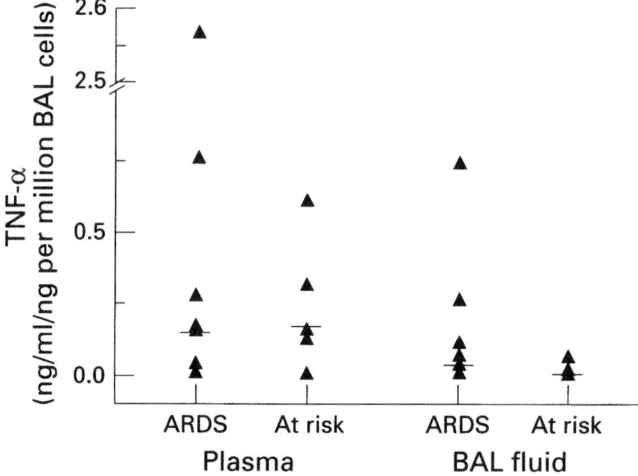

FIGURE 1.—TNF-α levels in the plasma and BAL fluid of patients with ARDS and those at risk of ARDS ($n = 10$). Protein levels in BAL fluid are adjusted to ng per million cells recovered by BAL. (Courtesy of Armstrong L, Millar AB: Relative production of tumour necrosis factor α and interleukin 10 in adult respiratory distress syndrome. *Thorax* 52:442–446, 1997, BMJ Publishing Group.)

lower than levels in at-risk patients (Fig 3). There was a significant correlation between IL-10 and TNF-α levels in BAL fluid, but not of survival of both ARDS and at-risk patients. The ratio of TNF-α to IL-10 in BAL fluid of ARDS patients was 3.52 and of at-risk patients was 0.85.

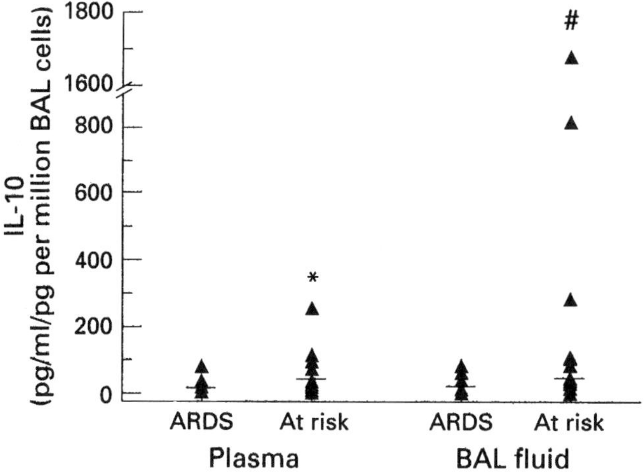

FIGURE 3.—IL-10 levels in the plasma and BAL fluid of patients with ARDS ($n = 10$) and those at risk of ARDS ($n = 16$). * p less than 0.05, median difference -17.5, 95% CI -52.4 to 1.31. * p less than 0.05, median difference -32.1: 95% CI -47.5 to 2.3 (Wilcoxon analysis). Protein levels in BAL fluid are adjusted to pg per million cells recovered by BAL. (Courtesy of Armstrong L, Millar AB: Relative production of tumour necrosis factor α and interleukin 10 in adult respiratory distress syndrome. *Thorax* 52:442–446, 1997, BMJ Publishing Group.)

Conclusion.—The pro- and anti-inflammatory imbalance, as measured by the ratio of TNF-α to IL-10, is significantly higher in ARDS patients than in at-risk patients.

▶ This article reports plasma and BAL levels of TNF and IL-10 in patients with or at risk for ARDS. Patients with ARDS had lower levels of IL-10 than those at risk for ARDS. However, there was no difference between the two groups with respect to the ability of alveolar macrophages to produce IL-10 in response to endotoxin stimulation in vitro. IL-10 is an "anti-inflammatory" cytokine which inhibits TNF synthesis. Low levels of IL-10 could contribute to increased levels of "pro-inflammatory" cytokines and thus contribute to the development of ARDS. However, the data is too preliminary to draw any firm conclusions.

L.C. Casey, M.D., Ph.D.

Acute Respiratory Distress Syndrome: CT Findings During Partial Liquid Ventilation
Meaney JFM, Kazerooni EA, Garver KA, et al (Univ of Michigan, Ann Arbor)
Radiology 202:570–573, 1997   4–12

Background.—Perflubron is a liquid ventilation agent used in neonates, children, and adults during partial liquid ventilation. Perflubron improves gas exchange and pulmonary function in patients with acute respiratory distress syndrome. A prospective multicenter study of partial liquid ventilation in adults is currently underway. Recent studies have described the appearance of lungs treated with partial liquid ventilation with perflubron on bedside chest radiographs. However, the radiopaque perflubron may obscure diagnostic information on plain radiographs.

Methods.—CT scans of 9 patients with acute respiratory distress syndrome who were treated with partial liquid ventilation with perflubron were reviewed. The patients were between 3 months and 75 years old. One to seven doses of perflubron were administered to each patient during a period of 1–8 days.

Results.—In 4 patients, the mean interval from administration of perflubron to scanning was 6.25 days, and the distribution of perflubron was gravity dependent. In another 4 patients, the mean interval from administration of perflubron to scanning was 16 days, and the distribution of perflubron was patchy. In 1 patient, the mean interval from administration of perflubron to scanning was 3 days, and the distribution of perflubron was homogeneous. Extraparenchymal perflubron was noted in intrathoracic lymph nodes in 4 patients, supraclavicular nodes in 2 patients, axillary nodes in 1 patient, and both the retroperitoneum and mediastinum in 2 patients. Perflubron was observed in a pneumatocele and the pleural space in 1 patient.

Discussion.—These findings of the appearance of lungs treated with partial liquid ventilation with perflubron indicate that the distribution of perflubron on CT scans is generally gravity dependent. The role of CT in patients treated with perflubron needs to be defined in larger studies.

▶ The distribution of the perfluorocarbon used in partial liquid ventilation was confirmed to be gravitationally dependent by the use of chest CT scans. This report details the chest CT findings in 9 patients with acute lung injury who were managed with partial liquid ventilation. The perflubron is much heavier than water and would be expected to be gravitationally distributed. The surprising finding was the presence of extraparenchymal perflubron, which was present in intrathoracic, supraclavicular, axillary, mediastinal, and retroperitoneal lymph nodes. One patient even had perflubron in the pleural space and in a pneumatocele.

R.A. Balk, M.D.

Additive Beneficial Effects of the Prone Position, Nitric Oxide, and Almitrine Bismesylate on Gas Exchange and Oxygen Transport in Acute Respiratory Distress Syndrome
Jolliet P, Bulpa P, Ritz M, et al (Univ Hosp, Geneva)
Crit Care Med 25:786–794, 1997 4–13

Background.—Several measures have been shown to improve arterial oxygenation in patients with acute respiratory distress syndrome (ARDS), including prone positioning, inhaled nitric oxide, and IV almitrine bismesylate. Each works by a different mechanism, which suggests that additional gains in oxygenation could be achieved by combining the techniques. The effects of these 3 interventions in combination on arterial oxygenation in patients with severe ARDS were studied.

Methods.—The randomized, controlled trial included 12 patients with ARDS and severe hypoxemia. The interventions studied, alone and in combination, were inhaled nitric oxide, 20 parts per million for 15 minutes, with the patient in the supine and the prone position; IV almitrine bismesylate, 1 mg/kg/hr for 60 minutes, with the patient in the prone position. The various single and combined approaches were studied in sequence, and measurements of hemodynamic, blood gas, and gas exchange were taken in response to each. Oxygenation was assessed in terms of PaO_2 or PaO_2/FIO_2 ratio.

Results.—Fifty-eight percent of patients had improved oxygenation in response to being turned to the prone position. Arterial oxygen saturation increased from 89% in the supine baseline condition to 92% in the nitric oxide, plus supine condition to 94% in the nitric oxide plus prone condition. A significant increase in arterial oxygen saturation and a significant reduction in the alveolar-arterial oxygen difference were achieved as well. Compared with baseline, almitrine bismesylate administration increased PaO_2/FIO_2. It also decreased the alveolar-arterial oxygen difference, compared with baseline and compared with the nitric oxide plus supine position. Although oxygenation was not improved by prone positioning alone, the nitric oxide plus almitrine bismesylate condition increased PaO_2/FIO_2 compared with the nitric oxide plus supine or prone condition.

Seven patients responded to prone positioning; this group had further improvement in PaO_2 with the combination of nitric oxide and almitrine bismesylate. In the same group, adding either nitric oxide or almitrine bismesylate did not further improve oxygenation. Almitrine bismesylate significantly improved heart rate and cardiac output. Nitric oxide significantly decreased and almitrine bismesylate significantly increased mean pulmonary arterial pressure. However, the latter increase was completely eliminated by nitric oxide. There were no changes in minute ventilation, respiratory system compliance, physiologic dead space, or $PaCO_2$.

Conclusions.—In combination, the 3 interventions studied—prone positioning, nitric oxide, and almitrine bismesylate—can significantly improve arterial oxygenation in patients with ARDS and severe hypoxemia. No harmful effects were apparent. Almitrine bismesylate increases mean pulmonary arterial pressure and right ventricular stroke work. Although these effects are lessened by nitric oxide, the combination approach should be used cautiously in patients with severe pulmonary hypertension or right ventricular failure.

► The prone position is known to allow recruitment of previously gravity-dependent alveoli, while making previously non–gravity-dependent lung tissue better perfused. Nitric oxide is known to cause dilation only in vessels perfusing ventilated alveoli. Almitrine bismesylate appears to potentiate the vasoconstriction of vessels perfusing poorly ventilated alveoli. Each of these modalities improves oxygenation in some patients with severe ARDS, but, unexplainably, not in all patients with severe ARDS. This study is an interesting demonstration of combinations of these modalities improving oxygenation to a greater degree than any single modality alone; it is some food for thought and reason for further investigations.

B.A. Shapiro, M.D.

Pulmonary Embolism

Efficacy and Safety of a Low-Molecular-Weight Heparin and Standard Unfractionated Heparin for Prophylaxis of Postoperative Venous Thromboembolism: European Multicenter Trial
Kakkar VV, Boeckl O, Boneu B, et al (Thrombosis Research Inst, London)
World J Surg 21:2–9, 1997
4–14

Objective.—Low–molecular weight heparins (LMWHs) have higher bioavailability but different pharmacokinetic properties, depending on the way they are prepared. The safety and efficacy of Clivarine, a second-generation LMWH, was compared with standard unfractionated heparin (UFH) in a randomized, double-blind multicenter trial.

Methods.—Either Clivarine, (1,750 anti-Xa IU) once daily plus a placebo injection 12 hours later, or UFH, (5,000 IU) every 12 hours, was administered subcutaneously to 665 and 677 abdominal surgery patients, respectively. The incidences of deep vein thrombosis (DVT) and pulmonary embolism (PE), bleeding complications, adverse events, and coagulation parameters were recorded.

Results.—Both products were equally effective. Deep vein thrombosis developed in 30 LMWH patients and in 28 UFH patients. Pulmonary embolism occurred in 1 LMWH patient and in 3 UFH patients. There were significantly fewer postoperative bleeding complications in the LMWH group than in the UFH group (8.3% vs. 11.8%, relative risk 0.7), including wound hematoma (4.4% vs. 7.7%) and bruising at the injection site (1.7% vs. 4.6%). Anti–factor Xa activity of 0.1 U/mL was constant in LMWH patients, but was not detected in UFH patients. Increases in transaminase, lactate dehydrogenase, and triglyceride levels were significantly lower in LMWH patients than in UFH patients.

Conclusions.—Clivarine (1,750 anti-Xa IU) daily was as effective as 10,000 IU of UFH daily in preventing DVT and PE, and resulted in significantly fewer bleeding complications.

▶ Most studies to date on LMWH have established its safety. The ES-SENCE trial has established its efficacy in reducing ischemic events in acute coronary syndromes. To date, no study has established a mortality reduction with LMWH.

J.E. Calvin, Jr., M.D.

J.E. Parrillo, M.D.

The Incidence of Deep Venous Thrombosis in ICU Patients

Marik PE, Andrews L, Maini B (Univ of Massachusetts, Worchester)
Chest 111:661–664, 1997   4–15

Introduction.—The incidence of deep vein thrombosis (DVT) in patients in the ICU has not been thoroughly evaluated. The incidence of DVT was assessed prospectively in a high-risk group of patients in an ICU who were receiving DVT prophylaxis. Risk factors and the effect of prophylactic regimens on the incidence of DVT were examined.

Methods.—Venous duplex scans were performed in 102 patients in the ICU between days 4 and 7 of hospitalization. Patients with clinical features suggestive of DVT, pulmonary embolism, or undiagnosed fever underwent follow-up duplex scans. Ventilation/perfusion scans were performed in patients with abnormal venous duplex scans. All patients underwent routine DVT prophylaxis with unfractionated heparin. Pneumatic compression boots were used for patients in whom heparin therapy was contraindicated. Patients were evaluated for risk factors for thromboembolism.

Results.—The mean age of the 102 patients was 65 years, and the mean length of ICU stay was 6 days. Ninety-four patients (92%) underwent DVT prophylaxis. Venous duplex scan detected DVT in 12 patients (12%). Eight patients had proximal clot extension, 4 with high-probability ventilation/perfusion scans. Two of 56 patients (3.6%) without symptoms of DVT had abnormal scan results. Six of 11 patients with leg swelling had DVT and 1 patient with unexplained fever had abnormal scan results. Deep vein thrombosis developed in 5 of 26 patients (19%) and 5 of 68 patients (7.4%), who received pneumatic compression and subcutaneous heparin, respectively (not a significant difference). None of the following factors increased the risk of DVT: cancer, previous DVT/pulmonary embolism, obesity, trauma, stasis changes, leg ulcer, claudication, mechanical ventilation, or surgery.

Conclusion.—The DVT occurrence was 12% in this cohort of high-risk patients receiving DVT prophylaxis in an ICU. Abnormal scans were detected in 3.6% of patients without signs or symptoms suggestive of DVT. Venous scans should be undertaken only in patients with suspected DVT or pulmonary embolism.

▶ This cohort study showed an incidence of DVT of 12% among patients submitting to venous duplex scans; most of the patients had signs and symptoms. It is disturbing that all these patients were receiving prophylaxis. Deep vein thrombosis remains an important complication in critically ill patients and should be sought out.

J.E. Calvin, Jr., M.D.

J.E. Parrillo, M.D.

The ECG in Pulmonary Embolism: Predictive Value of Negative T Waves in Precordial Leads—80 Case Reports
Ferrari E, Imbert A, Chevalier T, et al (Univ Hosp, Nice, France)
Chest 111:537–543, 1997   4–16

Introduction.—Because pulmonary embolism (PE) is difficult to detect, fewer than half of all cases are recognized while the patient is still alive. One of the first examinations to be performed in cases of suspected PE is the ECG, a test that appears to lack both specificity and sensitivity. A series of 80 consecutive patients hospitalized for PE were evaluated for the relationship between changes in ECG signs and angiographic and hemodynamic changes.

Methods.—The admission ECG and those performed during hospitalization were studied for ECG parameters, particularly heart rate, atrial and ventricular depolarization, and ventricular repolarization. At least 4 recordings were made each day for the first 3 days, then 1 per day for the duration of the hospital stay; at least 12 standard leads were recorded on all ECGs. The patient group included 47 men and 33 women, with a mean age of 65.4 years. Exclusion criteria were a history of cardiopulmonary disease that might modify the ECG, an absence of criteria allowing the massiveness of the PE to be assessed, and/or use of antiarrhythmic agents.

Results.—Initial angiography involving right heart catheterization confirmed the diagnosis of PE in all patients. In 59 cases, PE was classified as massive (defined as exhibiting a Miller index of more than 50% and/or a

TABLE 1.—Electrocardiographic Signs in Pulmonary Embolism

	Our Series, 1995 (n=80)	Cutforth et al.[1] 1958 (n=50)	Lenegre et al.[5] 1970 (n=37)	Stein et al.[12] 1975 (n=90)
T waves (—) from V_1 to V_4	68%	46%	89%	42%
S1 Q3 T3 pattern	50%	28%	52%	12%
Peripheral low voltage	29%	—	—	6%
Sinus tachycardia	26%† 36%†	—	90%	69%†
Complete or incomplete RBBB	22%	40%	24%	15%
Pulmonary P wave	5%	12%	—	6%
Normal ECG	9%	24%	10%	13%

Note: The prevalence of the ECG signs observed is classified by decreasing order of frequency and is compared with the results of other series in the literature.

*Incidence of tachycardia when heart rate considered is > 90 beats/min.

†Incidence of tachycardia when heart rate considered is > 100 beats/min.

Abbreviation: RBBB, right bundle branch block.

(Courtesy of Ferrari E, Imbert A, Chevalier T, et al: The ECG in pulmonary embolism: Predictive value of negative T waves in precordial leads—80 case reports. *Chest* 111:537–543, 1997.)

mean pulmonary artery pressure of greater than 30 mm Hg). Twenty-one were nonmassive. The initial ECG identified an interior ischemic pattern in 68% of patients, an S1 Q3 T3 pattern in 50%, low voltage in 29%, sinus tachycardia in 26%, incomplete right bundle branch block (RBBB) in 12%, complete RBBB in 10%, and pulmonary P wave in 5%; in 9% of patients the ECG results appeared normal (Table 1). The anterior ischemic pattern was present in 85% of patients with massive PE, but in only 19% of those with nonmassive PE (Table 2). Negative T waves on precordial leads were the ECG sign associated with the best sensitivity, specificity, positive predictive value, and negative predictive value. This subepicardial ischemic pattern was an even stronger marker of PE severity when it appeared as early as the first day; the more massive the PE, the earlier the onset of an anterior ischemic pattern. Reversibility of anterior T-wave inversion correlated with changes in PE.

Conclusion.—Among these patients hospitalized in a cardiology unit, the ECG pattern of inverted T waves in the precordial leads was the most frequent ECG sign of PE. This pattern is closely related to the initial

TABLE 2.—Incidence of ECG Abnormalities in Massive vs. Nonmassive Pulmonary Embolism

	Massive PE. %	Nonmassive PE. %
Sinus tachycardia	36	0
Anterior ischemic pattern	85	19
RBBB	22	24
S1 Q3 T3	54	54
Peripheral low voltage	36	36
Pulmonary P wave	7	0

Abbreviations: PE, pulmonary embolism; *RBBB*, right bundle branch block.

(Courtesy of Ferrari E, Imbert A, Chevalier T, et al: The ECG in pulmonary embolism: Predictive value of negative T waves in precordial leads—80 case reports. *Chest* 111:537–543, 1997.)

severity of PE, and its reversibility after thrombolysis indicates response to treatment.

▶ Anterior T wave inversion is not specific for pulmonary embolism, as it is also very common in coronary artery disease. However, when found in patients with pulmonary embolism, it is a sign of severity.

J.E. Calvin, Jr., M.D.

J.E. Parrillo, M.D.

Pneumonia

Evaluation of Outcome for Intubated Patients With Pneumonia Due to *Pseudomonas aeruginosa*

Rello J, Jubert P, Vallés J, et al (Autonomous Univ, Barcelona; Winthrop-Univ Hosp, Mineola, NY)
Clin Infect Dis 23:973–978, 1996   4–17

Background.—Many intubated patients develop ventilator-associated pneumonia. A debate exists, however, as to whether death in these patients results directly from the infection, or whether this type of pneumonia is a form of organ failure. These investigators studied patients with ventilator-associated pneumonia caused by *Pseudomonas aeruginosa* to determine whether their mortality rates were higher than those of patients with ventilator-associated pneumonia caused by other pathogens. They also assessed whether the Acute Physiological and Chronic Health Evaluation (APACHE) II scores were useful for estimating mortality rates in these patients.

Methods.—Cases (26 patients with ventilator-associated pneumonia caused by *P. aeruginosa*) were matched with controls (52 patients with ventilator-associated pneumonia caused by other pathogens). APACHE II scores were calculated for each patient 3 times: at admission, when pneumonia was first diagnosed, and 72 hours after treatment. Fiberoptic bronchoscopy or bronchoalveolar lavage was used to determine the microbiology of the pulmonary infiltrates.

Findings.—One of 12 matched controls died of pneumonia. Of the 26 cases, 6 died of pneumonia, and 2 died of cardiac complications; 18 had clinical resolution of the infection, but only 15 lived to be discharged. The mortality rate attributable to *P. aeruginosa* was 13.5%. The overall mortality rate of 42.3% was much higher than that predicted by the APACHE II scores at admission (28.1%). In the controls, however, predicted and observed APACHE II scores were similar (28.7% and 28.8%, respectively). In these cases, APACHE II scores did not differ at admission between the 6 patients who died of pneumonia and the 18 who had clinical resolution. However, once pneumonia developed, and after 72 hours of treatment, the APACHE II scores in these 2 groups differed significantly. Each patient who had an APACHE II score of 20 or more after 72 hours of treatment died.

Conclusions.—Patients with ventilator-associated pneumonia caused by *P. aeruginosa* were more likely to die than patients with ventilator-associated pneumonia caused by other pathogens. In these cases, the APACHE II score at admission was not an indicator of outcome, although a worsening APACHE II score after pneumonia set in was associated with a worse prognosis.

▶ Ventilator-associated pneumonia has a high associated morbidity and mortality. *Pseudomonas* infections are frequent causes of nosocomial infection and have a high degree of associated mortality, and this is particularly true when the *Pseudomonas* is the cause of the ventilator-associated pneumonia. This study evaluated 26 patients with *Pseudomonas aeruginosa* as the cause of ventilator-associated pneumonia to determine the usefulness of outcome prediction scores as a means to identify high-risk patients. The study used APACHE II scores and only included patients who were started on appropriate antibiotic therapy. A case–control format was used to identify a control group for comparison purposes. As expected, there was a high observed mortality in the *Pseudomonas*-infected patients with ventilator-associated pneumonia. More than 42% of these patients died during the hospital stay, and multiple organ failure was the primary cause of death. This mortality rate was in contrast to the APACHE II predicted mortality rate of 28% and the observed mortality rate of 28% among the case-matched control population. Six of the pneumonia deaths were believed by the authors to be directly related to the pneumonia. The increased, observed mortality rate in comparison with predicted mortality underscores a major area of concern in evaluating trials of therapy for hospital-acquired pneumonia. This concern deals with the important impact of a patient's underlying clinical condition, and factors that increase the risk of developing nosocomial infections in relationship to the actual effect of the complicating pneumonia on the ultimate outcome. Obviously, it may be difficult to attribute the observed increase in mortality to one of these particular entities. We also see that the APACHE II score may not have the power in the setting of this complex clinical situation to predict outcome, other than to conclude a high score that continues to increase despite therapy has a poor prognosis.

R.A. Balk, M.D.

Relationship of Microbiologic Diagnostic Criteria to Morbidity and Mortality in Patients With Ventilator-associated Pneumonia
Bregeon F, Papazian L, Visconti A, et al (Hôpital Sainte-Marguerite, Marseille, France)
JAMA 277:655–662, 1997
4–18

Background.—Although some authors suggest that patients with ventilator-associated pneumonia (VAP) diagnosed on positive protected specimen brush (PSB) culture have a worse prognosis than those with VAP diagnosed by other sampling procedures, this has never been demonstrated. Whether the mortality and morbidity of VAP defined by PSB culture differs from that of VAP defined by other sampling methods was investigated.

Methods. All patients with documented VAP during a 5-year period were included in the study. A total of 102 patients had VAP diagnosed by PSB culture, and 223 patients with VAP had it diagnosed by another sampling method. Patients were matched by diagnosis on admission, age, sex, date of admission, Acute Physiology and Chronic Health Evaluation II (APACHE II) score, and date of pneumonia onset. Seventy-six pairs were analyzed. The efficacy of matching was 81.9%.

Findings.—Mortality did not differ between groups. Fatality rates in the ICU were 38% in the PSB-positive group and 39.4% in the PSB-negative group. Hospital mortality was 41%. Mean duration of ventilation was 26 days, and mean length of ICU stay was 33 days in both groups.

Conclusions.—After adjustment for confounding factors, patients with VAP diagnosed by PSB had outcomes comparable to those diagnosed by other bacteriologic procedures. Thus, the conclusions of studies using PSB as the reference criterion for VAP can be extended to all VAP cases defined by the results of microbiological nonsurgical methods.

▶ This study supports those who believe there is no need to use invasive diagnostic and complex microbiologic studies to diagnose nosocomial pneumonia. This study used a case-matched cohort of patients who were identified during the same observation period, to compare the outcome of patients whose VAP was diagnosed using a positive PSB culture with those whose VAP was diagnosed using some other positive culture.

Analysis of the results demonstrated remarkable similarities between these 2 groups. No significant differences were observed in mortality, ICU mortality, hospital survival, days of ventilatory support, or length of ICU stay.

Unfortunately, this controversy continues and appears unlikely to be settled until we can design a multicenter, prospective, randomized trial that will control for the type of patient, underlying disease process, and treatment, as well as the diagnostic methodology used to diagnose the VAP.

R.A. Balk, M.D.

Scoring System for Nosocomial Pneumonia in ICUs

Kropec A, Schulgen G, Just H, et al (Univ Hosp, Freiburg, Germany)
Intensive Care Med 22:1155–1161, 1996   4–19

Background.—Nosocomial infections are a major health problem because of the associated cost, morbidity, mortality, and personal distress. The most common nosocomial infection in the ICU is pneumonia. Some studies of nosocomial pneumonia have reported mortality rates of 20% to 50%. One prevention strategy is to classify patients early after admission to the ICU according to risk for nosocomial pneumonia.

Methods.—In a 2-year prospective cohort study, 756 adult patients admitted to the ICU for at least 48 hours were followed until development of nosocomial pneumonia, discharge from ICU, or death.

Results.—Of the 756 patients, 129 developed nosocomial pneumonia; 106 of these developed it in the first 2 weeks. Multivariate analysis showed that male gender, urgent surgery, thorax drainage, neurological diseases, administration of antacids, partial pressure of oxygen > 110 mm Hg, administration of coagulation factors, and lack of infection on admission were independent risk factors. A scoring system was developed using a multivariate model to determine a predictive risk index for nosocomial pneumonia. The risk of developing nosocomial pneumonia ranged from 11% to 42.3%. The risk of developing nosocomial pneumonia for patients in the highest risk group was 7 times higher than for patients in the lowest risk group.

Discussion.—A predictive model was developed to classify patients in the ICU according to risk of developing nosocomial pneumonia. Patients in the higher-risk groups would probably benefit the most from prevention strategies. This predictive model is simple to use at bedside and had good predictive ability in the cohort from which it was derived. This model needs to be validated in other patient cohorts in ICUs in additional facilities.

▶ To address the problem of nosocomial pneumonia in the ICU patient, these authors prospectively evaluated 756 patients admitted to an ICU for more than 48 hours for the development of this complication. After identifying clinical parameters associated with an increased incidence of nosocomial pneumonia development, the authors went on to develop a scoring system to predict the risk of developing a nosocomial pneumonia over the following 2 weeks. This prediction tool now requires prospective evaluation and an assessment of its utility for the entire hospital stay, rather than 2 weeks, and its value in patients who require less than 48 hours of ICU care.

R.A. Balk, M.D.

Decrease in Nosocomial Pneumonia in Ventilated Patients by Selective Oropharyngeal Decontamination (SOD)

Abele-Horn M, Dauber A, Bauernfeind A, et al (Ludwig-Maximilians-Universität, München, Germany; City Hosp of Munich-Schwabing, Germany)
Intensive Care Med 23:187–195, 1997
4–20

Objective.—Selective decontamination of the digestive tract (SDD) is a technique to reduce bacterial colonization in the ICU and, thus, to reduce the rate of pneumonia and other infections. The use of only selective oropharyngeal decontamination (SOD) should be effective in eliminating potential pathogens and, thus, reducing colonization and infection rates. The effects of SOD on colonization and infection rates in ventilated ICU patients were investigated in a randomized, controlled trial.

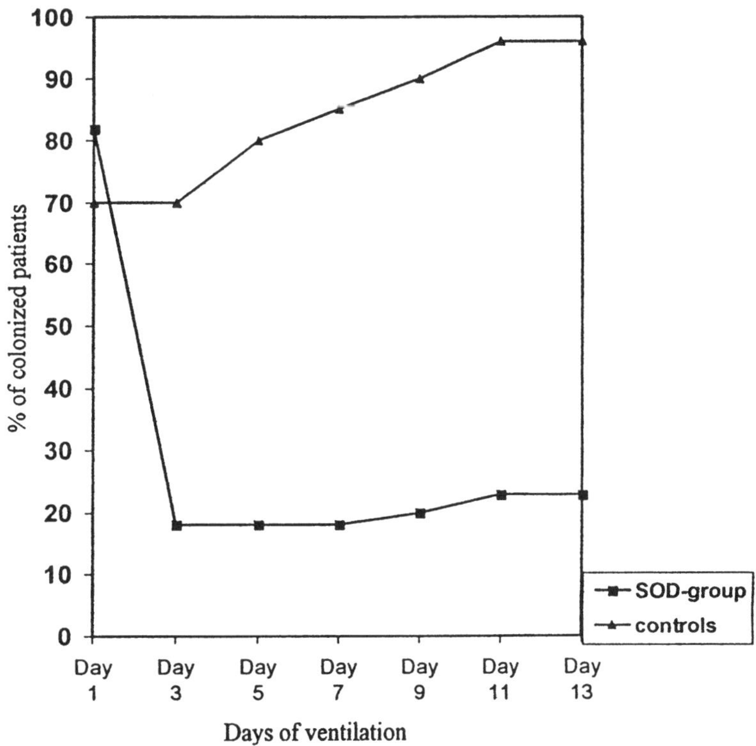

FIGURE 1.—Oropharyngeal colonization of both study and control groups during ventilation. (Courtesy of Abele-Horn M, Dauber A, Bauernfeind A, et al: Decrease in nosocomial pneumonia in ventilated patients by selective orpharyngeal decontamination (SOD). *Intensive Care Med* 23:187–195, 1997. Copyright Springer-Verlag 1997.)

Methods.—The study included 88 patients hospitalized on an emergency basis and intubated within 24 hours. Fifty were assigned to receive SOD, consisting of amphotericin B, colistin sulfate, and tobramycin applied to the oropharynx and systemic cefotaxime. The remaining 33 patients served as controls, receiving no antibiotics. Oropharyngeal specimens were obtained at admission, then twice a week and after extubation.

Results.—The SOD group had significant reductions in colonization (Fig 1). The infection rate was 77% in the SOD group vs. 22% in the control group. When colonization and pneumonia occurred, the major pathogen was *Staphylococcus aureus.* There were no significant differences between groups in terms of ICU days, duration of ventilation, and mortality. The average daily cost per patient for antibiotics was reduced in the SOD group. There were no problems with antibiotic resistance.

Conclusions.—In patients receiving mechanical ventilation, SOD effectively reduces rates of colonization and pneumonia, as well as total charges for antibiotics. There is no apparent effect on length of ICU stay, duration of ventilation, or mortality. More research is needed to clarify the clinical impact of the selection of *Staphylococcus aureus* by SOD.

▶ Here is yet another study touting the potential benefits of selective decontamination in the prevention of ventilator-associated pneumonia (VAP). It is similar in many aspects to its predecessors, showing a significant reduction in number of microorganisms, colonization rates, and incidence of pulmonary infections in the treated group. However, the selective decontamination used here involved only the oropharynx, with nonabsorbable antibiotic paste applied to the palate and lower lip. In this manner, the relatively high cost of decontaminating the digestive tract was avoided. Indeed, the study found that the total antibiotic charge was much lower for the decontaminated group than for the controls.

What good is selective decontamination in the prevention of VAP? Previous studies have shown that the gastropulmonary route does not play a significant role in the development of VAP. Still others have concluded that mortality in these patients is a reflection of the underlying disease process, and not primarily a result of the nosocomial pneumonia. In spite of demonstrating a reduction in VAP in this study, no significant differences were found in time spent receiving ventilatory support, number of ICU days, or mortality. As for the finding of lower total antibiotic cost in the treatment group, there are too many unanswered questions to allow this claim to go unchallenged. Total antibiotic cost is related to the incidence of use, type of antibiotic administered, and duration of therapy. These variables were either not well controlled or, at best, not well documented.

As with any study that does not unequivocally prove or disprove the stated hypothesis, the authors put out the call for further investigations. I, for one, do not see the need.

H. Nearman, M.D.

Usefulness of Quantitative Cultures of BAL Fluid For Diagnosing Nosocomial Pneumonia in Ventilated Patients
Jourdain B, Joly-Guillou M-L, Dombret M-C, et al (Hôpital Bichat, Paris)
Chest 111:411–418, 1997   4–21

Introduction.—Patients receiving mechanical ventilation can have complications with nosocomial bacterial pneumonias. In ventilated patients, classic clinical criteria for diagnosing pneumonia are unreliable. To establish microbiologic criteria for diagnosing nosocomial pneumonia, various techniques have been developed for obtaining respiratory specimens, including bronchoalveolar lavage (BAL), which is safe and samples a large area of lung parenchyma. In mechanically ventilated patients with suspected lung infection, the routine use of quantitative cultures of BAL fluid obtained with fiberoptic bronchoscopy was examined.

Methods.—In 84 patients who were mechanically ventilated for 48 hours or more, 141 episodes of suspected lung infection were found.

Microbiologic findings obtained with protected specimen brush were compared with those obtained using BAL fluid. A determination was made of their operating characteristics. Using different ways to report the results and over a range of values, the operating characteristics of BAL fluid cultures were determined.

Results.—There was a high level of qualitative agreement between BAL and protected specimen brush specimen cultures, as 83% of the organisms isolated in protected specimen brush specimens were recovered simultaneously from BAL fluid. There was a significant correlation between the results of quantitative BAL and protected specimen brush cultures. Based on the following criteria, pneumonia was diagnosed in 57 patients: protected specimen brush sample yielded 10^3 colony-forming units (CFU)/mL or more of at least 1 microorganism and/or at least 5% of cells contained intracellular bacteria on direct examination of BAL. An optimal threshold was the discriminative value of 10^4 CFU/mL, resulting in a specificity of 84.5% and a sensitivity of 82%.

Conclusions.—To diagnose pneumonia in ventilated patients, BAL fluid culture can offer a sensitive and specific means that may provide relevant information about the causative pathogens.

▶ The studies of Jourdain et al. and Luna et al. (Abstract 4–22) tackle aspects of the intense controversy surrounding the use of BAL in the diagnosis of ventilator-associated pneumonia and nosocomial pneumonia. Jourdain and colleagues demonstrate that BAL compares favorably to the results of protected specimen brushes when evaluated by direct examination, with greater than 5% of cells with intracellular organisms or with quantitative cultures of greater than 10^4 CFU/mL. This group of investigators have a record of advocating the use of invasive diagnostic studies to help make decisions whether to treat and with what antibiotic to treat a patient with nosocomial pneumonia or ventilator-associated pneumonia.

R.A. Balk, M.D.

Impact of BAL Data on the Therapy and Outcome of Ventilator-associated Pneumonia

Luna CM, Vujacich P, Niederman MS, et al (Univ of Buenos Aires, Argentina; Winthrop-Univ, Mineola, NY)
Chest 111:676–685, 1997   4–22

Introduction.—The course of mechanical ventilation can become complicated by hospital-acquired pneumonia. There is still controversy over the appropriate timing of antibiotic therapy and the most accurate way to diagnose this infection. Some studies indicate that antibiotic therapy itself is a risk factor for ventilator-associated pneumonia, leading investigators to conclude that antibiotic therapy decisions be guided by the results of bronchoscopically directed sampling. No previous study has examined the outcome of ventilator-associated pneumonia if antibiotics are prescribed

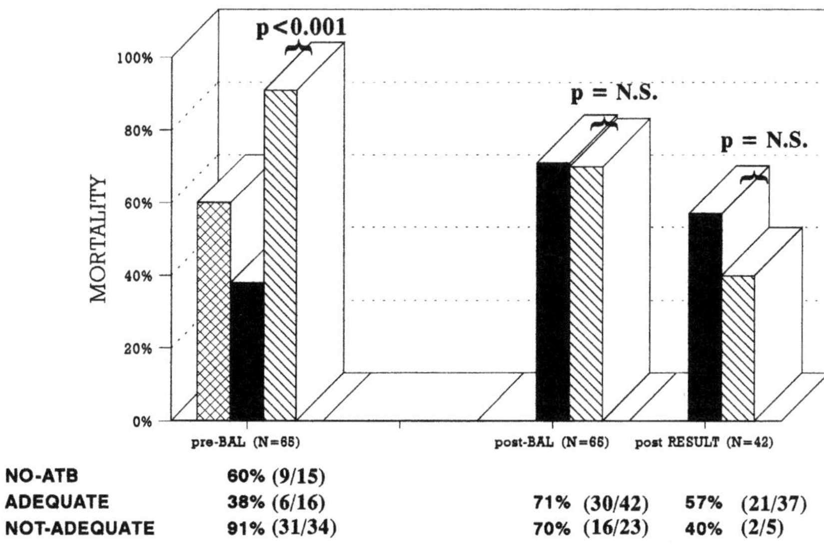

FIGURE 1.—Mortality rates are plotted in relation to the adequacy of antibiotic (*ATB*) therapy at 3 different times (pre–bronchoalveolar lavage [*pre-BAL*], post-BAL, and postresult). Statistical differences between adequate and inadequate therapy are present only at the pre-BAL time, when mortality was lower for patients receiving adequate therapy. (Courtesy of Luna CM, Vujacich P, Niederman MS, et al: Impact of BAL data on the therapy and outcome of ventilator-associated pneumonia. *Chest* 111:676–685, 1997.)

based on bronchoscopic diagnosis of ventilator-associated pneumonia rather than empirical evidence. In patients with clinically suspected ventilator-associated pneumonia, bronchoscopy with quantitative bronchoalveolar lavage (BAL) was performed, and a comparison was made as to the timing of antibiotic therapy.

Methods.—A total of 132 patients were studied who were hospitalized for more than 72 hours, were receiving mechanical ventilation, and had a new or progressive lung infiltrate with 2 of the following 3 clinical criteria for ventilator-associated pneumonia: an abnormal temperature, an abnormal leukocyte count, and purulent bronchial secretions. Within 24 hours of establishing a clinical diagnosis of a new episode of hospital-acquired, ventilator-associated pneumonia or progression of a prior episode of nosocomial pneumonia, bronchoscopy with BAL was performed. Antibiotics were administered to all patients: 107 before therapy and 25 immediately after.

Results.—Of the 132 patients studied, 67 were BAL negative and 65 were BAL positive, satisfying a microbiologic definition of ventilator-associated pneumonia. When compared with the BAL-negative patients, the positive patients had no differences in mortality, prior antibiotic use, and demographic features. Fewer of the negative patients (24 of 67) satisfied all 3 clinical criteria of ventilator-associated pneumonia than the positive patients (38 of 65). Before bronchoscopy, 50 positive patients

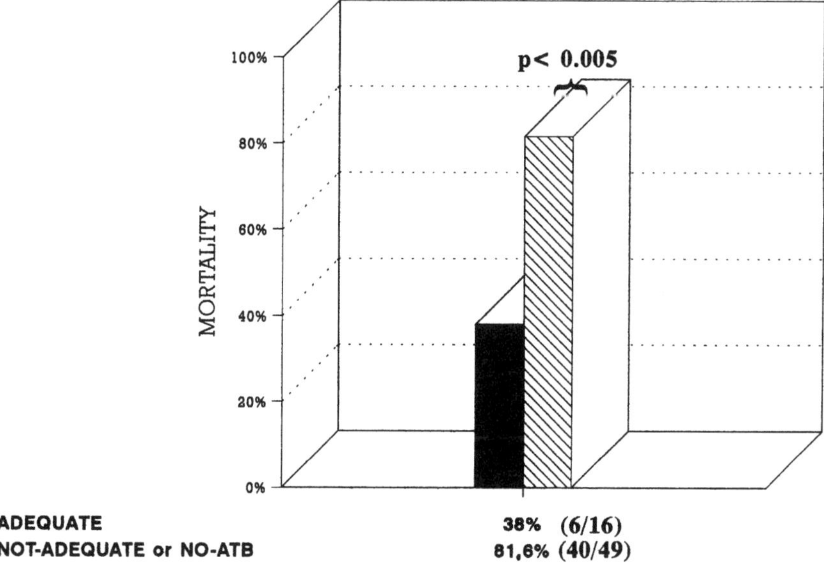

FIGURE 2.—For the 65 patients with a positive bronchoalveolar lavage (BAL) culture, the impact of the initial therapy, at the pre-BAL time, on the outcome was evaluated. Patients receiving adequate initial antibiotic (*ATB*) therapy had a significantly lower mortality rate than patients receiving either inadequate antibiotic therapy or no antibiotics. (Courtesy of Luna CM, Vujacich P, Niederman MS, et al: Impact of BAL data on the therapy and outcome of ventilator-associated pneumonia. *Chest* 111:676–685, 1997.)

received antibiotic therapy. For 16 patients, this therapy was adequate, as defined by the results of BAL, and the mortality rate was 38%. For 34 patients, this prior therapy was inadequate and the mortality rate was 91%. The mortality rate was 60% when no therapy was given (Fig 1). More patients received adequate therapy when changes were made after bronchoscopy, but the mortality rate was comparable to those who continued to receive inadequate therapy (Fig 2). Of the 65 BAL-positive patients, 46 died, and 23 died before the BAL results were known.

Conclusions.—Regardless of whether BAL cultures confirm the diagnosis of ventilator-associated pneumonia, patients with clinically suspected ventilator-associated pneumonia have a high mortality rate. Mortality rate is reduced when adequate antibiotic therapy is initiated before performing bronchoscopy. To influence survival, bronchoscopy information that defines the microbial etiology of ventilator-associated pneumonia can be too late.

▶ The overall benefit of the invasive diagnostic approach for nosocomial pneumonia and ventilator-associated pneumonia is addressed in this trial. This study contrasts the outcome of patients who were treated empirically with antibiotics vs. those treated when decisions were guided by the invasive diagnostic approach. All the patients were aggressively evaluated, and the initial empirical decisions concerning antibiotics were compared with subsequent management decisions based on the results of the invasive diagnostic studies. Based on the results of their study, these authors argue for early initiation of appropriate antibiotic therapy in patients with nosocomial and ventilator-associated pneumonia. Delaying the start of antibiotics until the results of the BAL are available or empirically initiating inappropriate antibiotic coverage were both associated with a poor outcome. The role of the invasive bronchoscopic approach appears to be limited to supporting the initial empirical antibiotic choices because, unfortunately, subsequent changes in the antibiotic coverage that are guided by the bronchoscopic results did not favorably influence patient outcome. In fact, this group had a worse outcome compared with the group who had early institution of appropriate antibiotic coverage.

R.A. Balk, M.D.

Prognostic Significance of Pathological Chest Radiography in Transplant Patients Affected by Cytomegalovirus and/or *Pneumocystis carinii*
Wilczek B, Wilczek HE, Heurlin N, et al (Karolinska Hosp, Stockholm; Huddinge Hosp, Sweden)
Acta Radiol 37:727–731, 1996
4–23

Background.—Pneumonia in immunosuppressed recipients of kidney and/or pancreatic grafts is associated with a 30% to 50% mortality. Most episodes of fever and pneumonia occur within 4 months of transplantation and are often caused by cytomegalovirus (CMV). Opportunistic organisms, such as *Pneumocystis carinii* (PC), have also occurred with increasing frequency in recipients of kidney transplants. The prognostic significance of chest film findings associated with CMV or PC infection or both was investigated.

Methods and Findings.—The pulmonary charts of 274 recipients of kidney and/or pancreatic grafts transplanted between 1987 and 1990 were reviewed. Ninety-two patients had positive laboratory findings for CMV or PC, or both. Only CMV was present in 77, both CMV and PC were present in 13, and only PC was present in 2. Chest films, obtained in 57 patients, were reviewed by 2 radiologists independently. Chest film findings were normal in 32 patients and abnormal in 25. Three patients showing pathologic changes had pleuritis only, and 22 had parenchymal infiltrations. None of the patients with CMV or PC, or both, and normal film results or pleuritis only died, compared with 9 with parenchymal infiltrations. Two of the patients who died had CMV only, 5 who died had both CMV and PC, and 2 who died had PC only. The overall mortality irrespective of radiologic findings did not exceed 3% in patients with CMV only, but rose to 38% in patients with both CMV and PC. Among patients with parenchymal infiltrations, the death rate for those with CMV only was 18%, and for those with both CMV and PC, it was 56%.

Conclusions.—Radiologic verification of pneumonia related to the infectious agent has some prognostic value. The prognosis for CMV pneumonia is more favorable than that for PC pneumonia.

▶ Radiographic findings often lag behind or are inconsistent with current clinical pictures. This study demonstrates that patients receiving solid organ transplants who have significant pulmonary infections may have no significant abnormalities noted on chest radiographs. However, it also demonstrates that the presence of radiographic abnormalities on chest films is associated with more severe disease processes and is a significant prognostic factor.

W.T. Peruzzi, M.D.

Stomach as a Source of Colonization of the Respiratory Tract During Mechanical Ventilation: Association With Ventilator-associated Pneumonia

Torres A, El-Ebiary M, Soler N, et al (Universitat de Barcelona)
Eur Respir J 9:1729–1735, 1996   4–24

Background.—Abnormal oropharyngeal and gastric colonization, in addition to the aspiration of their contents to the lower airways, are involved in the pathogenesis of ventilator-associated pneumonia. Ventilator-associated pneumonia can easily develop in patients with artificial airways with altered mechanical, cellular, or humoral defenses if aspiration or inoculation of microorganisms occur.

Risk Factors.—Risk factors for gastric colonization include changes in gastric juice secretion, alkalinization of gastric contents, administration of enteral nutrition, and presence of bilirubin. It is unclear how the colonized gastric reservoir is involved in the development of ventilator-associated pneumonia (Table 1).

The Role of the Stomach.—Randomized, controlled trials of selective gut decontamination and stress ulcer prophylaxis in the ICU have reported evidence supporting gastric involvement in the development of ventilator-associated pneumonia. In these trials, reducing the bacteria burden of the stomach lowered the rate of nosocomial respiratory infections. At least 3 other studies, however, have found no evidence of stomach involvement in pneumonia occurring during mechanical ventilation.

Prophylaxis.—Suggested prophylactic measures include jejunal feeding, acidifying enteral feeding, treating stress ulcers with sucralfate, preventing duodenal reflux with metoclopramide, and reducing gastric burden and bacterial translocation by selective digestive decontamination. Small bore nasogastric tubes and jejunal feeding can prevent gastroesophageal reflux. Positioning patients in a semi-recumbent position, checking tube cuff patency, and aspirating subglottic secretions can reduce aspiration of gastric contents.

TABLE 1.—Risk Factor and Recommended Prophylactic Measures to Prevent VAP in Relation to Gastric Reservoir

Risk factor	Intervention
Alkalinization	Sucralfate, acidification of enteral feeding, avoid antacids/H-2 blockers
Duodenal reflux	Metoclopramide, jejunal feeding
Gastric colonization	SDD, acidification of enteral feeding, jejunal feeding
Bacterial translocation	SDD (?), early treatment of haemodynamic instability
Gastro-oesophageal reflux	Small bore NGT, jejunal feeding
Aspiration of gastric contents	Semirecumbent position (45°), patency of tube cuff, aspiration of subglottic secretions.

Abbreviations: VAP, ventilator-associated pneumonia; *NGT,* nasogastric tube; *SDD,* selective digestive decontamination.

(Courtesy of Torres A, El-Ebiary M, Soler N, et al: Stomach as a source of colonization of the respiratory tract during mechanical ventilation: Association with ventilator-associated pneumonia. *Eur Resp J* 9:1729–1735, 1996.)

Discussion.—The exact role, if any, of the stomach as a source of microorganisms that can cause ventilator-associated pneumonia has not been determined. There is much evidence that the stomach may be involved in the development of these pulmonary infections.

▶ This paper reviews the literature concerning the hypothesis that the bacteria responsible for ventilator-associated pneumonia arise from the gastrointestinal tract. This has been a controversial subject of late, and most theorists are now leaning away from this argument. Nonetheless, colonization of the gastrointestinal tract with bacteria and microorganisms can be responsible for a number of potential complications that may befall a critically ill patient. The table gives the authors' recommendations for strategies designed to reduce the incidence of these complications.

R.A. Balk, M.D.

Severe Community-acquired Pneumonia in ICUs: Prospective Validation of a Prognostic Score

Leroy O, Georges H, Beuscart C, et al (Centre Hospitalier, Tourcoing, France; Lille Univ, France; Centre Hospitalier, Lens, France; et al)
Intensive Care Med 22:1307–1314, 1996   4–25

Background.—Community-acquired pneumonia is one of the most serious infectious diseases, in spite of the improvements in antibiotic treatment and the development of criteria for immediate hospitalization or admission to the ICU. Only a few studies have analyzed prognostic indicators of outcome for patients with severe community-acquired pneumonia in the ICU.

TABLE 4.—Predictors of ICU Mortality Based on Discriminant Analysis

Criteria	Value
Aspiration pneumonia	−0.37
Grading of sepsis ≥ 11	−0.2
Antimicrobial association	−0.01
Glasgow Coma Score ≥ 12+ mechanical ventilation (MV)	+0.09
Serum creatinine level ≥ 15 mg/l	+0.22
Chest involvement on X-ray ≥3 lobes	+0.28
Septic shock	+0.29
Bacteremia	+0.29
Initial MV	+0.29
Anticipated death <5 years	+0.31
SAPS ≥ 12	+0.49
Neutrophil count ≤3500/mm^3	+0.52
OSF score ≥2	+0.64
Delayed (> 12 h) MV	+0.67
Immunosuppression	+1.38
Ineffective initial antimicrobial therapy	+1.5

(Courtesy of Leroy O, Georges H, Beuscart C, et al: Severe community-acquired pneumonia in ICUs: Prospective validation of a prognostic score. *Intensive Care Med* 22:1307–1314, 1996. Copyright Springer-Verlag.)

Methods.—In a combined prospective and retrospective study, 335 patients admitted to the ICU with community-acquired pneumonia were studied to identify prognostic factors specific to pneumonia. An index was developed and validated in 125 consecutive patients with community-acquired pneumonia in the ICU. All patients were older than 16 years.

Results.—In the derivation group of 335 patients, 16 predictors of death were identified and assigned a point value from −0.37 to +1.5, according to their magnitude in the mortality model: aspiration pneumonia, grading

TABLE 5.—Mortality According to Mortality Risk Index in the Derivation and Validation Cohorts

	Non survivors	Survivors	Predictive value of:	Risk ratio	95% CI	P
Derivation cohort						
Score ≥2.5 (n = 72)	53	19	Death=74%	5.71	4.04 to 8.08	<0.001
Score <2.5 (n = 256)	33	223	Survival=87%			
Total (n = 328)	Sensitivity=62%	Specificity=92%				
Validation cohort						
Score ≥2.5 (n = 24)	22	2	Death=92%	6.61	4.01 to 10.9	<0.0001
Score <2.5 (n = 101)	14	87	Survival=86%			
Total (n = 125)	Sensitivity=61%	Specificity=98%				

(Courtesy of Leroy O, Georges H, Beuscart C, et al: Severe community-acquired pneumonia in ICUs: Prospective validation of a prognostic score. *Intensive Care Med* 22:1307–1314, 1996. Copyright Springer-Verlag.)

of sepsis greater than or equal to 11, antimicrobial combination, Glasgow score greater than 12 plus mechanical ventilation, serum creatinine greater than or equal to 15 mg/L, chest involvement on radiographs greater than or equal to 3 lobes, shock, bacteremia, initial mechanical ventilation, underlying fatal or rapidly fatal illness, Simplified Acute Physiology Score greater than or equal to 12, neutrophil count less than or equal to 3,500/mm^3, acute organ system failure score greater than or equal to 2, delayed mechanical ventilation, immunosuppression, and ineffective initial antimicrobial treatment (Table 4). An index was developed by adding the points for each patient. The cut-off value of this index was 2.5. In the validation group of 125 patients, an index of greater than or equal to 2.5 predicted death with a positive predictive value of 0.92, a sensitivity of 0.61, and a specificity of 0.98 (Table 5).

Discussion.—These results show that this prognostic index for patients admitted to the ICU with community-acquired pneumonia performs well. This index may help patient management. Further research is needed to develop a simplified index that will more accurately identify low-risk patients. A comparison of this index and an ICU prognosis-specific score will be performed.

▶ This is yet another predictive score for patients with pneumonia. This one is designed to predict mortality in patients with severe community-acquired pneumonia who require hospitalization in the ICU. The authors used univariate analysis to discern 20 variables that were significantly associated with outcome and then evaluated these variables in a new prospective cohort of patients admitted, with community-acquired pneumonia, to the ICU. For both components of their study, the authors used patients from the community or a nursing home and allowed patients to be admitted to the ICU, either directly or within 48 hours of hospital admission, for community-acquired pneumonia.

These predictors of mortality are very similar to those that common sense would dictate to be predictive of mortality. The results also display similarity to the recommendations from the American Thoracic Society concerning the clinical parameters that predict increased mortality from community acquired pneumonia.[1] The ATS predictors are easy to remember and do not involve the use of a calculator to tabulate a prediction score. There have also been other prediction scores which have received a lot of attention in the past year, and it would be interesting to compare the 2 scoring systems.[2] I would be interested to see this score used in other trials, to verify its utility as well as its ease of use, before we all go out and advocate this score as a means of assigning risk in our ICU pneumonia patients.

R.A. Balk, M.D.

References

1. Niederman MS, Bass JB Jr., Campbell GD, et al: Guidelines for the initial management of adults with community-acquired pneumonia: Diagnosis, assessment of severity, and initial antimicrobial therapy. *Am Rev Respir Dis* 148:1418–1426, 1993.
2. Fine MJ, Auble TE, Yealy DM, et al: A prediction rule to identify low-risk patients with community-acquired pneumonia. *N Engl J Med* 336:243–250, 1997.

Evaluation by Polymerase Chain Reaction of Cytomegalovirus Reactivation in Intensive Care Patients Under Mechanical Ventilation

Stéphan F, Méharzi D, Ricci S, et al (Hôpital Tenon, Paris)
Intensive Care Med 22:1244–1249, 1996   4–26

Introduction.—In immunocompromised patients, cytomegalovirus infection—especially cytomegalovirus pneumonia—is a major cause of illness and death. Patients with sepsis have had infection or reactivation of cytomegalovirus, with an incidence ranging from 20% to 96%. The virus can persist in the host as a latent infection after primary infection and has been known to reactivate to cause active infection. The hypothesis that critically ill, mechanically ventilated, nonimmunocompromised patients could experience reactivated latent cytomegalovirus in either lung or blood was tested by using an in vitro gene amplification technique, the polymerase chain reaction (PCR), and bronchoalveolar lavage.

Methods.—There were 23 nonimmunocompromised patients who were mechanically ventilated and who were anticytomegalovirus immunoglobulin G–positive. They were compared with a positive control group of 10 immunocompromised patients with active cytomegalovirus and a negative control group of 16 asymptomatic cytomegalovirus-seropositive nonimmunocompromised patients. Viral cultures and PCR were used to evaluate the presence of cytomegalovirus in blood and bronchoalveolar lavage. In 8 patients, sequential samples were evaluated.

Results.—A 290-bp fragment in the first exon of the immediate early 1 gene was amplified for PCR. A 268-bp fragment of the β-globin gene was concurrently amplified in all samples to exclude inhibitors of PCR amplification. In all 23 nonimmunocompromised, mechanically ventilated patients, viral cultures of blood and bronchoalveolar lavage were negative. In all samples, β-globin amplification was observed, but no cytomegalovirus DNA could be amplified in blood or bronchoalveolar lavage samples.

Conclusion.—No reactivation of cytomegalovirus in blood or lung was demonstrated in a series of critically ill patients under mechanical ventilation who were seropositive for cytomegalovirus.

▶ Cytomegalovirus (CMV) has recently been linked to the subsequent development of coronary artery disease. This article investigates the hypothesis of reactivation of latent CMV infection in patients with acute lung injury. Using sensitive and specific assays, the authors could find no evidence to support their hypothesis. Reactivation of latent CMV is not a major clinical concern in nonimmunocompromised ICU patients.

L.C. Casey, M.D., Ph.D.

Bronchoalveolar and Systemic Cytokine Profiles in Patients With ARDS, Severe Pneumonia and Cardiogenic Pulmonary Oedema

Schütte H, Lohmeyer J, Rosseau S, et al (Justus-Liebig Univ, Giessen, Germany)

Eur Respir J 9:1858–1867, 1996   4–27

Background.—Though cytokines are known to play a role in various types of inflammatory lung disease, there is ongoing debate regarding their pathogenetic significance and diagnostic value. Proinflammatory cytokines studied in this regard include interleukin-6 (IL-6), IL-8, and tumor necrosis factor-α (TNF-α). Levels of these cytokines in serum and bronchoalveolar lavage (BAL) fluid were studied for their ability to discriminate between different categories of patients with acute respiratory failure.

Methods.—Serum and BAL measurements of the 3 cytokines were made in 74 mechanically ventilated patients and 17 healthy controls. Thirty-eight patients were classified as having severe pneumonia (PN), 12 had acute respiratory distress syndrome (ARDS) in the absence of primary lung infection, 18 had ARDS in combination with pneumonia (PN+ARDS), and 6 had cardiogenic pulmonary edema (CPO). The ability of the cytokine findings to differentiate among these groups was assessed.

Results.—Patients with ARDS and/or PN had strikingly high BAL levels of IL-6 and IL-8, higher than in CPO patients or healthy controls. The presence or absence of lung infection, or the different categories of PN, could not be distinguished by the absolute quantities and time-course of these cytokines. Patients with ARDS and/or PN also had elevating serum levels of IL-6, with inconsistent elevations of IL-8. These patients also had elevated serum concentrations of TNF-α, though this cytokine was rarely detected in BAL fluid.

Conclusions.—Patients with ARDS and/or severe PN can be identified by their high BAL levels of IL-6 and IL-8 and serum concentrations of IL-8. Levels of TNF-α in BAL are not elevated. These findings can differentiate ARDS/PN from CPO. However, they cannot distinguish ARDS in the absence of lung infection from severe primary or secondary pneumonia, which apparently causes similar local and systemic inflammatory effects.

▶ The clinical definition of adult respiratory distress syndrome is a little sketchy here. The use of an accepted definition would have been preferred. Despite this limitation, profiling of patients' cytokine levels in blood and bronchial washings may prove useful to distinguish between cardiogenic and non-cardiogenic pulmonary edema and to determine which phase of the inflammatory response the patient is in.

J.E. Calvin, Jr., M.D.

J.E. Parrillo, M.D.

Tracheal and Airway Issues and Mechanical Ventilation

Prehospital Cricothyroidotomy by Physicians
Leibovici D, Fredman B, Gofrit ON, et al (IDF Med Corps; Meir Med Ctr; Tel Aviv Univ; et al)
Am J Emerg Med 15:91–93, 1997   4–28

Purpose.—Cricothyroidotomy may be used to gain control of the airway when intubation is not possible. The frequency with which this procedure is performed is unknown. This study reviewed the frequency and success rate of prehospital cricothyroidotomy.

Methods.—All prehospital cricothyroidotomies performed in Israel from 1991 to 1995 were identified by review of data from the national trauma registry. The review included the indications for cricothyroidotomy, the technical difficulty of the procedure, and the surgical skills of the physicians.

Results.—Twenty-nine cricothyroidotomies were performed in Israel during the study period. They accounted for 3.3% of all prehospital airway management procedures performed during that time. The patients (median age was 10 years) had a median Glasgow Coma Scale score of 4 and a median Revised Trauma Score of 7. Fifty-five percent of the patients died. Intubation was tried before cricothyroidotomy, usually repeatedly, in 83% of patients. The major indications for cricothyroidotomy were intubation failure with no apparent anatomical distortion and traumatic distortion of the pharynx and larynx.

The success rate of cricothyroidotomy was 90%. Surgeons, anesthesiologists, and intensive care specialists had a success rate of 100%; however, this was not significantly higher than the 83% success rate for all other specialties. All 29 physicians performing the procedure had completed training in Advanced Trauma Life Support (ATLS), but only 3 had done the procedure before. Cricothyroidotomy failed to establish the airway in 3 patients, resulted in minor bleeding in 2, and was complicated by an air leak around the cannula in 1 patient.

Conclusions.—With ATLS training, physicians can successfully perform emergency cricothyroidotomy in the field. The success rate is high and complication rate low, regardless of physician specialty. Cricothyroidotomy should be used for trauma patients in whom endotracheal intubation is impossible. This is a better option than repeated attempts at intubation, which may be detrimental.

► This study examines the experience with performance of cricothyroidotomy between October 1991 and April 1995 in the prehospital setting in Israel. A total of 29 cricothyroidotomies were performed during this period.

The physicians performing them were divided into 2 groups: group 1 consisted of surgeons, anesthesiologists, otolaryngologists, thoracic surgeons, plastic surgeons, obstetricians, and intensive care specialists; group 2 included general practitioners, internists, cardiologists, and pediatricians. It is important to note that all of the physicians who performed cricothyroidotomies underwent training through a certified ATLS course. Although the success rate in group 1 surgeons was 100%, the overall success rate of 89.6% was not significantly different. This indicates that simple training through a short trauma life support course is quite adequate for teaching physicians to perform cricothyroidotomies. Because airway management can be quite difficult in many patients and precious time can be lost during multiple attempts at intubation, this study indicates that simple training of physicians in both surgical and nonsurgical fields in cricothyroidotomies would be quite beneficial. The procedure could be performed quickly by these physicians with excellent success and low complication rates.

R.V. Rege, M.D.

Percutaneous Tracheostomy: A Cost-effective Alternative to Standard Open Tracheostomy
McHenry CR, Raeburn CD, Lange RL, et al (Case Western Reserve Univ, Cleveland, Ohio)
Am Surg 63:646–652, 1997   4–29

Background.—Percutaneous tracheostomy has become increasingly popular in recent years, based on reports suggesting that it could be done in the ICU more quickly, with less expense, and with less morbidity than

---

TABLE 2.—Cost Analysis for Patients Who Underwent Percutaneous ($n = 19$) vs. open ($n = 23$) Tracheostomy as the Sole Procedure in the Operating Room

Cost for operating time		Number of Patients (Total Cost)	
Time (minutes)	Cost per Unit	Percutaneous	Open
≤30	$370	18 ($6,660)	3 ($1,110)
30–60	$672	1 ($672)	16 ($10,752)
≥60	$974	0 (0)	4 ($3,896)
		19 ($7,332)	23 ($15,758)
Equipment costs			
Percutaneous			$ 707
Open			$ 685
Mean operating room cost/patient (combined cost for operating room time and equipment)			
Percutaneous			$1,093
Open			$1,370

(Courtesy of McHenry CR, Raeburn CD, Lange RL, et al: Percutaneous tracheostomy: A cost-effective alternative to standard open tracheostomy. *Am Surg* 63:646–652, 1997.)

TABLE 3.—Complication Rates for Percutaneous Tracheostomy

References	Year	Number of Patients with Percutaneous Tracheostomy	Morbidity (%)	Mortality (%)
Hazard et al.[3]	1991	22	25	0
Griggs et al.[4]	1991	153	3.9	0
Ivatury et al.[5]	1992	61	20*	1.6
Ciaglia and Graniero[9]	1992	170	10	0
Shrager et al.[11]	1994	400	5	0.25
Toursarkissian et al.[12]	1994	141	21†	0.7
Barba et al.[6]	1995	27	3.7	3.7
Cobean et al.[7]	1996	65	38‡	1.5
Fernandez et al.[8]	1996	162	6	0

*10% intraoperative/immediate postoperative and 10% late postoperative.
†11% intraoperative, 8% perioperative, and 2% late complications.
‡22% intraoperative, 9% early postoperative, and 7% late postoperative.
(Courtesy of McHenry CR, Raeburn CD, Lange RL, et al: Percutaneous tracheostomy: A cost-effective alternative to standard open tracheostomy. *Am Surg* 63:646–652, 1997.)

open tracheostomy. In 1993, the authors' institution began using percutaneous dilational tracheostomy as a minimally invasive alternative to standard open tracheostomy. Percutaneous tracheostomy was compared with open tracheostomy in terms of safety, operative time, and cost.

Methods.—The retrospective analysis included 74 patients undergoing percutaneous tracheostomy over a 28-month period and 109 patients undergoing open tracheostomy over the preceding 12 months. The 2 groups were compared in terms of indications, length of procedure, morbidity, and cost.

Results.—The indications for tracheostomy were chronic ventilator dependence, 66% and 53%; airway protection, 26% and 39%; laryngeal dysfunction, 3% and 6%; and facial trauma, 8% and 2% for the percutaneous group and the open group, respectively. The procedure took a mean of 21 minutes in the percutaneous group and 46 minutes in the open group. Perioperative morbidity was 3% with percutaneous tracheostomy vs. 9% with open tracheostomy. Mean operating room costs were $1,093 vs. $1,370 per patient, respectively (Table 2).

Conclusions.—Percutaneous tracheostomy has become a useful alternative to standard open tracheostomy. It is simple, quick, and less expensive than the open procedure. Experience has demonstrated lower morbidity as well (Table 3). For most patients, the percutaneous procedure is the preferred approach to elective tracheostomy.

▶ While the percutaneous tracheostomy technique has been around for over forty years, this is really only the second decade that it has been employed in a practical manner in ICU patients. This article is important in that the authors who are surgeons unequivocally endorse the procedure as the preferred approach for most patients requiring tracheostomy. They found the procedure to be safe, more convenient, and less expensive than standard tracheostomy in the patients they evaluated. When surgical departments are reporting these results, it is safe to say the procedure has attained a level of general acceptance. I think that, soon, most other surgical intensivists will recommend percutaneous tracheostomy as the procedure of choice for most ICU patients. There are still many questions to be answered about percutaneous tracheostomy, including when to use the bronchoscope and what to do in patients requiring high levels of positive pressure, but we are witnessing a bona fide innovation in the practice of critical care medicine.

C.M. Franklin, M.D.

Bacteraemia Following Percutaneous Dilational Tracheostomy
Teoh N, Parr MJA, Finfer SR (Royal North Shore Hosp, Sydney, NSW)
Anaesth Intensive Care 25:354–357, 1997   4–30

Background.—Percutaneous tracheostomy using a guidewire is a popular technique with several important advantages over traditional surgical tracheostomy. The nature of percutaneous tracheostomy suggests that it might be associated with a significant incidence of bacteremia. Some patients undergoing this procedure have risk factors for endocarditis or intravascular prostheses. A prospective study of bacteremia following percutaneous dilational tracheostomy is reported.

Methods.—On the basis of clinical observations of episodes suggesting bacteremia, the authors began obtaining peripheral blood samples for culture after each percutaneous tracheostomy. One hundred six consecutive procedures performed over 18 months were analyzed to determine the incidence of bacteremia and the causative organisms.

Results.—About 10% of blood samples taken after tracheostomy were culture positive, compared with 7% of other blood cultures take from the same population of ICU patients (odds ratio, 1.64). *Staphylococcus aureus* was present in 7% of posttracheostomy cultures, compared with 3% of other cultures (odds ratio, 2.43). The remaining positive posttracheostomy cultures grew organisms that were also cultured from the patients' tracheal secretions. Administration of antibiotics at the time of tracheostomy made no significant difference in the likelihood of positive blood cultures.

Conclusions.—This study finds a 10% incidence of bacteremia after percutaneous dilational tracheostomy. The infecting organisms seem to come from the patients' trachea or skin. The authors do not currently recommend antibiotic prophylaxis for patients with intravascular catheters in situ, but do for patients at risk for endocarditis or intravascular graft infection.

▶ This is one of the first reports of bacteremia as a common complication of percutaneous dilational tracheostomy. While it does not appear to be a deterrent to performing the procedure, the report suggests that patients with abnormal heart valves or surgically implanted foreign bodies may need antibiotic prophylaxis when percutaneous dilational tracheostomy is contemplated.

C.M. Franklin, M.D.

Influence of Gender and Endotracheal Tube Size on Preextubation Breathing Pattern
Epstein SK, Ciubotaru RL (Tufts Univ, Boston)
Am J Respir Crit Care Med 154:1647–1652, 1996   4–31

Introduction.—A rapid and shallow breathing pattern (increased respiratory rate/tidal volume [f/VT]) is frequently seen in intubated patients who fail weaning trials. This pattern can be caused by an imbalance between work of breathing and respiratory muscle capacity. But, despite an elevated f/VT, some women and patients with narrow endotracheal tubes (ETTs) are often successfully extubated. The influences of gender and ETT size on the f/VT measured before extubation were examined in a study of 218 ICU patients.

Methods.—Study participants were 136 men and 82 women. These 2 groups were similar in clinical characteristics at the start of mechanical ventilation and in etiologies of respiratory failure. All patients had a f/VT measured through an oral ETT (off of ventilatory support) during 1 minute of spontaneous respiration at the onset of a weaning trial designed to culminate in extubation. The decision to initiate weaning and extubation was based primarily on clinical judgment. Extubation success or failure was examined for differences between men and women and between ETT sizes (less than or equal to 7 mm vs. greater than 7 mm internal diameter).

Results.—With 6 exceptions (all men who were subsequently successfully extubated), all patients satisfied the general extubation criteria. Men and women differed in the spontaneous pattern of breathing, measured at the onset of the weaning trial. Women had a significantly higher f/VT, lower tidal volumes, and a higher respiratory rate, and were 2.5 times as likely as men to have a respiratory rate greater than 35 breaths/min during spontaneous breathing. A smaller internal diameter ETT was associated with a substantially higher f/VT among women. For the entire study population, patients with less than or equal to 7 mm internal diameter tubes were nearly 3 times more likely to have a f/VT greater than or equal to 100. Men and women had a similar likelihood of successful extubation (83% and 87%), but men were more likely to require reintubation. Multiple linear regression analysis identified both female gender and smaller ETT size (but not extubation outcome) as being independently correlated with f/VT.

Conclusion.—Women have a more rapid and shallow breathing pattern before extubation from mechanical ventilation, and this pattern is more pronounced among women with small ETTs. This finding was independent of extubation outcome. In a population with a high pretest probability of extubation success, the false negative rate of elevated F/VT may be increased.

▶ This article looks at pattern of ventilation as a predictor of successful extubation. The authors have demonstrated that endotracheal tube size, as would be predicted, affects pattern of ventilation; however, they also demonstrated that gender may have some part to play as well. This article illustrates that it is important to differentiate cause-and-effect relationships from clinical or statistical associations. In this case, they highlight the fact that factors aside from detrimental work of breathing and respiratory muscle fatigue may result in alteration of a measurement used as an indicator of respiratory reserves.

W.T. Peruzzi, M.D.

Criteria for Extubation and Tracheostomy Tube Removal for Patients With Ventilatory Failure

Bach JR, Saporito LR (Univ Hosp, Newark, NJ; Kessler Inst for Rehabilitation, West Orange, NJ)
Chest 110:1566–1571, 1996

4–32

Introduction.—Criteria for ventilator weaning have been described in the literature, but no comparable standards exist for tracheostomy tube removal. A prospective study of extubation/decannulation attempts tested the hypothesis that an important parameter may be the patient's ability to create expiratory airflow to clear secretions.

Methods.—The study population consisted of 49 consecutive patients with primarily neuromuscular ventilatory insufficiency. Forty-three had failed to respond to conventional weaning, and 6 were weaned but had tracheostomy tubes that could not be removed during the acute hospitalization. Thirty-four ventilator users needed 24-hour ventilatory support. Successful decannulation was defined as extubation or removal of the tracheostomy tube and closure of the tracheostomy site, with continuous use of noninvasive intermittent positive pressure ventilation (IPPV) and assisted coughing as needed, and without respiratory distress or blood gas deterioration for a period of at least 2 weeks. Variables examined as potential predictors of successful extubation or decannulation were age, extent of predecannulation ventilator use, vital capacity, and peak cough flows (PCF).

Results.—The only predictor of successful extubation and decannulation was the ability to generate PCF greater than 160 L/min. All those for whom greater than 160 L/min of PCF could be achieved had a successful attempt, whereas no patient with PCF less than 160 L/min was successfully extubated or decannulated. Four patients had PCF of 160 L/min; attempts were successful in 2 and failed in 2. The extent of need for ventilatory support was not important for successful extubation or decannulation. Seven of 14 patients who failed decannulation attempts were discharged from the hospital with tracheostomy tubes. Fiberoptic laryngoscopy, followed by surgery in some patients, relieved obstructing upper airway lesions in the remaining 7 patients.

Conclusion.—The ability to safely extubate or decannulate patients with neuromuscular conditions is related to the assisted PCF, but not to patient age, ventilator-free breathing time, duration or extent of ventilator need, or vital capacity. The cutoff PCF is 160 L/min.

▶ The authors have investigated factors that determine the ability to discontinue artificial airway use primarily in patients with neuromuscular disease processes. They have demonstrated that a peak cough flow is statistically associated with an ability to remain free of an artificial airway, even if noninvasive positive pressure ventilation is required. This study helps to define a way to predict a need for an important life-support device in critically ill patients. However, it must be understood that these data apply primarily to patients who have neuromuscular disease processes, but relatively normal parenchymal lung function. Therefore, additional data will be required before more generalized application of this predicator can be reliably applied.

W.T. Peruzzi, M.D.

Reduced Airway Resistance and Work of Breathing During Mechanical Ventilation With an Ultra-thin, Two-stage Polyurethane Endotracheal Tube (the Kolobow Tube)
Velarde CA, Short BL, Rivera O, et al (George Washington Univ, Washington, DC; Natl Heart, Lung and Blood Inst, Bethesda, Md)
Crit Care Med 25:276–279, 1997   4–33

Background.—Premature neonates are usually intubated with small endotracheal tubes of 2.5–3.0 mm in internal diameter, which significantly increases airway resistance. The work of breathing needed to overcome this resistance may not be significant while infants are receiving high ventilatory support, but they may not be able to tolerate the extra work of breathing after they are breathing spontaneously through the tube. Dr. Kolobow and associates have designed a new endotracheal tube of polyurethane that is reinforced with a flat stainless steel wire. This new tube has ultrathin walls of 0.2 mm, which gives the tube a larger internal diameter than conventional tubes of the same external diameter.

Methods.—A comparison was made between dynamic pulmonary function tests of the Kolobow endotracheal tube and tests of conventional endotracheal tubes with similar external diameters. Adult rabbits were intubated with a conventional endotracheal tube, then paralyzed and placed on a mechanical ventilator. Ventilatory settings were adjusted to achieve standard arterial blood gases. After a 60-minute stabilization period, pulmonary function tests were measured (period 1), the conventional tube was replaced with the Kolobow tube, and the pulmonary function tests were measured again (period 2). Peak inspiratory pressure was decreased to match the tidal volume measured during ventilation with the conventional tube. When the desired tidal volume was obtained, pulmonary function tests were again measured (period 3). Flows were unchanged and the length of both types of endotracheal tube was the same.

Results.—The Student's *t* test was used to compare the mean values of airway resistance with the work of breathing from period 1 to period 3. A 59% reduction in total airway resistance and a 45% reduction in the work of breathing was noted.

Discussion.—These findings indicate that the ultrathin Kolobow endotracheal tube can significantly decrease airway resistance and the work of breathing. These reductions may improve ventilatory mechanics in very small premature infants. The Kolobow tube is being tested in high-frequency ventilation and intratracheal pulmonary ventilation. This tube may have potential value in liquid ventilation, because it is made of polyurethane and is not subject to erosion by perfluorocarbons.

▶ The authors have developed an endotracheal tube with a steel wire–reinforced ultrathin wall that permits the internal diameter to be significantly greater than that of conventional endotracheal tubes of the same size. This permits a decrease in the resistance to air flow, which translates into a decrease in the work of breathing for the intubated patient. This represents a significant advance in endotracheal tube design. It has important implications in terms of the decreased work of breathing and also for critical care procedures (i.e., bronchoscopies) in which the internal diameter of the endotracheal tube is important.

W.T. Peruzzi, M.D.

Influence of Airway Pressure on Minimum Occlusive Endotracheal Tube Cuff Pressure

Guyton DC, Barlow MR, Besselievre TR (Univ of Mississippi, Jackson)
Crit Care Med 25:91–94, 1997   4–34

Background.—Tracheal ischemic complications are associated with excessive pressure from an endotracheal tube cuff on the tracheal mucosa. Although the use of high-volume, low-pressure endotracheal tube cuffs has significantly lowered the rate of cuff-induced tracheal ischemia complications, some patients are still at risk for these complications. In vitro studies of the high-volume, low-pressure cuff have reported that the minimum occlusive pressure increases as peak inflation pressure increases. The effect of airway pressure on minimum occlusive pressure has not been analyzed in vivo.

Methods.—In a prospective study, the in vivo relationship between peak inflation pressure and minimum occlusive pressure of a high-volume, low-pressure endotracheal tube cuff was analyzed in 15 adult patients receiving mechanical ventilation and general anesthesia. After general anesthesia was established, the endotracheal tube cuff was deflated and reinflated until the tracheal seal was reestablished by auscultation. Fluid-filled transducers were used to determine peak inflation pressure and minimum occlusive pressure, and airway pressure proximal to the endotracheal tube and cuff pressure through the pilot tube were recorded simultaneously.

Results.—The peak inflation pressure was 12.1–43.7 mm Hg. The peak inflation pressure was associated with a minimum occlusive pressure of 2.2–39.7 mm Hg. Minimum occlusive pressure increased in a linear fashion over the range of measured peak inflation pressure values.

Discussion.—A cuff pressure of 25 mm Hg corresponded to a peak inflation pressure of 35.3 mm Hg. Patients with higher peak inflation pressures may have a risk of ischemic tracheal injuries. even when proper cuff inflation techniques are used. Awareness of the linear relationship between peak inflation pressure and minimum occlusive pressure is useful for identifying patients at risk for tracheoesophageal fistulas, tracheal stenosis, and other cuff-induced tracheal ischemia complications.

▶ Iatrogenic tracheal injury secondary to short- and long-term airway management has been a significant concern of the medical community since the advent of the cuffed endotracheal tube. Cuff pressures have long been thought to be an indicator of the risk of tracheal injuries associated with tracheal intubation. This study raises questions regarding "safe" cuff pressure limits. It is becoming evident that the precise relationship between endotracheal or tracheostomy cuff pressures and the risk of tracheal injury is blurred. This topic needs a good deal more investigation, especially in light of the variable lung pathologic conditions for which these devices are used.

W.T. Peruzzi, M.D.

Laryngotracheal Stenosis After Intubation or Tracheostomy in Patients With Neurological Disease

Richard I, Giruad M, Perrouin-Verbe B, et al (Universitaire de Nantes, France)
Arch Phys Med Rehabil 77:493–496, 1996   4–35

Introduction.—Prolonged use of an endotracheal tube vs. tracheostomy is the topic of several investigations that have provided conflicting results. The incidence of airway complications in patients with neurologic problems after translaryngeal intubation, tracheostomy, or both, was evaluated retrospectively.

Methods.—The medical records of 315 consecutive patients with neurologic problems were examined for data regarding the type of artificial airway, duration of intubation, and use of nocturnal ventilation. All patients with abnormal findings on tomograms or flow-volume loop analysis underwent tracheolaryngoscopy. The tracheolaryngoscopy reports were reviewed for evidence of stenosis. Stenosis that was lethal or required surgical intervention was classified as severe. If the stenosis was successfully treated medically or by local means, it was considered benign.

Results.—Fifty-five percent of patients underwent intubation only for a mean of 17 days; 3% underwent tracheostomy only; and 42% underwent intubation for a mean of 13 days, then tracheostomy. Of 20% of patients with stenosis, one fourth had severe stenosis. Fifteen percent of patients died because of tracheal complications. The incidence of stenosis was significantly higher in patients who underwent tracheostomy vs. intubation only. Severe stenosis was experienced in significantly more patients who underwent tracheostomy than in patients who underwent intubation only. There was no significant association between the length of intubation or timing of tracheostomy and the incidence of stenosis.

Conclusion.—Transtracheal intubation is associated with significantly lower rates of stenosis and severe stenosis than is tracheostomy. The decision to perform tracheostomy must be made while taking this risk and that of immediate complications into consideration. Longer periods of intubation should be used before resorting to tracheostomy, if weaning is not successful.

▶ The debate over prolonged use of an endotracheal tube vs. tracheostomy has existed for more than 4 decades. This article provides an excellent review of the available data and appropriately places the debate in an historical perspective. As this is a retrospective study, it only tells us what happens at this institution after the patients are received. We have no information concerning the tracheostomy techniques used, the airway care provided in an attempt to minimize glottic damage, etc. Although this retrospective study may not impact the debate itself, it provides an excellent review of the issue.

B.A. Shapiro, M.D.

Mortality Is Directly Related to the Duration of Mechanical Ventilation Before the Initiation of Extracorporeal Life Support for Severe Respiratory Failure

Pranikoff T, Hirschl RB, Steimle CN, et al (Univ of Michigan, Ann Arbor)
Crit Care Med 25:28–32, 1997
4–36

Background.—Mechanical ventilation can result in irreversible lung injury, which may lead to death from severe acute respiratory failure. Respiratory problems are the major cause of mortality in patients undergoing extracorporeal life support (ECLS). These investigators examined whether previous mechanical ventilation plays a role in the survival of patients undergoing ECLS who have severe acute respiratory failure.

Methods.—Extracorporeal life support was used to manage 36 patients with severe respiratory failure (estimated 90% mortality rate). The following respiratory parameters were similar in all patients before ECLS: peak inspiratory pressure averaged 56 ± 16 cm H_2O, positive end-expiratory pressure averaged 14 ± 6 cm H_2O, and the respiratory rate averaged 23 ± 10 breaths/min. Extracorporeal life support was initiated from 1 to

TABLE 2.—Patient Survival Data According to Days of
Pre-ECLS Ventilation

Pre-ECLS Ventilation (days)	N	Recovered	Survived	% Survival
1–2	11	9	8	72.7
3–4	8	6	6	75.0
5–6	5	2	1	20.0
≥7	12	3	3	25.0

Abbreviation: N, number of patients.

(Courtesy of Pranikoff T, Hirschl RB, Steimle CN, et al: Mortality is directly related to the duration of mechanical ventilation before the initiation of extracorporeal life support for severe respiratory failure. *Crit Care Med* 25:28–32, 1997.)

17 days after the start of mechanical ventilation and set at a peak inspiratory pressure of 30 cm H_2O, a positive end-expiratory pressure of 10 cm H_2O, and a respiratory rate of 6 breaths/min. Patients who discontinued ventilation and breathed room air for 24 hours were determined to have recovered lung function, and those who were discharged from the hospital were determined to have survived.

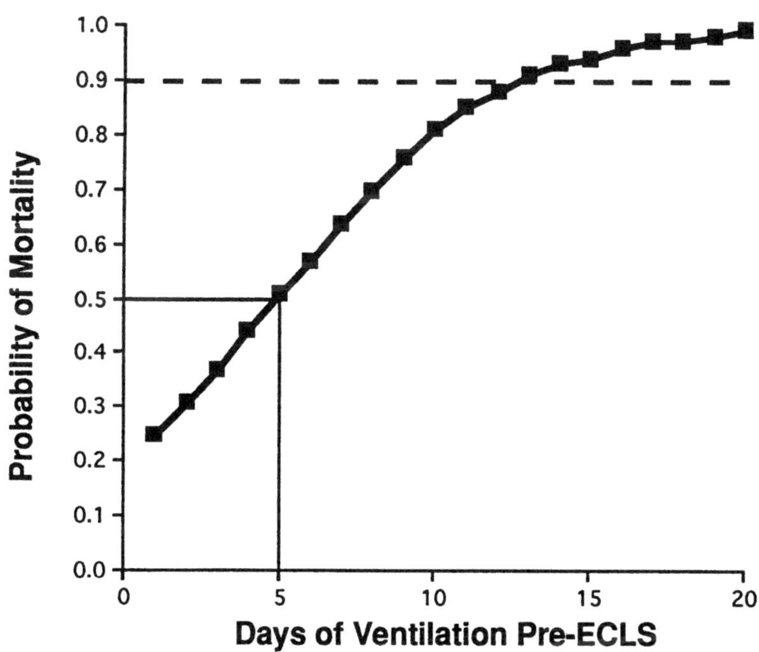

FIGURE 1.—Probability of mortality for each day of pre-ECLS ventilation. The *solid line* indicates the duration of mechanical ventilation where the mortality rate is 50%. The *dotted line* indicates 90% mortality. (Courtesy of Pranikoff T, Hirschl RB, Steimle CN, et al: Mortality is directly related to the duration of mechanical ventilation before the initiation of extracorporeal life support for severe respiratory failure. *Crit Care Med* 25:28–32, 1997.)

Findings.—Of the 36 patients, only 20 (56%) recovered lung function, and only 18 of 36 (50%) survived. Of the 18 who died, ECLS had been discontinued in almost two thirds because of irrecoverable pulmonary parenchymal damage and end-stage lung disease. Table 2 shows that a shorter period of ventilation before ECLS was associated with much better survival. Regression analysis of mortality as a function of ventilation duration pre-ECLS (Fig 1) also supported this association, with a predicted mortality rate of 50% after only 5 days of mechanical ventilation.

Conclusions.—Mechanical ventilation before ECLS is associated with a poor outcome, and the prognosis worsens as the length of ventilation increases. Thus, patients with severe acute respiratory failure should begin ECLS as soon as possible, within 5 days of starting mechanical ventilation.

▶ Despite the negative results from the NIH-sponsored ECMO trial of the 1970s, there are still some centers that believe this technique has utility in the severely compromised patient with acute lung injury.[1] The surgical group at the University of Michigan has been one of the centers that has continued to use this salvage technique for those younger individuals with acute lung injury who display diffuse infiltrates, reduced compliance, and unresponsive oxygenation and shunt abnormalities, despite "optimum support" using high levels of PEEP and ventilatory support. This population of severely injured patients has a reported mortality rate at this center that exceeded 90%, whereas, with the use of ECLS, the mortality rate has been reduced to 50%. These authors have now addressed the question of whether the pre-ECLS ventilatory strategy and time may have adversely affected the eventual outcome from the acute lung injury.

To answer this question, Dr. Pranikoff et al. have retrospectively reviewed their last 36 patients who were treated with ECLS to compare the pre-ECLS ventilatory support time with eventual outcome. The results are depicted in Table 2 and graphically displayed in Fig 1. The longer the patient was managed on ventilatory support before the institution of ECLS, the worse the ultimate outcome. This observation could support the notion that ventilator-induced lung injury (or hindrance of recovery) could be potentially responsible for this reduction in recovery from injury and survival. The majority of the patients were initially managed at other centers, and there are no data on the peak or end-inspiratory plateau pressures, F_iO_2, or mode of ventilation used for this initial period of ventilatory support. Further, this was not a randomized, controlled trial, and the authors are using historical survival data, which may not be representative of survival from acute lung injury at this center in 1998. In addition, we are not given any data concerning the pre-ECLS ventilatory support strategies, and there was no defined ventilatory management protocol that was used for the pre-ECLS management. The reported causes of death in this group of patients were predominantly progressive respiratory failure and fibrosis. This result is in contrast to other large populations of patients with acute lung injury, who died primarily of recurrent bouts of sepsis and/or multiple organ failure or dysfunction.[2] If fibrosis, or the fibroproliferative phase of acute lung injury, was responsible for a majority of the deaths, we also would like to discover how corticosteroids were used in this setting and what affect they may have had on the ultimate outcome of these patients.

This study presents some interesting observations and supplies a rationale for the conduct of a prospective trial to answer this important question of the effect of the type of ventilatory support on recovery from severe acute lung injury.

R.A. Balk, M.D.

References

1. Zapol WM, Snider MT, Hill JD, et al. Extracorporeal membrane oxygenation in severe acute respiratory failure: A randomized prospective study. *JAMA* 242:2193–2196, 1979.
2. Montgomery AB, Stager C, Carrico CJ, et al: Causes of mortality in patients with the adult respiratory distress syndrome. *Am Rev Respir Dis* 132:485–489, 1985.

The Effects of Long-term Prone Positioning in Patients With Trauma-induced Adult Respiratory Distress Syndrome
Fridrich P, Krafft P, Hochleuthner H, et al (Univ of Vienna; Trauma Hosp "Lorenz Böhler," Vienna)
Anesth Analg 83:1206–1211, 1996   4–37

Introduction.—Prone positioning has been found to improve arterial oxygenation in some patients with acute respiratory failure, but there are no reports of the long-term effects of repeated turns between supine and prone position. A prospective study was designed to evaluate gas exchange, lung mechanics, and hemodynamic variables during repeated, long-term prone positioning in a group of patients with multiple trauma and severe adult respiratory distress syndrome (ARDS).

Methods.—During a 30-month study, severe ARDS developed in 31 patients who met additional entry criteria: an Injury Severity Score greater than 16 and partial pressure of arterial oxygen PaO_2/fraction of inspired oxygen (FIO_2) less than 200 mm Hg at inverse ratio ventilation with positive end-expiratory pressure (PEEP) greater than 8 cm H_2O for more than 24 hours. A protocol was followed in which sedated or paralyzed patients were turned from supine to prone at noon, then turned back to the supine position at 8 AM the next day. The protocol was continued until either recovery or death, as long as patients met entry criteria at the 11 AM evaluation.

Results.—Data from 20 patients were available for analysis. In this group, the mean duration of ventilation was 30 days; a mean of 8 days was spent in the prone position. In addition to ARDS, renal failure was present in 2 patients and impaired liver function in 5. Documented cycles of prone/supine turning numbered 148; in 11, patients had to be returned early to the supine position (hemodynamic instability accounted for 6 cases). A significant improvement in oxygenation variables was observed each time the patients were placed prone. After the first turn from supine,

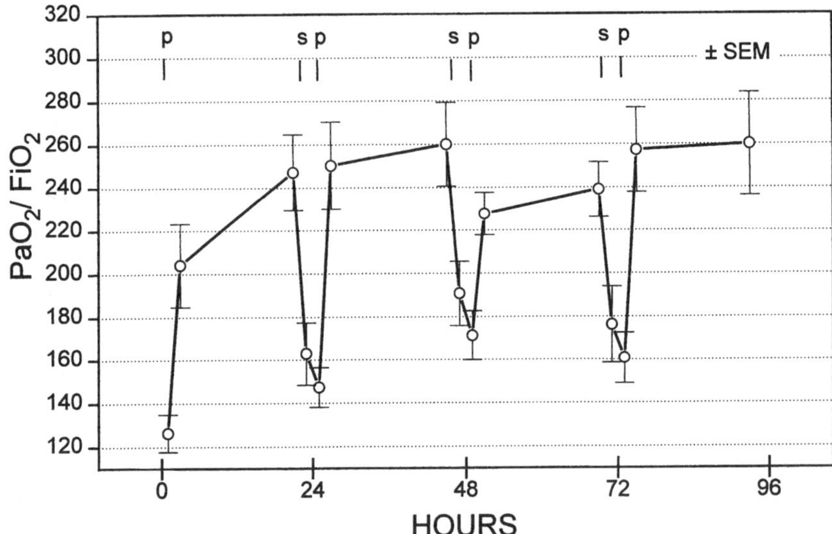

FIGURE 1.—Course of partial pressure of arterial oxygen (*PaO₂*/fraction of inspired oxygen (*FiO₂*) during the first 4 study cycles. *Abbreviations:* S (supine) and *p* (prone) indicate the points of turning. (Courtesy of Fridrich P, Krafft P, Hochleuthner H, et al: The effects of long-term prone positioning in patients with trauma-induced adult respiratory distress syndrome. *Anesth Analg* 83:1206–1211, 1996.)

mean PaO₂ increased from 97 to 152 mm Hg, mean intrapulmonary shunt (Qva/Qt) decreased from 30.3 to 25.5, and the mean alveolar-arterial oxygen difference decreased from 424 to 339 mm Hg (Fig 1). Short periods in the supine position were needed for nursing care, medical evaluation, and interventions. Although the improvements gained during prone positioning were lost when patients were turned supine, a return to prone position within 4 hours allowed these gains to be reproduced. Eleven patients recovered quickly with use of the prone position, but 9 required 10 turns or more.

Conclusion.—Prone positioning of patients with trauma-induced severe ARDS led to significant improvements in lung function. Beneficial effects of the prone condition were lost to some extent when the supine position was required for a period. The turning maneuver must be performed carefully to avoid complications.

▶ This study lends credence to the postulate that the prone position improves oxygenation in patients with severe ARDS for reasons other than making previously gravity-dependent lung non–gravity dependent, and vice versa.

B.A. Shapiro, M.D.

Prone Position in Mechanically Ventilated Patients With Severe Acute Respiratory Failure

Chatte G, Sab J-M, Dubois J-M, et al (Hôpital de la Croix Rousse, Lyon, France)
Am J Respir Crit Care Med 155:473–478, 1997   4–38

Objective.—The mechanical ventilation settings required in patients with severe acute respiratory failure are potentially toxic and dangerous. Anything that can be done to lower the levels of fractional concentration of inspired oxygen (FIO_2) and/or positive end-expiratory pressure in these patients would be helpful. It has been suggested that turning patients with adult respiratory distress syndrome to a prone position can improve oxygenation. The effects of prone positioning in patients with severe acute respiratory failure were studied.

Methods.—The study included 32 consecutive patients with severe acute respiratory failure, defined as a partial pressure of arterial oxygen PaO_2/FIO_2 of 150 or less. In each case, the impairment of oxygenation was unrelated to either left ventricular failure or atelectasis. The patients were studied 1 hour before, 1 and 4 hours during, and 1 hour after being placed in the prone position. The mean PaO_2/FIO_2 values at those times were 103, 158, 159, and 128, respectively. Patients who had at least a 20 mm Hg–improvement in PaO_2/FIO_2 after 1 hour in the prone position were considered responders.

Results.—Seventy-eight percent of patients responded to being placed in the prone position and 22% did not. Two of the 7 nonresponders could not tolerate the prone position and had to be returned to the supine position before the 4 hours was up. Complete data were available on 23 responders: 43% had their PaO_2/FIO_2 return to baseline value when they were returned to the supine position; the other 57% of responders had sustained improvement in oxygenation. The improvement could be repeated by returning patients to the prone position. Complications of prone positioning included minor skin injury and edema; 2 cases of apical atelectasis; and 1 case each of catheter removal, catheter compression, extubation, and transient supraventricular tachycardia.

Conclusion.—For some patients with severe acute respiratory failure, changing from the supine to the prone position can improve oxygenation. This is an efficient and simple technique that is far less invasive and expensive that other measures, such as extracorporeal or IV oxygenation. Although turning patients is not difficult, it does require some forethought, as well as sufficient personnel, to ensure patient safety.

▶ This study clearly demonstrates that oxygenation is improved by the prone position in many patients with severe acute respiratory failure. The study also shows that this procedure is occasionally accompanied by some significant mishaps. To their credit, the authors point out that the procedure is very personnel intensive and should only be considered as an alternative to more invasive means of improving oxygenation, such as extracorporeal techniques. I believe that is a statement worth emphasizing.

B.A. Shapiro, M.D.

Effects of Various Timings and Concentrations of Inhaled Nitric Oxide in Lung Ischemia-Reperfusion

Murakami S, for the Paris-Sud University Lung Transplantation Group (Paris-Sud Univ; Kanazawa Univ, Japan; Harvard Med School, Boston)
Am J Respir Crit Care Med 156:454–458, 1997   4–39

Purpose.—There is evidence that nitric oxide (NO) is a central modulator of ischemia-reperfusion injury. Experiments using inhaled NO in models of lung ischemia-reperfusion have given conflicting results—some have shown a preventive effect, others a worsening effect, and others no effect. The disagreement could stem from differences in the timing of administration or the concentration of inhaled NO. The effects of different timings and concentrations were studied in a rat model.

Methods.—Isolated perfused rat lungs were prepared and subjected to 1 hour of ischemia followed by 1 hour of blood reperfusion. Different combinations of NO dose and timing were studied: 30 ppm during ischemia, 30 or 80 ppm started immediately at reperfusion, and 30 ppm given 15 minutes after the start of reperfusion. The effects of these combinations on total pulmonary vascular resistance (PVR), coefficient of filtration (K_{fc}), lung wet/dry weight ratio (W/D), and lung myeloperoxidase activity (MPO) were assessed.

Findings.—Giving NO during ischemia left K_{fc} and MPO unchanged, compared to no NO treatment. However, PVR was reduced significantly. Given in a dose of 30 ppm during early or delayed reperfusion, NO decreased PVR, W/D, K_{fc}, and MPO. At the 90 ppm dose, PVR and MPO decreased but W/D and K_{fc} did not.

Conclusions.—Given in a dose of 30 ppm immediately at or after the beginning of reperfusion, NO reduces ischemia-reperfusion–induced injury in isolated rat lungs. Giving the same dose during ischemia, or an 80-ppm dose during reperfusion, has no such protective effect. The mechanism of this effect probably involves polymorphonuclear neutrophil inhibition, rather than vasodilation.

▶ Nitric oxide may have both a beneficial and detrimental role in the setting of the inflammatory injury that may result from ischemia-reperfusion. Data suggest that inhaled NO, if given in high doses during the period of reperfusion, may worsen the injury. This trial investigated the effect of both doses of inhaled NO and timing on the injury that results from ischemia-reperfusion in an isolated perfused rat lung model. During the period of ischemia, the use of inhaled NO decreased the PVR, but did not produce other demonstrable benefits. The use of a lower dose of inhaled NO, 30 ppm, during the reperfusion phase was associated with improved PVR, W/D lung weight

ratio, K_{Fc}, and MPO. The beneficial effects on W/D weight and K_{Fc} were not noted with the use of the higher dose of inhaled NO, 80 ppm. Unfortunately, I'm not sure that these data help sort out the issues concerning the potential beneficial effects of inhaled NO in humans with or at risk for acute lung injury. We are still in need of well-designed, multicenter, controlled, blinded trials in a well-defined population of patients with acute lung injury to help settle the question as to whether or not there is a place for inhaled NO in the management of these critically ill patients.

R.A. Balk, M.D.

Combining Partial Liquid Ventilation With Nitric Oxide to Improve Gas Exchange in Acute Lung Injury

Houmes R-JM, Hartog A, Verbrugge SJC, et al (Erasmus Univ Rotterdam, The Netherlands)
Intensive Care Med 23:163–169, 1997   4–40

Introduction.—During acute lung injury, the presence of increased surface tension at the alveolar air-liquid interface leads to hypoxemia. By filling the lung with a fluid, such as perfluorocarbon, that is able to maintain gas exchange, this air-liquid interface could be eliminated. It was hypothesized, that after increasing the area of gas exchange at end-expiration by partial liquid ventilation, oxygenation may be further enhanced with the administration of nitric oxide by inhalation, resulting in lower pulmonary artery pressures. During incremental dosages of perflubron, increasing concentrations of nitric oxide were administered to investigate the effects on gas exchange, oxygen transport, and hemodynamics in pigs.

Methods.—Lung lavage was used on 6 pigs with induced acute lung injury so that they could be surfactant depleted to a partial pressure of oxygen in arterial blood of less than 100 mm Hg. Four incremental doses of 5 mL/kg perflubron were administered. The animals received 0, 10, 20, 30, 40, and 0 parts per million (ppm) of nitric oxide between each dose. After each dose of perflubron and after each nitric oxide concentration, measurements were taken of blood gases, hemodynamic parameters, and oxygen delivery.

Results.—A dose-dependent increase in partial pressure of oxygen in arterial blood resulted with perflubron. Additional nitric oxide inhalation resulted in a further significant increase in partial pressure of oxygen in arterial blood at each perflubron dose, with a maximum effect at 30 ± 10 ppm of nitric oxide. A significant decrease in mean pulmonary artery pressure resulted with the perflubron dose of 5 mL/kg, and with higher nitric oxide concentrations, it decreased further.

Conclusions.—Without having any deleterious effect on measured systemic hemodynamic parameters, partial liquid ventilation can be com-

bined with nitric oxide administration and results in a cumulative effect on arterial oxygenation and decreases pulmonary artery pressure.

▶ This pig model of surfactant depletion after lung lavage was used to evaluate successive doses of 5 mL/kg perflubron for partial liquid ventilation coupled with progressively increasing doses of inhaled nitric oxide (0, 10, 20, 30, 40 ppm) to evaluate their synergistic effects on experimental acute lung injury. The combination of these 2 therapies appeared to have increased benefit on gas exchange and reduction in pulmonary artery pressure. The clinical value of this maneuver, however, remains to be seen. For now, these results fall into the category of interesting observation and highlight the idea that multiple therapies may be combined in the management of severe acute lung injury.

R.A. Balk, M.D.

Hypoxic Pulmonary Vasoconstriction in Nonventilated Lung Areas Contributes to Differences in Hemodynamic and Gas Exchange Responses to Inhalation of Nitric Oxide

Benzing A, Mols G, Brieschal T, et al (Univ of Freiburg, Germany)
Anesthesiology 86:1254–1261, 1997   4–41

Introduction.—Inhalation of nitric oxide is known to decrease pulmonary artery pressure and intrapulmonary right-to-left shunt in patients with the acute respiratory distress syndrome. Ventilation-perfusion matching also improves, and hypoxic pulmonary vasoconstriction in lung areas with low ventilation-perfusion ratios is a physiologic mechanism of such improvement. Almitrine has enhanced hypoxic pulmonary vasoconstriction in nonventilated lung areas, which has increased the respiratory response to inhaled nitric oxide. The respiratory response to inhaled nitric oxide may be decreased with attenuation of hypoxic pulmonary vasoconstriction in nonventilated lung areas.

Methods.—A total of 11 patients with acute respiratory distress syndrome who were treated by veno-venous extracorporeal lung assist were studied. At a fraction of inspired oxygen of 1.0, the patients' lungs were ventilated. Mixed venous oxygen tension was adjusted to 4 levels of 47, 54, 64, and 84 mm Hg by varying extracorporeal blood flow. To prevent changes in mixed venous carbon dioxide tension, extracorporeal gas flow was adjusted. Before, during, and after 15 parts per million of nitric oxide, hemodynamic and gas exchange variables were measured.

Results.—A progressive decrease in lung perfusion pressure and pulmonary vascular resistance index and an increase in intrapulmonary shunt resulted by increasing partial oxygen pressure in mixed venous blood from 47 to 84 mm Hg. There was no change in cardiac index or mixed venous carbon dioxide tension. At high partial oxygen pressure in mixed venous blood, the nitric oxide–induced reduction in lung perfusion pressure was smaller, but nitric oxide–induced decrease in intrapulmonary shunt was

independent of the baseline partial oxygen pressure in mixed venous blood. Arterial mixed venous oxygen tension increased more and arterial oxygen saturation increased less at high, compared with low, partial oxygen pressure in mixed venous blood in response to nitric oxide.

Conclusions.—Hypoxic pulmonary vasoconstriction in nonventilated lung areas modifies the hemodynamic and respiratory response to nitric oxide in patients with acute respiratory distress syndrome. The nitric oxide–induced decrease becomes more pronounced in progressive decrease in lung perfusion pressure as the hypoxic pulmonary vasoconstriction strengthens. In intrapulmonary shunt, the nitric oxide–induced decrease is independent of partial oxygen pressure in mixed venous blood over a wide range of partial oxygen pressure in mixed venous blood levels. By virtue of its location on the oxygen dissociation curve, the effect of nitric oxide on the arterial oxygen tension varies with the level of partial oxygen pressure in mixed venous blood.

▶ This interesting physiologic observation in 11 consecutive patients with acute respiratory distress syndrome treated with venovenous bypass emphasizes the important role hypoxic vasoconstriction plays in gas exchange and pulmonary hemodynamics. The ability of high mixed venous oxygen tensions to overcome the hypoxic pulmonary vasoconstriction in nonventilated lung units may explain, in part, the increased shunting observed in patients with sepsis. This physiologic response may be helpful in guiding future trials of inhaled nitric oxide, which exerts its beneficial effect on vessels supplying the ventilated lung units.

R.A. Balk, M.D.

Randomized, Prospective Trial of Bilevel Versus Continuous Positive Airway Pressure in Acute Pulmonary Edema

Mehta S, Jay GD, Woolard RH, et al (Brown Univ, Providence, RI)
Crit Care Med 25:620–628, 1997   4–42

Introduction.—It has been shown that continuous positive airway pressure (CPAP) given by face mask can reduce the need for endotracheal intubation in patients with acute pulmonary edema. By alternating between higher inspiratory and lower expiratory positive airway pressures, bilevel positive airway pressure might provide an inspiratory assist in addition to the benefits of CPAP. The effects of bilevel and CPAP on ventilation, acidemia, and dyspnea in patients with acute pulmonary edema were compared.

Methods.—The randomized, controlled trial included 27 patients with acute pulmonary edema. All had dyspnea, tachypnea, tachycardia, accessory muscle movement, bilateral rales, and radiographic signs of congestion. All patients received standard therapy. In addition, 13 patients received nasal CPAP, 10 cm of water. The other 14 received nasal bilevel positive airway pressure in a spontaneous/timed mode that combined

Permissive Hypercapnia With and Without Expiratory Washout in Patients With Severe Acute Respiratory Distress Syndrome

Kalfon P, Rao GSU, Gallart L, et al (Natl Inst of Mental Health and Neurosciences, Bangalore, India; Hosp Universitari del Mar, Barcelona, Spain)
Anesthesiology 87:6–17, 1997   4–43

Objective.—Acute respiratory distress syndrome (ARDS) produces a substantial reduction in aerated lung parenchyma. The resulting high inflation pressures required when normal tidal volume (VT) is administered leads to lung volutrauma. Ways to reduce the partial pressure of carbon dioxide while maintaining low VT would improve ventilation of ARDS patients. Prospectively, the efficacy of expiratory washout (EWO) for reducing the partial pressure of carbon dioxide was assessed, and the effects on airway pressures were quantified in patients with severe ARDS treated by using the permissive hypercapnia ventilatory strategy.

Methods.—Extension of lung hyperdensities was measured in 7 patients with severe ARDS using a thoracic CT scan. Hemodynamic and respiratory variables were determined at baseline and between each study phase. Respiratory status was calculated by dividing the patient's VT by the corresponding airway pressure on the PV curve. A positive-end expiratory pressure (PEEP) equal to the opening pressure was administered, respiratory rate was set at 18 breaths per min, and inspiratory/expiratory ratio was fixed at 33%. VT was reduced until the end-expiratory plateau pressure reached 25 cm of water. On day 2, a 3-phase study was begun (Fig 1).

Results.—The partial pressure of carbon dioxide decreased significantly (76 versus 53 mmHg), pH increased significantly (7.20 versus 7.34) during permissive hypercapnia with EWO, and the partial pressure of oxygen increased significantly (205 vs. 296 mm Hg). The reduction in partial pressure of carbon dioxide was attended by a significant 26% increase in end-inspiratory plateau pressure and a significant 29% increase in mean tracheal pressure. In addition, cardiac index decreased significantly by 20%, heart rate by 9%, mean pulmonary arterial pressure by 11%, right ventricular stroke work index by 25%, and true pulmonary shunt by 24%. At the same time, systemic vascular resistance index increased significantly by 22%, arteriovenous oxygen difference by 32%, and oxygen extraction ratio by 29%.

Conclusion.—Whereas EWO during permissive hypercapnia reduces the partial pressure of carbon dioxide and increases pH, it also increases airway pressures and lung volume in ARDS patients already at risk of lung volutrauma. PEEP must be monitored in these patients.

▶ An impressive demonstration that EWO will significantly reduce the $PaCO_2$ in patients with ARDS receiving permissive hypercapnia. Although the authors present a compelling argument for CO_2 clearance of endotracheal and tracheal gases as the mechanism by which EWO reduces $PaCO_2$,

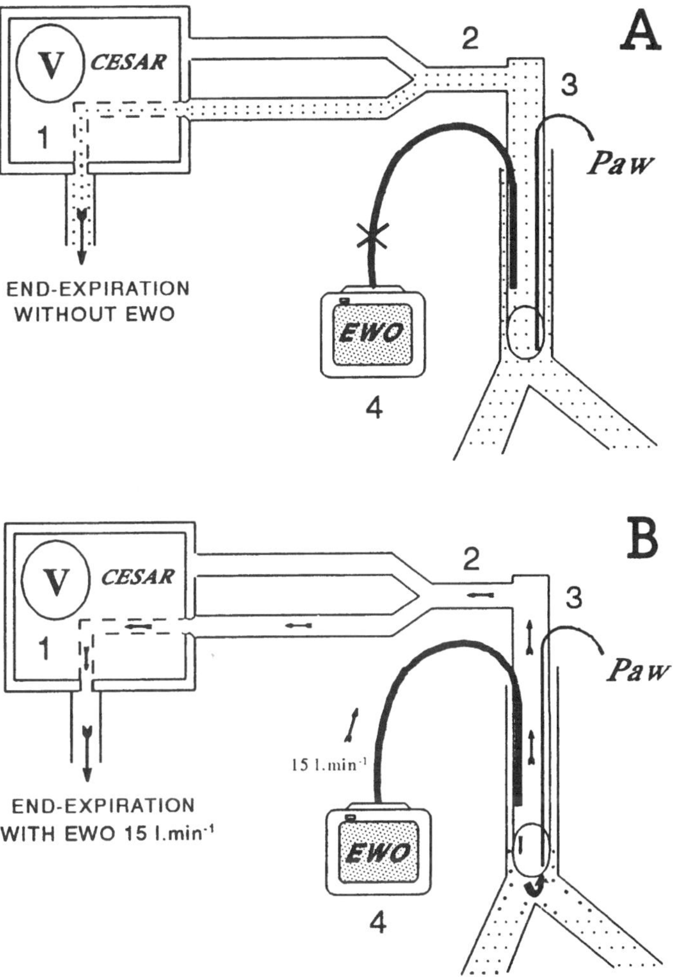

FIGURE 1.—The prototype ventilator equipped with expiratory washout (EWO). (**A**) end-expiration without EWO. (**B**) end-expiration with EWO 15 L/min: carbon dioxide has been removed entirely from "prosthetic" dead space. In addition, a distal washout effect is shown below the distal tip of the EWO channel of the endotracheal tube (see comments in the discussion). 1 = César ventilator, 2 = connecting tube between the Y-piece and the endotracheal tube, 3 = Mallinckrodt Hi-Lo Jet endotracheal tube, 4 = EWO prototype connected to the proximal channel of the endotracheal tube, Paw = distal channel of the endotracheal tube that allows airway pressure monitoring. (Courtesy of Kalfon P, Rao GSU, Gallart L, et al: Permissive hypercapnia with and without expiratory washout in patients with severe acute respiratory distress syndrome. *Anesthesiology* 87:6–17, 1997. Copyright American Society of Anesthesiologists, Inc. Used with permission of Lippincott-Raven Publishers.)

that is by no means the only plausible explanation. Changes in airway dynamics and lung volume may also be playing a major role. The appeal of all tracheal gas insufflation techniques is simplicity. This approach deserves further investigation, but is not yet ready for routine clinical application.

B.A. Shapiro, M.D.

Comparison of Pressure- and Flow-triggered Pressure-Support Ventilation on Weaning Parameters in Patients Recovering From Acute Respiratory Failure

Tütüncü AS, Çakar N, Çamci E, et al (Univ of Istanbul, Turkey)
Crit Care Med 25:756–760, 1997   4–44

Introduction.—Before the inspiratory flow is delivered to the patient during partial mechanical ventilatory support, a set trigger sensitivity has to be reached. There is some debate over the impact of the triggering systems (pressure-trigger or flow-trigger) on weaning parameters. In some studies, work of breathing has been shown to decrease with a flow-trigger system in comparison with a pressure-trigger system. Little is known about the effects on patients who do not have chronic obstructive pulmonary disease. The effects of flow-triggered and pressure-triggered ventilation systems on weaning parameters were compared in patients without chronic obstructive pulmonary disease.

Methods.—Sixteen orotracheally intubated patients, recovering from acute respiratory failure of various causes but without chronic obstructive pulmonary disease, were studied. They received randomized application of flow-triggered and pressure-triggered pressure-support ventilation at 75% and 100% ventilatory support levels in each triggering system. In all patients, 4 conditions were applied for 30 minutes each. Measurements were taken of ventilatory, respiratory, and hemodynamic data. An esophageal probe and a flow sensor between the "Y" piece of the ventilatory circuit and the endotracheal tube were used to measure the weaning parameters, with pressure and volume signals directed to a computerized respiratory monitor. To decrease the work of breathing performed by the patient to zero, peak airway pressures were applied during both pressure-triggered and flow-triggered pressure-support ventilation with a ventilator. With each triggering system, partial ventilatory support was applied at 75% of the peak airway pressures achieved during full ventilatory support.

Results.—Among the 4 experimental conditions, total ventilation volumes, arterial blood gas data, and hemodynamics did not differ. There was a significant increase in the work of breathing, rapid shallow breathing index, and esophageal pressure during partial ventilatory support with both triggering systems when compared with full ventilatory support. There were comparable weaning parameters between pressure- and flow-triggered pressure-support ventilation during the condition of ventilatory support. For work of breathing, pressure-triggered ventilation was 0.38 ± 0.24 J/L, and flow-triggered ventilation was 0.42 ± 0.26 J/L.

Conclusions.—In patients recovering from acute respiratory failure of various etiologies without chronic obstructive pulmonary disease, the application of either a pressure- or flow-triggered system during pressure-support ventilation with the ventilator did not significantly affect short-term changes in gas exchange, inspiratory workload, and respiratory mechanics.

▶ It has been generally accepted that flow-triggered breaths require less work of breathing than pressure-triggered breaths. This has been shown for both patients with and without chronic obstructive pulmonary disease (COPD).[1, 2] This study measures work of breathing with both systems in 16 stable mechanically ventilated patients, none of whom have COPD. The authors find no difference between the 2 systems with regard to work of breathing, weaning parameters, and tracheal occlusion pressure. There are several explanations for these findings. One possibility is that none of these patients had significant expiratory flow limitation. Theoretically, flow-triggering might be preferred in these patients who are at risk for dynamic hyperinflation. A more likely possibility is that the pressure-triggering design of the Servo 300 has been significantly improved. Reduced time delay to pressure-trigger a breath enhances responsiveness and may contribute to reduced work of breathing. A recent review suggests that differences in inspiratory work of breathing may be ventilator as well as triggering related.[3] With recent improvements in mechanical ventilators, differences between flow- and pressure-triggered breaths may now be minimal.

M.R. Silver, M.D.

References

1. Sassoon CSH, Lodia R, Rheeman CH, et al: Inspiratory muscle work of breathing during flow-by, demand-flow, and continuous-flow systems in patients with chronic obstructive pulmonary diseases. *Am Rev Respir Dis* 145:1219–1222, 1992.
2. Sassoon CSH, Giron AE, Ely E, et al: Inspiratory work of breathing on flow-by and demand-flow continuous positive airway pressures. *Crit Care Med* 17:1108–1114, 1989.
3. Sassoon CSH, Gruer SE: Characteristics of the ventilator pressure- and flow-trigger variables. *Intensive Care Med* 21:159–168, 1995.

Passive Mechanics of Lung and Chest Wall in Patients Who Failed or Succeeded in Trials of Weaning
Jubran A, Tobin MJ (Edward Hines Jr VA Hosp, Hines, Ill; Loyola Univ, Hines, Ill)
Am J Respir Crit Care Med 155:916–921, 1997   4–45

Background.—The authors have found that, among patients with chronic obstructive pulmonary disease, pulmonary mechanics get worse in those who fail a trial of weaning from mechanical ventilation compared with those who are successfully extubated. This suggested that patients in whom weaning fails may have more problems with pulmonary mechanics than are apparent before the trial of weaning is done. The passive mechanics of the respiratory system, lung, and chest wall in patients who did and did not tolerate a trial of weaning from mechanical ventilation was investigated.

Methods.—The study included 12 patients with chronic obstructive pulmonary disease (COPD) who failed a trial of spontaneous breathing and 12 who were successfully weaned from mechanical ventilation. In both groups, detailed measurements of the resistance and elastance of the total respiratory system, lung, and chest wall were performed during passive ventilation at the usual ventilator settings. Possible differences in lung and chest wall mechanics were sought.

Results.—Respiratory system, lung, and chest wall resistances were similar between groups. The results were also similar when resistances were considered in components derived from ohmic resistance and visco-elastic behavior/time–constant inhomogeneities. Static elastance and dynamic intrinsic positive end-expiratory pressure of the respiratory system and the respective lung and chest wall components were similar, as were dynamic elastances of the respiratory system and chest wall. Patients who did not tolerate a trial of weaning had increased dynamic lung elastance. However, the values overlapped considerably between groups.

Conclusion.—In patients with COPD receiving passive ventilation, the mechanics of the respiratory system, lung, and chest wall during passive ventilation cannot predict which patients will pass and which will fail a trial of weaning. Although dynamic lung elastance is increased in patients who fail weaning as a group, this value is not a reliable indicator of whether individual patients will be able to breathe on their own. None of the other mechanical characteristics studied are significantly different between groups.

▶ The search continues for tests that can predict whether a ventilator patient will breathe spontaneously. This study shows that measuring passive mechanics of the lung and chest wall is not the answer.

B.A. Shapiro, M.D.

Impact of Positive End-expiratory Pressure on Chest Wall and Lung Pressure–Volume Curve in Acute Respiratory Failure

Mergoni M, Martelli A, Volpi A, et al (Azienda Ospedaliera de Parma, Italy; Azienda Ospedaliera di Verona, Italy)
Am J Respir Crit Care Med 156:846–854, 1997   4–46

Objective.—Setting ventilator patterns, according to measurements of respiratory mechanics, can have a significant impact on the outcomes of patients with acute respiratory distress syndrome, studies have found. It is generally assumed that the total respiratory system pressure-volume (P-V) curve—obtained through supersyringe lung inflation—is primarily an indicator of the elastic behavior of the lung, unaffected by the elastic properties of the chest wall. However, even though the P-V curve has been extensively used in clinical practice, this assumption has never been tested. Patients with acute respiratory failure (ARF) were studied to determine whether chest-wall mechanics could influence the shape of the total respiratory system P-V curve and, thus, alter ventilatory settings.

Methods.—Thirteen patients with ARF were studied. The supersyringe method and esophageal balloon technique were used to draw total respiratory system (P-Vrs), lung (P-VL), and chest wall (P-VCW) curves. The curves were remeasured at varying levels of positive end-expiratory pressure (PEEP) from 0 to 15 cm of water. The starting compliance, inflation compliance, and end compliance were derived from each P-V curve. The effects of chest wall mechanics on the P-Vrs were analyzed, particularly on the lower inflection point (LIP) of the curve.

Results.—At a PEEP of 0, all patients showed an LIP on the P-Vrs curve, with a mean value of 7.5 cm of water. Two patients showed an LIP only on the P-VL curve, 7 had an LIP only on the P-Vw curve, and 4 had an LIP on both the P-VL and P-Vw curves. Under conditions of PEEP, the LIP disappeared, suggesting a volume-related mechanism for the LIP on the P-VL and P-Vw curves. High-level PEEP was associated with an upper inflection point (UIP) on both the P-Vrs and P-VL curves, with mean values of 12 and 9 cm of water, respectively; this finding suggested alveolar overdistention. As PEEP increased, so did PaO_2. However, this increase became significant only in patients with an LIP on the P-VL curve: from 70.5 to 117.5 mm Hg, compared with 91–122 mm Hg for patients without an LIP on the P-VL curve.

Conclusions.—In mechanically ventilated patients with ARF, chest wall mechanics can significantly influence the LIP appearing on the P-Vrs curve. Only patients with an LIP on the lung P-V curve—and not on the chest wall curve—showed improved PaO_2 with PEEP. The lung may be overdistended and a UIP may appear at high levels of PEEP. At least with the patient in supine position, measurement of P-Vrs alone may give misleading results in setting the level of PEEP. However, by showing the inflection volume above which a UIP may develop, this measurement can help to prevent excessive alveolar overdistention.

▶ The quest for "best" PEEP in the patient with ARF seems to be moving toward a definition that encompasses an emphasis on pulmonary mechanics. The rationale for ventilation within the linear portion of the respiratory system P-V curve makes good physiologic sense. Using this approach, enough PEEP is applied so that end-expiratory volume does not encroach on the lower, less compliant part of the curve. Tidal volume cycling on the upper, less compliant part of the curve is avoided to minimize the risk of alveolar overdistention. This study attempts to partition total respiratory system mechanics into the lung and chest wall components. Interestingly, the authors found that the lower inflection point on the total respiratory PV curve may be determined by chest wall, rather than lung mechanics. Increasing PEEP in these patients was shown to increase the compliance of the chest wall (and total respiratory system), but not to result in recruitment of underventilated lung spaces or to increase PaO_2. Further investigation is needed to determine the cause of abnormal chest wall mechanics, as well as its potential contribution to the pathophysiology of ARF.

H. Nearman, M.D.

with survival rates of similar studies. There is a need for further prospective, randomized trials of algorithm-controlled conventional vs. high-frequency oscillatory ventilation in ARDS. At this time, the use of high-frequency oscillatory ventilation in adults should be considered investigational.

▶ Modern strategies for supporting ventilation and oxygenation in patients with severe lung disease include (1) recruitment of all available alveoli, (2) avoidance of alveolar overdistention, (3) decreasing FIO_2 to 60% or less, and (4) keeping the partial pressure of arterial carbon dioxide to less than 60 mm Hg, if possible. A number of strategies have been put forth to accomplish these goals, using traditional volume preset or volume variable positive pressure ventilators. This limited study demonstrates that high-frequency oscillatory ventilation can be used to accomplish the above goals, and can maybe do it better. Further study is definitely warranted.

B.A. Shapiro, M.D.

Tracheal Pressure Triggering a Demand-flow Continuous Positive Airway Pressure System Decreases Patient Work of Breathing

Messinger G, Banner MJ (Univ of Florida, Gainesville; Tel-Aviv Med School, Israel)

Crit Care Med 24:1829–1834, 1996

Introduction.—In a previous study using an in vitro lung model, the authors demonstrated a significant decrease in work of breathing during spontaneous ventilation with continuous positive airway pressure using tracheal pressure triggering. Compared with both conventional pressure and flow-by triggering, airway pressure was increased for part of the inspiratory cycle during tracheal pressure triggering, yielding an effect similar to pressure-support ventilation. These findings were confirmed in a prospective study of 14 patients with acute respiratory failure.

Methods.—Patients were 6 men and 8 women, ranging in age from 31 to 84. All were studied using the same ventilator. Patients were breathing spontaneously at an FIO_2 of 0.30 to 0.40 and received 5 cm H_2O of continuous positive airway pressure. The 3 different methods of triggering the ventilator were employed in random order. For each respiratory and hemodynamic parameter, 5 measurements were recorded for 1 minute and averaged.

Results.—Total work of breathing was significantly decreased during tracheal pressure triggering compared with both conventional pressure and flow-by triggering. The decrease in imposed work of breathing was 83% with tracheal pressure triggering compared with conventional pressure triggering. Compared with the other 2 methods, delivered inspiratory flow rate and tidal volume were significantly increased during tracheal pressure triggering. The small, but significant, increases in tidal volume with tracheal pressure triggering may not be clinically important. Tracheal pressure triggering decreased systolic blood pressure, the index of rapid shallow breathing, and the pressure-time product per breath. None of the 3 triggering methods significantly altered minute ventilation, the ratio of inspiratory time to total cycle time, diastolic blood pressure, heart rate, or oxygen saturation.

Conclusion.—Compared with conventional pressure and flow-by triggering, the total work of breathing decreased by approximately 40% during tracheal pressure triggering the ventilator "ON." This finding was consistent in all study participants, and the same results should occur with other commonly used ventilators.

▶ This study compares tracheal pressure measurement as a trigger for delivery of mechanical breaths with conventional methods of ventilator triggering. The authors found that initial pressure triggering resulted in more efficient ventilator triggering and decreased work of breathing. However, as the authors point out, measuring tracheal pressures with catheters inserted into the airway or with specially designed endotracheal tubes, while relatively straightforward to accomplish, presents problems in maintaining patency of the pressure monitoring system. This requires vigilance, or else adverse affects could occur due to system occlusion. The primary consideration in this circumstance is whether or not the improvement in imposed work of breathing results in sufficiently great clinical benefit to merit standard utilization of this technique. Additional study will be necessary in various patient populations to further define this question.

W.T. Peruzzi, M.D.

Comparison of Assisted Ventilator Modes on Triggering, Patient Effort, and Dyspnea
Leung P, Jubran A, Tobin MJ (Edward Hines Jr VA Hosp, Hines, Ill; Loyola Univ, Hines, Ill; Suburban Hosp, Hinsdale, Ill)
Am J Respir Crit Care Med 155:1940–1948, 1997   4–50

Introduction.—Calculations performed on a small number of representative breaths have been used in studies of patient-ventilator interaction, but some patients have difficulty in triggering the ventilator and representative breaths may not convey the true nature of patient-ventilator interaction. Four ventilator modes were compared to determine the relative efficacy of graded levels of pressure support and intermittent mandatory ventilation in reducing patient effort and dyspnea.

Methods.—During 4 ventilator modes, a comparison was made for 11 ventilator-dependent patients. The modes were assist-control ventilation, intermittent mandatory ventilation, pressure support, and a combination of intermittent mandatory ventilation and pressure support.

Results.—Inspiratory pressure-time product was decreased by progressive increases in intermittent mandatory ventilation and pressure support. With pressure support, reductions in pressure-time product were greater than with intermittent mandatory ventilation at lower but proportional levels of maximal assistance. Greater reductions in pressure-time product were achieved during intervening breaths and during mandatory breaths, when pressure support of 10 cm H_2O was added to a given level of intermittent mandatory ventilation. During intervening breaths, this additional unloading during mandatory breaths was proportional to the decrease in respiratory drive. With assist-control ventilation, maximal unloading occurred with a fivefold decrease in pressure-time product when compared with unassisted breathing. Decreases in pressure-time product were confined to the posttrigger phase. There was a correlation of pressure-time product of the post-trigger phase and decrease in respiratory drive. Despite marked changes in drive and intrinsic positive end-expiratory pressure, effort during the trigger phase remained constant. With all modes, ineffective triggering occurred. With increasing levels of assistance as a result of the accompanying decrease in drive and increase in volume, wasted pressure-time product increased. Shorter respiratory cycle times and expiratory times and higher positive end-expiratory pressure were seen in breaths preceding nontriggering efforts. This probably indicates that neural-mechanical asynchrony resulted from inspiratory activity beginning prematurely before elastic recoil pressure had fallen to a level that could be overcome by a patient's muscular effort.

Conclusion.—Progressive decreases in inspiratory muscle effort and dyspnea occurred with increases in the level of ventilator assistance, which were accompanied by increases in the rate of ineffective triggering.

▶ Does increasing the level of positive pressure ventilation (frequency or pressure) diminish dyspnea and the patient's efforts to spontaneously breath? This fundamental question has been asked and answered in numerous studies over the past 20 years. The answer is yes. This article describes an extremely sophisticated study of this fundamental question, and the answer remains yes.

B.A. Shapiro, M.D.

A Randomized, Controlled Trial of Protocol-directed Versus Physician-directed Weaning From Mechanical Ventilation
Kollef MH, Shapiro SD, Silver P, et al (Washington Univ, St Louis; Barnes-Jewish-Christian Hosps Health System, St Louis)
Crit Care Med 25:567–574, 1997   4–51

Introduction.—The gradual reduction of ventilatory support and its replacement with spontaneous ventilation is the definition of weaning from mechanical ventilation, yet there is controversy on how it should be performed. The efficacy of a protocol to wean patients from mechanical ventilation was compared with the traditional practice of physician-directed weaning. Using the protocol guidelines, the authors hypothesized

TABLE 5.—Scores and Outcomes

Group	No. of Patients With a Given Weaning Score						
	0	1	2	3	4	5	6
Died prior to the beginning of weaning (9)				2	2	3	2
Died due to mechanical failure (3)			1	1		1	
Transferred to another site (7)		1		2	2	1	1
Died prior to completing the 42-day weaning period (15)			2	2	4	5	2

(Courtesy of Gluck EH, Corigian L: Predicting eventual success or failure to wean in patients receiving long-term mechanical ventilation. *Chest* 110:1018–1024, 1996.)

Methods.—On admission, patient histories (including ventilator histories) were obtained, along with assessments of the levels of electrolytes, serum calcium, magnesium, phosphorus, white blood cells, hemoglobin, albumin, total protein, transferrin, oxygen intake, carbon dioxide production, respiratory quotient, and dead space/tidal volume. Patients were then enrolled in a weaning protocol that involved an increasing duration of pressure support ventilation during the day, with complete rest at night. Forty-two days after the study enrollment (which was 3 times the duration of the weaning protocol), successfully weaned patients were compared with those remaining ventilator dependent. The parameters predicting successful weaning in this group were then applied prospectively to a new group of 72 patients.

Findings.—Static compliance, airway resistance, the dead space to tidal volume ratio, $PaCO_2$, and the frequency/tidal volume were the only parameters meeting fale-positive and false-negative requirements for the scoring system. A score exceeding 3 was associated with failure to wean, and a score of less than 3 predicted successful weaning. A score of 3 was not predictive. The scoring system had a sensitivity of 100%, a specificity of 91%, positive predictive value of 83%, and a negative predictive value of 100%. None of the individual parameters was as reliable as the overall scoring system (Table 5).

Conclusions.—Generally available admission parameters can be combined in a scoring system to predict whether patients can eventually be weaned from mechanical ventilation. The current scoring system resulted in no false-negative results and an acceptable number of false-positive results.

▶ This study uses outcomes analysis to determine factors that will be predictive of successful withdrawal of mechanical ventilatory support for patients admitted to long-term ventilator facilities. The authors have developed a scoring system that could be useful in not only long-term ventilator support units, but also acute care facilities in terms of decisions regarding the timing of patient transfers to long-term ventilator units. Further assessment that nurses and respiratory therapists could safely and effectively wean most patients from mechanical ventilation.

Methods.—Of the 356 patients requiring mechanical ventilation, 179 were randomized into the protocol-directed group and 178 were randomized into the physician-directed weaning from mechanical ventilation. The duration of mechanical ventilation from tracheal intubation until discontinuation of mechanical ventilation was measured. Need for reintubation, length of hospital stay, hospital mortality rate, and hospital costs were also analyzed.

Results.—For the protocol-directed group, the median duration of mechanical ventilation was 35 hours, compared with 44 hours for the physician-directed group. Significantly shorter durations of mechanical ventilation were seen with the patients randomized to protocol-directed weaning. The rate of successful weaning was significantly greater for patients receiving protocol-directed weaning. For the 2 treatment groups, the hospital mortality rates were similar, with the protocol-directed group having a 22.3% mortality rate and the physician-directed group having a 23.6% mortality rate. Patients in the protocol-directed group saved $42,9609 on hospital costs, compared with the patients in the physician-directed group.

Conclusion.—Extubation occurred more rapidly with protocol-guided weaning of mechanical ventilation by nurses and respiratory therapists than with physician-directed weaning.

▶ I have always been mystified by the pervasive reluctance of physicians to accept protocol-directed ventilator weaning in the ICU. To my knowledge, no credible evidence has ever been presented that suggests the practice may be dangerous, whereas numerous studies suggest the practice is safe and perhaps advantageous. This study is a welcome addition to the increasing evidence in favor of protocols for respiratory therapists and nurses to perform ventilator weaning.

B.A. Shapiro, M.D.

Predicting Eventual Success or Failure to Wean in Patients Receiving Long-term Mechanical Ventilation

Gluck EH, Corgian L (Vencor Hosp, Northlake, Ill; Finch Univ, Chicago; Rush-Presbyterian-St Luke's Med Ctr, Chicago)
Chest 110:1018–1024, 1996   4–52

Background.—Centers devoted solely to the care of patients requiring long-term ventilator support are being established nationwide to handle the increasing numbers of such patients. Although this strategy significantly reduces the cost of care, further cost-saving means are needed. Allocating services to patients most likely to benefit from them is one such means. Whether the ultimate ability of a patient to wean himself from prolonged ventilatory support can be predicted at the time of admission to a long-term ventilator center was determined.

and validation of this scoring system will better define its applicability in various clinical settings.

W.T. Peruzzi, M.D.

Proportional Assist Ventilation in Acute Respiratory Failure: Effects on Breathing Pattern and Inspiratory Effort
Navalesi P, Hernandez P, Wongsa A, et al (Montreal Gen Hosp; Sir Mortimer B Davis Jewish Gen Hosp, Montreal; Montreal Chest Hosp Ctr; et al)
Am J Respir Crit Care Med 154:1330–1338, 1996   4–53

Introduction.—Proportional assist ventilation (PAV) differs from other forms of assisted ventilation by applying pressure in proportion to volume (volume assist, VA) and flow (flow assist FA), thus, regulating the amount of ventilatory support provided in proportion to identified respiratory abnormalities. There are few reports, however, on the effects of PAV. A study of 8 patients with acute respiratory failure examined the effects of varying the level of VA on breathing pattern, inspiratory effect, and work of breathing and the interaction between VA and FA.

Methods.—The patients were intubated and mechanically ventilated. All were clinically stable for the 12 to 24 hours preceding the study and could tolerate limited periods of decreased ventilatory support. After a brief period of hyperventilation, respiratory system elastance (Ers) and resistance (Rrs) were determined using the end-inspiratory occlusion method during constant flow inflation. Ventilator settings were selected to match the breathing pattern parameters noted during a preliminary spontaneous breathing (SB) trial. Four levels of VA (20%, 40%, 60%, and 80% of the patient's Ers) were applied for 5-minute periods in random order. For each of these settings, a fixed amount of FA (50% Rrs) was added for an additional 5 minutes.

Results.—Compared with SB, VA increased tidal volume, whereas as respiratory rate (RR) fell slightly or was stable. There was a small, nonsignificant increase in minute ventilation. Addition of FA further increased tidal volume and significantly reduced RR, resulting in unchanged minute ventilation. An increase in VA led to a graded reduction in inspiratory effort, which was further reduced by the addition of FA. Although VA decreased the elastic work of breathing, resistive work tended to increase; thus, the fall in total work was less than anticipated. The addition of FA significantly reduced resistive work and total work at each VA setting.

Discussion.—Proportional assist ventilation is a means of improving the breathing pattern while reducing inspiratory effort in patients with acute respiratory failure. By adjustment of VA and FA, the patient's elastic and resistive work can be reduced in proportion to the level of assistance set on

HFOV alone (33.6 ± 21.5 mm Hg). PaO_2 increased steadily in both groups during the course of the experiment, with no further significant differences detected. By the end of the study, PaO_2 was 328 ± 80 mm Hg in perflubron-treated animals, and 331 ± 164 mm Hg in animals receiving HFOV alone. $PaCO_2$ and pH did not differ among treatment groups at any time during the study.

Conclusions.—Partial liquid ventilation is an effective adjunct to HFOV in providing oxygenation following acute lung injury. Although the final PaO_2 achieved in this study did not differ between the 2 treatment groups, oxygenation improved more rapidly in animals treated with perflubron and HFOV than it did in those receiving HFOV alone. The perflubron–HFOV combination may allow ventilation and oxygenation at lower airway pressures because of the ability of the compound to facilitate expansion of alveoli and to decrease the incidence of intrapulmonary shunting.

▶ The use of new methods of support and treatment for acute lung injury is taken to a new level in this trial of high-frequency oscillation plus liquid ventilation in a piglet model of acute lung injury. The combination of the 2 modalities was associated with more rapid improvement in oxygenation. This result sets the stage for future trials that may combine multiple approaches to treatment or support. One may envision a future trial of high-frequency oscillation plus partial liquid ventilation, inhaled nitric oxide, and prone positioning. The difficulty will come in determining if all of these interventions are truly necessary and which of them are the beneficial maneuvers.

R.A. Balk, M.D.

Randomized, Controlled Trial of Selective Digestive Decontamination in 600 Mechanically Ventilated Patients in a Multidisciplinary Intensive Care Unit

Verwaest C, Verhaegen J, Ferdinande P, et al (Univ Hosp Gasthuisberg, Leuven, Belgium)
Crit Care Med 25:63–71, 1997   4–56

Introduction.—Antimicrobial decontamination typically is performed to prevent nosocomial infections (usually of the respiratory tract) by eliminating potentially pathogenic micro-organisms colonizing in the intestinal tract. The mortality benefit of this practice is not clear. The clinical effectiveness of 2 selective decontamination regimens were compared with the clinical effectiveness of a conventional antibiotic regimen in patients likely to receive mechanical ventilation for at least 48 hours.

Methods.—A total of 660 consecutive patients were randomized to receive 1 of the following: conventional antibiotic regimen (control group A); oral and enteral ofloxacin–amphotericin B (group B); or oral and enteral polymyxin and E-tobramycin–amphotericin B (group C). The treatment groups received systemic antibiotics for 4 days—ofloxacin and cefotaxime for groups B and C, respectively. Data were collected regarding colonization and primary and secondary infection rate, ICU mortality rate, emergence of antibiotic resistance, length of hospital stay, and antimicrobial agent expenses.

Results.—Patients in group A had significantly more infections, secondary lower respiratory tract infections, and urinary tract infections. Patients in group C had significantly more gram-positive bacteremias than patients in group A. For all groups, infection at the time of admission was the most significant factor for subsequent infections. The ICU mortality rate was similar in all groups and was not related to primary or secondary infection. Significantly increased antimicrobial resistance was observed in both treatment groups, compared with control group A. The cost of antimicrobial agents was comparable in control group A and group C, and was one third less in group B.

Conclusion.—Selective decontamination added substantially to the cost of ICU care and did not improve survival. The emergence of multiple antibiotic-resistant micro-organisms causes definite changes in the ecology of environmental, colonizing, and infecting bacteria that should be weighed when considering selective digestive decontamination.

▶ Selective digestive decontamination (SDD) has been advocated by a number of investigators for more than 15 years. Although the pharmaceutical regiments for reducing microbial colonization have varied, the fundamental principle hasn't. Prophylactic administration of parenteral and enteral antibiotics does reduce microbiological colonization. This appears to be true in both medical and surgical ICU patients. In trauma, head injury, and general medical ICU patients, SDD also appears to reduce infection rates. Proponents of SDD believe that, in certain settings, SDD also is associated with reduced ICU length of stay, ICU costs, ICU mortality, or hospital mortality. This has been much more difficult to prove to intensivists.

This study compares the original regimen proposed by Soutenbeek et al.[1] (oral and enteral polymyxin E tobramycin-amphotericin B combined with IV cefotaxime) with another regimen (oral and enteral ofloxacin-amphotericin B with IV ofloxacin) with no SDD. In this large, randomized, controlled study of 600 mechanically ventilated patients, SDD once again reduced the colonization rates of different mucosae with potentially pathogenic microorganisms. Both regimens reduced bronchial aspirate, oropharynx, and gastric mucosa colonization rates significantly. Only the ofloxacin regimen significantly reduced colonization rates of the urinary tract and rectal mucosa.

Because nearly a third of these ICU patients were infected at the time of admission, the authors examined the effect of SDD on secondary infections. The ofloxacin regimen, but not the control or cefotaxime regimens, was associated with a significant reduction in the number of secondary infections. Selective digestive decontamination did not reduce the incidence of pulmonary infections. Neither SDD regimen was associated with a reduction in the ICU length of stay. In fact, the cefotaxime regimen was associated with a significantly increased ICU length of stay, compared with the control

The Outcome of Prolonged Mechanical Ventilation in Elderly Patients: Are the Efforts Worthwhile?

Meinders AJ, van der Hoeven JG, Meinders AE (Univ Hosp Leiden, The Netherlands)

Age Ageing 25:353–356, 1996

4–58

Background.—It has been generally accepted that elderly patients derive less benefit from intensive therapy than younger patients do, and that increasing age is a risk factor for mortality in the hospital. The acceptability of using age alone as a predictor of quality of life and mortality, in the process of choosing appropriate treatment options, however, has recently been called into question. Few studies have specifically addressed the relationship between prolonged mechanical ventilation and outcome in elderly patients. Risk factors for mortality in the hospital were determined, in this retrospective study, in elderly patients subject to protracted mechanical ventilation.

Methods.—Records were reviewed for 181 patients age 70 years or older, who received mechanical ventilation at a single university hospital for more than 3 days between 1970 and 1990. Demographic and medical data, including APACHE III scores, were collected.

Results.—The median age of research subjects was 75 years, and patients spent a mean of 12 days (range, 4–102 days) on mechanical ventilation. The overall rate of mortality in-hospital was 57.5%. Mortality rate increased with increasing APACHE III scores, and APACHE III scores were significantly lower for survivors than they were for nonsurvivors ($P < 0.001$). An admission diagnosis of cardiac arrest ($P < 0.001$) or shock in the ICU ($P = 0.006$) was positively, and significantly, correlated with risk of in-hospital mortality. Age; duration of either the ICU stay or of mechanical ventilation; preadmission diagnoses other than cardiac arrest; and ICU complications, excluding shock, were not significant predictors of in-hospital mortality.

Conclusions.—The mortality rate of patients age 70 years or older who receive prolonged mechanical ventilation appears to be independent of chronic health status and age. Rather, diagnosis at admission and acute complications in the ICU are more significant predictors of patient outcome.

▶ Over a 20-year period, there were 181 patients admitted to an ICU and requiring mechanical ventilation for more than 3 days. The survival rate was 42.5%. This is comparable with the 41% to 78% survival rate for the elderly in other similarly designed studies.[1, 2] Not surprisingly, the occurrence of shock in the ICU did portend a worsened survival rate (5 of 77 survivors vs. 35 of 104 nonsurvivors). Increasing APACHE III score also correlated with increased mortality. Age, days of mechanical ventilation, and the need for acute hemodialysis did not correlate with mortality.

This study does little to help the clinician at the bedside. Many intensivists recognize that the hospital mortality in elderly patients requiring mechanical ventilation for more than 3 days is at least 50%. Although it is possible to select patients more likely to survive,[3] this selection process excludes the majority of patients. For the majority of patients, it is important to define the goals and limits of care. Because it is unlikely that the physician will ever be able to say the mortality rate for a given patient will always be 100%, patients will continue to require individualized plans of care. Although the concept of futility as being a very low probability of survival has been advocated,[4] it has not been institutionalized in the ICU.[5] As health care resources for all patients diminish, physicians will increasingly be called on to determine the most cost-effective strategy for managing this patient population.

M.R. Silver, M.D.

References

1. Cohen IL, Lambrinos J, Fein IA: Mechanical ventilation for the elderly patient in intensive care: Incremental charges and benefits. *JAMA* 269:1025–1029, 1993.
2. Elpern E, Larson R, Douglas P, et al: Long-term outcome for elderly survivors of prolonged ventilator assistance. *Chest* 96:1120–1124, 1989.
3. Gracey DR, Hardy DC, Naessens JM, et al: The Mayo ventilator-dependent rehabilitation unit: A 5-year experience. *Mayo Clin Proc* 72:13–19, 1997.
4. Schneiderman LJ, Jecker NS, Jonsen AR: Medical futility: Its meaning and ethical implications. *Ann Intern Med* 112:949–954, 1990.
5. Waisel DB, Truog RD: The cardiopulmonary resuscitation-not-indicated order: Futility revised. *Ann Intern Med* 122:304–308, 1995.

Safety and Yield of Transbronchial Biopsy in Mechanically Ventilated Patients
O'Brien JD, Ettinger NA, Shevlin D, et al (Washington Univ, St Louis)
Crit Care Med 25:440–446, 1997   4–59

Background.—Many patients undergoing mechanical ventilation because of respiratory failure develop pulmonary infiltrates. Although open-lung biopsy can identify the causal organism, many physicians hesitate to use this method in such critically ill ventilated patients. These investigators report their experience with another sampling method, transbronchial biopsy, in identifying pulmonary infiltrates and influencing patient management.

Methods.—A total of 71 patients receiving mechanical ventilation who developed diffuse pulmonary infiltrates underwent 83 instances of fiberoptic bronchoscopy with transbronchial biopsy. Variables examined included the histologic correlation between samples obtained with transbronchial biopsy and other methods, and whether a change in the patient's management occurred based on the transbronchial biopsy results.

Findings.—Most patients had received a lung transplant (n = 34) or were immunocompromised (n = 17). No deaths or episodes of sepsis or pneumonia occurred that were related to the procedure. The most significant procedure-related complications were pneumothorax (which occurred in 10 patients without preexisting chest tubes), transient oxygen desaturation to less than 90% (7 patients), hypotension (6 patients), and bronchial hemorrhage of more than 30 mL (5 patients). Biopsy specimens yielded a specific diagnosis in about one third of cases. Results of the transbronchial biopsy caused changes in patient management (typically starting or discontinuing antimicrobial agents or corticosteroids) in 41% of cases. However, the mortality rate of the patients whose medical regimen changed did not differ significantly from that of patients who continued on their same medical course. Comparisons of the results from transbronchial biopsy with those from open-lung biopsy or autopsy showed complete agreement in 11 of 13 samples. In the other 2 instances, transbronchial biopsy had not retrieved sufficient material.

Conclusions.—Transbronchial biopsy was a reasonably safe procedure in these ventilated patients with diffuse pulmonary infiltrates. Its results led to management changes in slightly under half the patients, and its agreement with histologic findings from other biopsy techniques was good. The authors suggest that the ideal candidate for transbronchial biopsy should be hemodynamically stable with adequate oxygenation and without severe pulmonary hypertension or an uncorrectable bleeding diathesis. Transbronchial biopsy should be undertaken only after less invasive tests are tried (unless a tissue diagnosis is considered necessary), and only if the results of the procedure could affect the patient's medical management.

▶ This study examines the impact of performing transbronchial biopsies (TBBx) in mechanically ventilated patients. Before examining the results, it is important to consider the clinical population studied. Except for diffuse infiltrates in the transplanted lung of single-lung transplanted patients, all patients had diffuse bilateral infiltrates. Initially, 210 patients underwent bronchoscopy without TBBx. Useful clinical information, obviating the need for a TBBx, was obtained in 100 patients. Of the remaining 110 patients, 39 did not undergo TBBx for reasons including patient refusal and increased risk (e.g., uncorrectable bleeding diathesis, inability to oxygenate during bronchoscopy, MAP less than 60 mm Hg, suspicion of severe pulmonary hypertension). Nearly half of the patients undergoing TBBx (34/71) were status-post lung transplantation. There were patients with coagulopathies who received fresh frozen plasma before TBBx. There were several patients who underwent TBBx with platelet counts between 50,000 and 100,00 cells/mm^3. Several patients with elevated BUN levels received desmopressin acetate.

Patients who underwent TBBx had an average of 9.5 biopsies per patient. Lung transplant patients had significantly more biopsies (12.3 per patient) than nontransplant patients (6.0 per patient). C-arm fluoroscopy was used for all patients. Of the 29 specific histologic diagnoses found, 18 of 29 were infectious, including 5 of 18 with CMV. The authors report that changes in management directly attributable to the TBBx results occurred in roughly 60% of the nontransplant population and 26% in the transplant population.

The incidence of pneumothorax was 14.3% for the entire patient population, which was significantly higher than the 5% rate in nonventilated patients.[1] In 13 of 110 patients, chest tubes were already in place, so the incidence of pneumothorax might be greater than 14%. Clinically significant was the higher rate of pneumothoracies for the nontransplant group (18.9%) than for the transplant group (6.5%). Major bleeding (more than 30 mL of blood) occurred in 5 patients, with 1 patient having more than 100 mL of blood. This patient did not have any coagulation abnormalities before the procedure. No deaths were directly attributable to the biopsy.

Should TBBx be performed in mechanically ventilated patients with diffuse infiltrates and negative bronchoscopy with lavage and brushing? This report from a skilled group of clinicians indicates that it is feasible, although it is associated with a complication rate at least 3 times that of spontaneously breathing patients. Although management decisions were impacted less frequently, for patients after lung transplant, TBBx appears preferable to open-lung biopsy. For critically ill nontransplant patients, clinicians should recognize the increased likelihood of complications if they choose to perform TBBx in this patient population. Because this report describes the outcomes in patients with diffuse bilateral infiltrates, the results are not directly applicable to nontransplant patients requiring mechanical ventilation with localized infiltrates.

M.R. Silver, M.D.

Reference

1. Fulkerson WJ: Fiberoptic bronchoscopy. *N Engl J Med* 311:511–515, 1984.

Reproducibility of Quantitative Cultures of Endotracheal Aspirates From Mechanically Ventilated Patients
Bergmans DCJJ, Bonten MJM, De Leeuw PW, et al (Univ Hosp Maastricht, The Netherlands)
J Clin Microbiol 35:796–798, 1997   4–60

Objective.—When ventilator-associated pneumonia is suspected, the diagnosis is often made by quantitative cultures of specimens obtained bronchoscopically. However, this approach is expensive and carries the potential for adverse effects. A simpler, less expensive method is quantitative culture of endotracheal aspirates. Although studies have shown that this technique correlates well with bronchoscopy, there are no data on the reproducibility of quantitative cultures of endotracheal aspirates. A quantitative analysis of endotracheal aspirates from mechanically ventilated patients was reported.

Methods.—The 2-day study included 21 patients receiving mechanical ventilation who required 5 or more endotracheal suctionings per day. Samples were obtained every 2 to 6 hours, for a total of 140 endotracheal aspirates. The reproducibility of quantitative cultures of these aspirates was studied.

Results.—The quantitative culture results showed a median variation of 12.3%, corresponding to 0.7 log CFU/mL. The amount of variation was unaffected by the time between samples. Eighty-two percent of specimens showed at least 10^5 CFU/mL of pathogens in consecutive cultures. The results of semiquantitative culture correlated well with those of quantitative culture. However, the results of quantitative culture correlated poorly with the number of polymorphonuclear neutrophils on Gram's stain.

Conclusion.—This study establishes the reproducibility of quantitative cultures from endotracheal aspirates. This technique may be of value in the diagnosis of ventilator-associated pneumonia. Further study is needed to correlate the results of quantitative cultures from endotracheal aspirates with bronchoscopically obtained specimens.

▶ In approaching the patient with ventilator-associated pneumonia, some advocate empirical antibiotic therapy, whereas others insist on invasive specimen acquisition and the use of quantitative culture techniques to assist with interpretation. Most clinicians have concern regarding the validity of a deep tracheal suction specimen, for fear that the culture will only demonstrate colonizing bacteria rather than a true pathogen.

If this technique proves to be reproducible and valuable on further study, it would enhance management by identifying the offending organisms and the antibiotics to which they are susceptible. On the other hand, there are still those who believe that the whole problem of ventilator-associated pneumonia is overrated and that the major impact on mortality arises from the patient's underlying disease.

R.A. Balk, M.D.

A Survey of Emergency Airway Management in the United Kingdom
Ratnayake B, Langford RM (St Bartholomew's Hosp, London)
Anaesthesia 51:908–911, 1996   4–61

Introduction.—Several techniques and protocols have been used to perform cricothyrotomy and transtracheal ventilation. A postal questionnaire was used to determine the availability of equipment for this procedure, experience with its use, and the prevalence of education for airway management.

Methods.—A postal survey was mailed to all tutors of the Royal College of Anesthesia in the United Kingdom and Northern Ireland. The tutors were questioned about their own or their colleagues' experience with cricothyrotomy, equipment used, availability of equipment for emergency airway management in various sites within the hospital, method of ventilation, complications, outcome, and resources for education and type of education.

Results.—Of 263 hospitals to which the questionnaire was mailed, 197 (74.9%) responded. Emergency airway equipment was present in 60%, 90%, 89.4%, and 87.1%, respectively, of general operating theater sites;

ear, nose, and throat theaters; obstetric theaters; and accident/emergency theaters. Of departments that responded, 57% had had experience with cricothyrotomy. The rate at which equipment was used was as follows: 58.6% Portex Minitrach, 8.5% William-Cook, 1.5% Shirley, and 1.5% Rapitrach. The most commonly improvised cricothyrotomy device used was the 14-G IV cannula. The complication rate for the Portex-Minitrach device was 65%. Over half the complications were serious; they represented 17.1% total failure to cannulate, 20.7% multiple attempts to cannulate, 8.5% pneumothorax, and 7.3% severe bleeding. The major complication rate for the William-Cook device was 27.3%; for the 14-G IV cannula, it was 22.2%.

Of attempted cannulations, 75% of patients eventually achieved successful airway management with full recovery. Of the remaining patients, 9.6% had partial recovery and 15.4% died. Of responding anesthetic departments, 14.2% had formal emergency airway management education, 73.6% had informal education, and 12% had no education.

Conclusion.—Cricothyrotomy is valuable and emergency equipment should be readily available in anesthetic and resuscitation areas. This technique is associated with a high complication rate that may be improved with proper education and equipment.

▶ This article bolsters the stance that an essential part of emergency airway management is the ability to appropriately establish a surgical entrance to the airway. The cricothyroidotomy is universally considered the preferred emergency entrance procedure and a number of "devices" have been developed to supposedly facilitate the procedure. This article clearly demonstrates that training in the use of these devices is essential.

B.A. Shapiro, M.D.

Comparison of A-mode Ultrasound and Computed Tomography: Detection of Secretion in Maxillary and Frontal Sinuses in Ventilated Patients
Lucchin F, Minicuci N, Ravasi MA, et al (Ospedale Civile de Rovigo, Italy; Univ of Padova, Italy; Gen Hosp, Rovigo, Italy; et al)
Intensive Care Med 22:1265–1268, 1996   4–62

Background.—Paranasal sinusitis in critically ill, intubated patients receiving mechanical ventilation is a serious infection that may result in sepsis. The diagnosis of paranasal sinusitis is based on results of the culture of purulent matter from sinus cavities and is supported by technical images of sinus secretions. Computed tomography gives good definition of sinus cavity contents, even when only axial slides are used. It would be useful to have a diagnostic technique for detecting sinus secretion that overcomes the problems of transportation and mobility of patients admitted to the ICU.

Methods.—There were 50 consecutive critically ill patients in comas who were receiving mechanical ventilation and who needed cerebral CT

Continuous End-tidal Carbon Dioxide Monitoring During Normofrequent Jet-ventilation

Bach LF, Wanner-Olsen H, Andersen BN, et al (Viborg Hosp, Denmark)
Acta Anaesthesiol Scand 40:1238–1241, 1996   4–64

Background.—The close correlation between end-tidal and arterial partial pressures of PCO_2 in patients and animals receiving spontaneous or mechanical ventilation and anesthetization is well known. It is also recognized that end-tidal and arterial PCO_2 do not correlate during high-frequency jet-ventilation because of the slow response time of carbon dioxide analyzers and the small tidal volumes delivered during high-frequency jet-ventilation. There is less information about low-frequency or normal frequency jet-ventilation, but it has been assumed that if the end-tidal–arterial carbon dioxide gradient is tidal-volume dependent, no differences should be seen among normal frequency jet-ventilation, intermittent positive pressure ventilation, or spontaneous breathing. However, Capan et al. detected significant gradients in dogs.

Methods.—Continuous end-tidal carbon dioxide measurements were compared with $PaCO_2$ measurements in 19 adult patients. The original air sampling line and the suction catheter were wrapped together with aluminum foil to make continuous monitoring of end-tidal carbon dioxide possible, then they were placed in the trachea 4–5 cm proximal to the carina.

Results.—The values for end-tidal carbon dioxide and $PaCO_2$ were paired for each patient. Pearson's product moment correlation was applied, and significant agreement ($r = 0.836$; $P < 0.001$) was found. This showed that the methods were closely correlated. The difference against the mean scatter diagram revealed a mean difference of 0.50 kPa and limits of agreement of–0.52–1.53 kPa. This confirmed that measurements of end-tidal carbon dioxide and $PaCO_2$ are equally valuable in monitoring healthy patients during normal frequency jet-ventilation.

Discussion.—A continuous method of monitoring end-tidal carbon dioxide in patients during normal frequency jet-ventilation and IV anesthesia administration is described. This technique is inexpensive because equipment already available is used. This method may be useful in patients with diseased lungs.

▶ The authors have devised and tested a means of monitoring end-tidal CO_2 concentrations during normal frequency jet-ventilation under general anesthesia. The method described appears to be useful and accurate in determining end-tidal CO_2 levels under stable intraoperative conditions. However, one must always be cognizant of the fact that this will likely not be the case in the face of hemodynamic instability or in patients with significant pathologic lung conditions. The authors' conclusion that end-tidal CO_2 monitoring by this method could supplant arterial CO_2 measurements in such patients must be interpreted cautiously because of the potential errors introduced by cardiopulmonary instability.

W.T. Peruzzi, M.D.

Accurate Measurement of Intrinsic Positive End-expiratory Pressure: How to Detect and Correct for Expiratory Muscle Activity
Zakynthinos SG, Vassilakopoulos T, Zakynthinos E, et al (Athens Univ, Greece)
Eur Respir J 10:522–529, 1997

4–65

Background.—It has recently been reported that expiratory muscle contraction during expiration increases end-expiratory alveolar pressure independently of dynamic hyperinflation. This results in overestimation of intrinsic positive end-expiratory pressure (PEEPi). When determining actual PEEPi produced by dynamic hyperinflation, it is unclear how much of this overestimation of PEEPi should be subtracted from measured PEEPi.

Methods.—There were 12 adult patients with acute respiratory failure. A comparison was made between PEEPi during spontaneous breathing using the end-expiratory airway occlusion technique (PEEPi,occl) and static PEEPi measured with end-expiratory airway occlusion during simulation of spontaneous breathing with the ventilator (PEEPi,st). The PEEPi,st was regarded as the gold standard for PEEPi,occl. Full mechanical ventilation was resumed when patients could not sustain spontaneous breathing. Spontaneous breathing was simulated by manipulating the variables of the ventilator. The PEEPi,st corresponding to PEEPi,occl was measured. Patients were divided into 2 groups according to the presence or absence of an expiratory rise in gastric pressure (*P*ga), a rapid decrease in end-expiratory *P*ga at the beginning of inspiration (*P*ga,exp,rise), and abdominal muscle electromyographic activity. Group 1 consisted of patients actively expiring, and group 2 consisted of patients passively expiring.

Results.—In group 1, PEEPi,occl was higher than PEEPi,st. PEEPi,occl – *P*ga,exp,rise and PEEPi,st were very similar; the mean difference was 0.03 cmH$_2$O, and limits of agreement were–0.48 to +0.53 cmH$_2$O. In group 2, PEEPi,occl and PEEPi,st were similar.

Discussion.—These findings show that, in patients who are breathing spontaneously and actively expiring, actual PEEPi,st can be determined by subtracting *P*ga,exp,rise from PEEPi,occl. In patients passively expiring, actual PEEPi,st can be accurately measured by the airway occlusion technique.

▶ The authors have demonstrated that active exhalation in patients receiving mechanical ventilator support can result in an erroneous estimation of intrinsic PEEP levels. In addition, they have devised guidelines to assist in more accurately estimating the intrinsic PEEP level in this circumstance. Because intrinsic PEEP levels may be significant in patients with severe lung disease who require mechanical ventilatory support, these data shed important light on how to better obtain this clinical information.

W.T. Peruzzi, M.D.

Estimation of Occlusion Pressure During Assisted Ventilation in Patients With Intrinsic PEEP

Conti G, Cinnella G, Barboni E, et al (Hôpital Henri Mondor, Creteil, France)
Am J Respir Crit Care Med 154:907–912, 1996   4–66

Introduction.—Determination of the occlusion pressure ($P_{0.1}$), although of potential usefulness as a predictor of successful weaning from ventilation in patients with chronic obstructive pulmonary disease (COPD), has required a maneuver with special equipment. An easier technique was proposed when a close correlation was found between $P_{0.1}$ assessed with the conventional occlusion technique and the magnitude of the inspiratory depression in the first 100 ms required to activate the inspiratory trigger mechanism. The validity of this proposed method was assessed in ventilated patients showing variable levels of intrinsic positive end-expiratory pressure.

Methods.—The first part of the study included 16 patients with COPD. Values of $P_{0.1}$ measured with the conventional technique were compared with those obtained during occlusion of the demand valve. The patients were studied during acute exacerbations caused by bronchopulmonary infections (13 patients) or by postoperative failure (3 patients). Seventeen additional patients, 11 with COPD and 6 with other diagnoses, participated in a comparison of the different slopes observed on the airway tracings and on the esophageal pressure tracing used to assess $P_{0.1}$.

Results.—Findings of the first part of the study indicated good agreement and a highly significant correlation between the 2 methods of measuring the airway occlusion pressure. In the second group of patients, results showed a good correlation and good agreement between respective data obtained from the airway and the esophageal pressure curves, taking into account the timing of both inspiratory muscle activation and of the demand valve system.

Discussion.—In patients with various levels of dynamic hyperinflation and intrinsic positive end-expiratory pressure, occlusion pressure can be easily and reliably estimated from airway pressure tracing during assisted breathing. The technique does not cause discomfort, and analysis of the airway pressure signal might be easily incorporated into ventilator monitoring software.

▶ The authors have looked at an indicator of inspiratory drive and how this indicator can be measured with reasonable reliability from airway pressure tracings during pressure support ventilation. This provides additional information that may assist in further assessment of patients' respiratory reserves during mechanical ventilatory support.

W.T. Peruzzi, M.D.

Comparison of the Effects of Heat and Moisture Exchangers and Heated Humidifiers on Ventilation and Gas Exchange During Weaning Trials From Mechanical Ventilation

Le Bourdellès G, Mier L, Fiquet B, et al (Hôpital Louis Mourier, Colombes, France; INSERM, Paris)
Chest 110:1294–1298, 1996   4–67

Background.—The use of heat and moisture exchangers (HME) to warm and humidify inspired gases in intubated patients receiving ventilatory support is increasing. However, these devices create dead space that may change the alveolar ventilation, which may impair the efficiency of spontaneous ventilation (SV) during weaning trials from mechanical ventilation. The effects of HMEs and heated humidifiers (HHs) on ventilation and gas exchange during weaning trials from mechanical ventilation were studied.

Methods.—Fifteen patients were assessed with an HME and HH used in random order during weaning trials in SV with inspiratory pressure support. The minute ventilation, tidal volume, and respiratory rate were recorded, and arterial blood was obtained for blood gas analysis.

Findings.—The HME was associated with a significantly greater minute ventilation than the HH, which reflected an increased respiratory rate. Tidal volume was unchanged for both devices. There was a greater $PaCO_2$ value with HME than with HH, which indicated an insufficient alveolar ventilation response to the increase in dead space. Arterial PO_2 increased with the HME, but was not significantly greater than the HH value, possibly because the HME had a positive end-expiratory pressure effect.

Conclusions.—The use of an HME may change the outcome of weaning trials, especially in very weak patients. The increase in minute ventilation resulting from the added dead space may result in an overload of respiratory work. Until additional research is completed, physicians should be aware that HMEs may be unsuitable for patients who are difficult to wean.

▶ Cost containment is a serious consideration in all health care environments today. It is, however, critical to also consider how less expensive devices may affect therapeutic outcomes. This study demonstrates the potential adverse effects of a less expensive system of airway humidification. Although this may not cause significant clinical problems in the majority of patients, some very marginal patients may have adverse outcomes. This study illustrates the need to be cognizant of these matters and the need to be vigilant in watching for them.

W.T. Peruzzi, M.D.

Significant Reduction in Minute Ventilation and Peak Inspiratory Pressures With Arteriovenous CO_2 Removal During Severe Respiratory Failure

Tao W, Brunston RL Jr, Bidani A, et al (Univ of Texas, Galveston; Shriners Burns Inst, Galveston, Tex)
Crit Care Med 25:689–695, 1997

4–68

Introduction.—About 150,000 patients in the United States are affected by adult respiratory distress syndrome, which is primarily treated by mechanical ventilation, a technique aimed at restoring normal blood gases. Mechanical ventilation, however, causes iatrogenic injury to the lungs, and survival may be improved by extracorporeal membrane oxygenation, a modified form of cardiopulmonary bypass, but the procedure is costly and complex. Using extracorporeal membrane oxygenation devices that do not depend on a pump simplifies the use and reduces the cost. A commercially available, low-resistance membrane oxygenator for extracorporeal CO_2 removal in sheep after severe smoke inhalation injury was used to evaluate the effect of such an arteriovenous gas exchange treatment on the reduction of ventilatory requirements during acute respiratory failure.

Methods.—There were 5 adult female sheep instrumented with femoral and pulmonary arterial catheters who had LD_{50} level cotton smoke inhalation injury via a tracheostomy under halothane anesthesia. The animals were systemically heparinized 24 hours after smoke inhalation injury for cannulation of the left carotid artery and common jugular vein to construct a simple arteriovenous shunt. Within the arteriovenous shunt, a membrane gas exchanger was interposed. At the time of complete recovery from anesthesia, blood flow produced by the arteriovenous pressure gradient was unrestricted. Measurements were taken of CO_2 removal by the gas exchanger. Stepwise 20% reductions in ventilator support were made hourly.

Results.—Over the 6-hour study period, the mean blood flow through the arteriovenous shunt ranged from 1,154 ± 82 mL/min (25% cardiac output) to 1,277 ± 38 mL/min (29% cardiac output). Across the gas exchanger, the pressure gradient was always less than 10 mm Hg. At 6 hours of arteriovenous CO_2 removal, maximum arteriovenous CO_2 removal was 102.0 ± 9.5 mL/min, allowing minute ventilation to be reduced from the baseline of 10.3 ± 1.4 L/min to 0.5 ± 0.0 L/min while maintaining normocapnia. There was also a decrease of peak inspiratory pressure from 40.8 ± 2.1 to 19.7 ± 7.5 cm H_2O). At maximally reduced ventilator support, partial pressure of arterial oxygen was maintained at more than 100 mm Hg. As a result of arteriovenous shunting, mean arterial pressure and cardiac output did not change significantly.

Conclusion.—Significant reduction in minute ventilation and peak inspiratory pressure, without hypercapnia or the complex circuitry and monitoring required for conventional extracorporeal membrane oxygenation, resulted with extracorporeal CO_2 removal using a low-resistance gas exchanger in a simple arteriovenous shunt. To minimize ventilator-induced barotrauma and volutrauma during severe respiratory failure, arteriove-nous CO_2 removal can be applied as an easy and cost-effective treatment.

▶ A primary goal of positive pressure ventilation is to facilitate CO_2 removal via the lungs. It stands to reason that when positive-pressure ventilation potentially threatens to initiate or facilitate lung injury, it may be advantageous to provide for CO_2 excretion via a corporeal system other than the lungs. Many approaches to extra-lung CO_2 excretion have been introduced in the past 30 years. Although most of these techniques successfully excrete CO_2, concerns regarding complications, expense, and lack of improved outcome data have prevented widespread acceptance. Extracorporeal approaches such as extracorporeal membrane oxygenation and extracorporeal CO_2 removal are being utilized clinically, but they are presently limited to specific patient populations and/or specific medical centers.

This study reports on the efficacy of CO_2 removal using a low-resistance arteriovenous gas exchange device. There must be clinical studies before this device can be considered simpler, safer, or more desirable than existing techniques.

B.A. Shapiro, M.D.

Cisapride Improves Gastric Emptying in Mechanically Ventilated, Critically Ill Patients: A Randomized, Double-blind Trial

Heyland DK, Tougas G, Cook DJ, et al (St Joseph's Hosp, Hamilton, Ont, Canada; McMaster Univ, Hamilton, Ont, Canada)
Am J Respir Crit Care Med 154:1678–1683, 1996   4–69

Objective.—Early enteral nutrition has several important benefits in critically ill patients. However, many clinicians wait until signs of bowel function occur before starting enteral feeding; this can result in delays of 3 to 7 days. Intolerance of enteral feeding by critically ill patients may be related to delayed gastric emptying. The effects of cisapride on gastric emptying in this patient population were evaluated.

Methods.—The study sample comprised 72 patients receiving mechanical ventilation who were expected to remain in the ICU for more than 48 hours. The patients' average age was 54 years; 39% were women. The patients' mean simplified acute physiology score was 9.5. Forty-seven percent were surgical patients, and 83% were receiving narcotics. On day 1, within 72 hours after ICU admission, all patients received 1.6 g of acetaminophen suspension via nasogastric tube. Gastric emptying was assessed by measuring plasma acetaminophen levels in blood samples taken 30 to 180 minutes later. On day 2, gastric emptying was measured again after administration of cisapride, 20 mg, or placebo. The maximal plasma concentration on day 2 was subtracted from the value on day 1 to assess the change in gastric emptying.

Results.—The day 2 minus day 1 maximal plasma concentration was 49 µmol/L in patients receiving cisapride vs. 12 µmol/L in those receiving

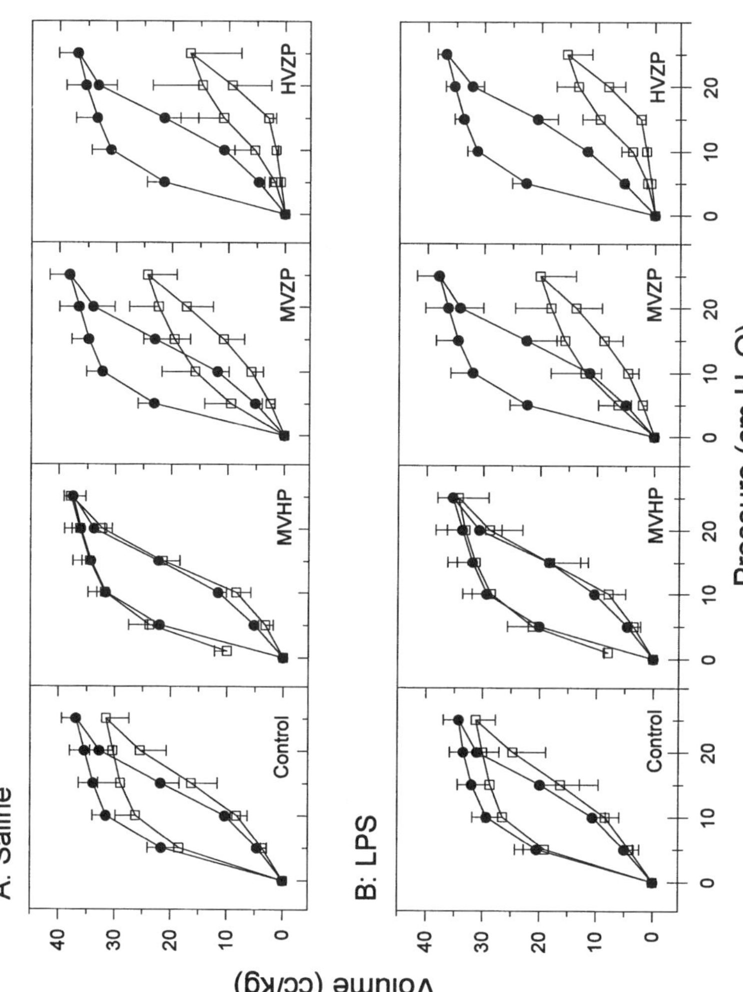

FIGURE 1.—Static compliance curves of the lungs prior to ex vivo ventilation (*black circles*) and after 2 hours of ex vivo ventilation (*open squares*). A significant rightward shift developed in both zero positive end-expiratory pressure (PEEP) groups (*P* less than 0.005 for moderate volume, zero PEEP [*MVZP*] and high volume, zero PEEP [*HVZP*], whereas no shift was observed in the presence of 10 cm of PEEP for either saline- or lipopolysaccharide-treated lungs. *MVHP* indicates moderate volume, high PEEP. (Reproduced from *The Journal of Clinical Investigation*, courtesy of Tremblay L, Valenza F, Ribeiro SP, et al: Injurious ventilatory strategies increase cytokines and *c-fos* m-RNA expression in an isolated rat lung model. *J Clin Invest* 99:944–952, 1997, by copyright permission of The Rockefeller University Press.)

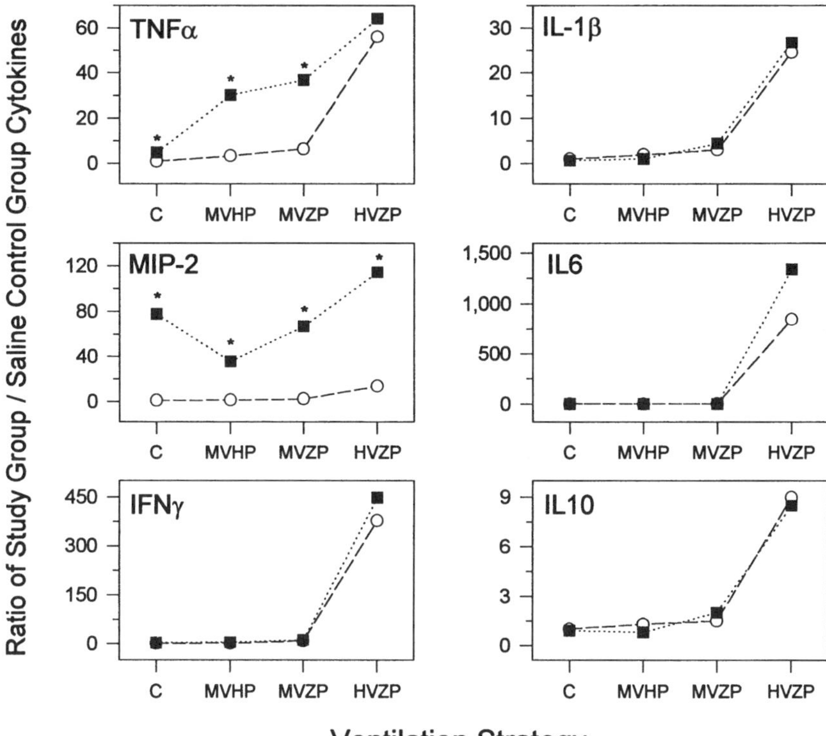

Ventilation Strategy

FIGURE 4.—Ratio of study group bronchoalveolar lavage cytokine concentrations relative to saline-treated controls. Lipopolysaccharide (*black squares*) pretreatment resulted in significantly increased levels of tumor necrosis factor–α for 3 of the ventilatory strategies (i.e., an approximately fivefold increase for controls, an approximately 30-fold increase for moderate volume, high positive end-expiratory pressure [PEEP] [*MVHP*], and an approximately 37-fold increase for moderate volume, zero PEEP [MVZP]), as compared with saline-treated controls (*open circles*). Lipopolysaccharide also increased levels of MIP-2 for all 4 ventilatory strategies, whereas no significant changes were seen with the other 4 cytokines assessed. As interleukin (*IL*)-6 and interferon-γ (*IFN*γ) were undetectable in saline-treated controls, an arbitrary value of 1 was assigned to allow comparison. *Asterisk* indicates *P* less than 0.05 vs. saline-treated group. *INF-α* indicates tumor necrosis factor–2; *MVHP*, moderate volume, high positive end-expiratory pressure; *MVZP*, moderate volume, zero positive end-expiratory pressure. (Reproduced from *The Journal of Clinical Investigation*, courtesy of Tremblay L, Valenza F, Ribeiro SP, et al: Injurious ventilatory strategies increase cytokines and c-*fos* m-RNA expression in an isolated rat lung model. *J Clin Invest* 99:944–952, 1997, by copyright permission of The Rockefeller University Press.)

described. The controls of lipopolysaccharide (LPS)-treated rats were ventilated using 4 different strategies of varying tidal volume (V_t) and positive end-expiratory pressure (PEEP):

1. V_t = 7 mL/kg, 3 PEEP (control)
2. V_t = 15 mL/kg, 10 PEEP (MVHP)
3. V_t = 15 mL/kg, zero PEEP (MVZP)
4. V_t = 40 mL/kg, zero PEEP (HVZP)

Measurements included lung compliance, lung lavage cytokines that are thought to be inflammatory (tumor necrosis factor–α [TNFα], IL-1β, IL-6, interferon-γ chemotactic (MIP-2), or anti-inflammatory (IL-10), serum cytokines (TNFα, IL-1β) and transcribed TNFα and c-*fos*. The last is thought to be a representative immediate-early response gene with a stretch responsive promoter. Static compliance curves were similar between controls and MVHP, both in vivo and ex vivo (Fig 1). Both groups without PEEP (MVZP and HVZP) showed significant reduction in compliance. These results were strikingly similar, regardless of whether or not the animals received LPS. Lung lavage cytokines were most elevated in the HVZP group, whether or not the animals received LPS. The LPS administration did result in increased lung lavage cytokine levels in all groups (Fig 4). High volume, zero pressure resulted in the highest messenger RNA c-*fos* levels, although all experimental groups had reduced transcription after administration of LPS.

If human responses are similar to rat responses, the clinical implications of this report are significant. First and foremost is the observation that mechanical ventilation can alter lung cytokine and gene expression. This may explain why patients with ARDS go on to have and die from multiple organ dysfunction syndrome (MODS). If this is true, then use of low-to-moderate tidal volumes coupled with some PEEP may prevent the overall clinical deterioration often seen in patients with ARDS. Cytokine biology remains complex and not completely understood. From the measurements made at one point in time in this study, it is not possible to generalize about either the progression of cytokine expression or the interactions between various mediators and host response. Nevertheless, this article adds to the growing concern that inappropriate mechanical ventilation, with either large tidal volumes, or now possibly zero PEEP, may be deleterious both to lung function and overall clinical condition.

M.R. Silver, M.D.

Reference

1. Bezzant TB, Mortesen JD: Risks and hazards of mechanical ventilation: A collective review of published literature. *Dis Mon* XL:581–640, 1994.

Chronic Obstructive Pulmonary Disease

Outcomes Following Acute Exacerbation of Severe Chronic Obstructive Lung Disease
Connors AF Jr, for the SUPPORT Investigators (Case Western Reserve Univ, Cleveland, Ohio)
Am J Respir Crit Care Med 154:959–967, 1996   4–71

Background.—The mortality rate associated with chronic obstructive pulmonary disease (COPD), a leading cause of death in the United States, is increasing. However, there is relatively little information on the long-term outcomes of patients hospitalized with an acute exacerbation of COPD. Such outcomes were investigated and the relationship between patient characteristics and length of survival determined.

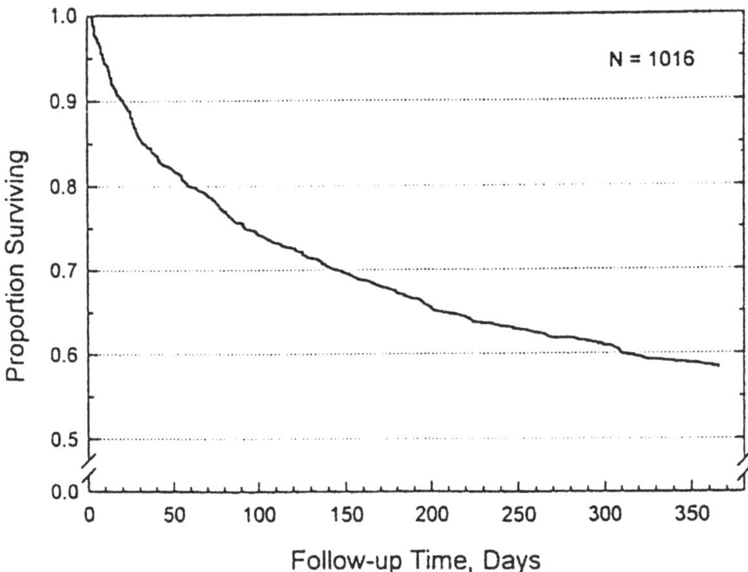

FIGURE 1.—One-year survival for 1,016 patients with severe acute exacerbation of chronic obstructive pulmonary disease. The Kaplan-Meier survival estimates over the 365 days after study entry are shown. Although moderate hospital mortality (11%) was seen, there was considerable mortality in the months after the index admission. (Courtesy of Connors AF Jr, for the SUPPORT Investigators: Outcomes following acute exacerbation of severe chronic obstructive lung disease. *Am J Respir Crit Care Med* 154:959–967, 1996. Official Journal of the American Thoracic Society. Copyright 1996 American Lung Association.)

Methods and Outcomes.—A cohort of 1,016 adults admitted to a total of 5 hospitals with an exacerbation of COPD and a partial pressure of arterial carbon dioxide (Pa$_{CO_2}$) of 50 mm Hg or more was studied prospectively. Although only 11% of the patients died in the hospital, the mortality rates were 20% at 60 days, 33% at 180 days, 43% at 1 year, and 49% at 2 years. The median length of the index hospitalization was 9 days, with a median cost of $7,000. In the 6 months after discharge, 446 patients were readmitted a total of 754 times. At 6 months, only 26% were alive and had good-to-excellent quality of life. Illness severity, body mass index, age, prior functional status, partial pressure of arterial oxygen/fraction of inspired oxygen, congestive heart failure, serum albumin, and the presence of cor pulmonale were independently associated with survival time (Fig 1).

Conclusion.—Hospital admission for exacerbation of COPD with a Pa$_{CO_2}$ of 50 mm Hg or more is associated with a moderate risk of death in the hospital, but a substantial risk of death in the months thereafter. Readily available clinical information can be used to predict the probability of survival.

▶ The authors of this substudy of the Study to Understand Prognoses and Preferences for Outcomes and Risks of Treatment trial evaluated 1,016 adult patients hospitalized for an acute exacerbation of COPD with a Paco$_2$ of 50 mmHg or more, and found that the mortality rate was 11% during the index admission. During the subsequent follow-up, it was observed that the mortality rate increased from 20% at 60 days to 49% after 2 years. In addition, at 6 months only 26% of the patients were found to be alive and having a good, very good, or excellent quality of life. The clinical parameters that appeared to be related to survival included severity of illness, body mass index, age, prior functional status, partial pressure of arterial oxygen/fraction of inspired oxygen, congestive heart failure, serum albumin, and the presence of cor pulmonale.

These data highlight the dramatic impact the onset of acute respiratory failure has on patients with COPD. Although their ability to survive the index hospitalization appears to be high, the outlook for long-term survival and, importantly, survival with a good-to-excellent quality of life, is much less frequent. This information should be used by physicians to counsel patients with hypercapnic respiratory failure so that they can get their affairs in order and begin to make end-of-life decisions.

R.A. Balk, M.D.

Small Airway Closure and Positive End-expiratory Pressure in Mechanically Ventilated Patients With Chronic Obstructive Pulmonary Disease
Guerin C, LeMasson S, de Varax R, et al (Centre Hospitalier Lyon-Sud, Pierre-Bénite, France; McGill Univ, Montréal)
Am J Respir Crit Care Med 155:1949–1956, 1997   4–72

Introduction.—There may be some benefit to administering positive end-expiratory pressure (PEEP) to patients with chronic obstructive pulmonary disease (COPD) with acute respiratory failure and expiratory flow limitation. Small airway closure is often present during tidal breathing in the supine position in patients with (COPD), leading to decreased lung compliance and impaired gas exchange. In a group of patients with (COPD) and acute respiratory failure, the effects of (PEEP) on small airway closure and recruitment of atelectatic alveoli were assessed.

Methods.—In 10 supine, sedated, and paralyzed patients with (COPD) and acute respiratory failure, the effects of (PEEP) on alveolar recruitment and closing volume were studied. Positive end-expiratory pressure was applied at 0, 5, 10, and 15 cm H_2O. Inflation static volume-pressure curves were constructed.

Results.—No recruitment of previously atelectatic lung units occurred with PEEP, after the static volume-pressure curves obtained at different PEEP levels were superimposed on each other. An inflection point was exhibited by the static volume-pressure curves, which should reflect the critical pressure required to reopen all closed airways. The opening volume is reflected by the corresponding lung volume. Lung volume was 0.71 L above the relaxation volume of the respiratory system, on average. Dynamic hyperinflation was exhibited by all patients. The end-expiratory lung volume was 0.54 L above the respiratory system with zero PEEP.

However, there was cyclic reopening and closing of small airways with each breathing cycle, as a result of the end-expiratory lung volume on the zero PEEP was below lung volume in 7 patients. This was accompanied by mechanical stresses on the peripheral airways that may lead to low-volume barotrauma. By increasing the end-expiratory lung volume to lung volume by means of PEEP, such barotrauma may be prevented.

Conclusions.—There are no atelectatic lung units that can be recruited with PEEP in supine mechanically ventilated patients with COPD. To prevent opening and collapse of some small airways, which could lead to lung injury, the end-expiratory lung volume should be increased to lung volume by adjusting PEEP.

▶ This very interesting study evaluated 10 patients with COPD and acute respiratory failure to assess whether there was evidence of dynamic hyperinflation from the generation of intrinsic PEEP. The study also evaluated whether there was evidence of alveolar and small airway collapse during the expiratory cycle. The repetitive opening and closing of these small airways and alveoli could result in the production of barotrauma, or possibly even acute lung injury. The authors found that at zero PEEP, there was evidence of increased airways resistance and pulmonary compliance that was associated with the development of intrinsic PEEP, and there was no evidence of atelectasis, but actually close-to-normal lung volume. During the assessment of the pressure-volume curves used to establish whether recruitment was taking place, it was noted that there was evidence to support successive opening and closing of lung units until there was approximately 15 cm H_2O of PEEP applied.

The results of this trial would support the judicious use of PEEP in the management of COPD patients who are receiving ventilatory support. There must be careful dosing of the PEEP and continuous monitoring of the effect to avoid worsening gas exchange, producing barotrauma, or creating adverse hemodynamic effects.

R.A. Balk, M.D.

Controlled Expiration in Mechanically-ventilated Patients With Chronic Obstructive Pulmonary Disease (COPD)

Aerts JGJV, van den Berg B, Bogaard JM (Erasmus Univ, Rotterdam, The Netherlands)

Eur Respir J 10:550–556, 1997   4–73

Background.—In patients with severe chronic obstructive pulmonary disease (COPD), flow limitation can affect lung emptying. It has long been suspected, but never verified, that controlling expiratory flow can counteract airway compression leading to flow limitation. This study evaluated the effects of an external resistor on lung emptying in mechanically ventilated patients with COPD.

Methods.—The study included 6 patients on mechanical ventilation for acute respiratory failure caused by an exacerbation of their COPD. With the patients sedated and paralyzed, the effects of an external resistor—a carousel with holes of different sizes attached to the expiratory outlet of the ventilator—were assessed. The effects of the resistor on respiratory mechanics were analyzed. The interruptor method was used to detect airway compression and to compute isovolume pressure-flow curves. The study used a turbulent resistor at the highest resistance level that did not increase end-expiratory lung volume. In all patients, this level of resistance generated external positive end-expiratory pressure (PEEP).

Results.—During controlled expiration, total PEEP levels were unchanged at both settings. However, intrinsic PEEP levels dropped significantly, from 0.96 to 0.53 kPa. On analysis of expiratory flow-volume curves, flows were significantly reduced during the first 40% of the expired volume and increased during the last 60%. There was no change in end-expiratory lung volumes during either setting, so the flow increases reflected a reduction in effective resistance. The interruptor method showed airway compression during unresisted expiration in all patients. However, airway compression became undetectable once the resistor was applied.

Conclusions.—External resistance to expiration may reduce effective expiratory resistance in patients with COPD receiving ventilatory support. The resistor counteracts airway compression without increasing end-expiratory lung volume. This study did not demonstrate any effects on gas exchange; more research is needed.

▶ In the early 1970s, mechanical ventilators had an expiratory retard valve, the purpose of which was to limit exhalation in patients with COPD. Like many new dials and buttons on ventilators, things are added because they can be done and not because there are data supporting a specific need or usefulness. Sometimes when things are added but not needed, people find uses for which they were not intended. For instance, playing with the expiratory retard valve resulted in the discovery of PEEP and its ability to improve oxygenation in patients with ARDS. This article provides data showing that the use of an expiratory retard valve can decrease expiratory resistance by counteracting airway compression without causing an increase in end-expiratory lung volume. Look for the next generation of mechanical ventilators to have an expiratory retard valve.

L.C. Casey, M.D., Ph.D.

Miscellaneous

Treatment of Refractory Acute Allograft Rejection With Aerosolized Cyclosporine in Lung Transplant Recipients

Keenan RJ, Iacono A, Dauber JH, et al (Univ of Pittsburgh, Pa; State Univ of New York, Stony Brook)
J Thorac Cardiovasc Surg 113:335–341, 1997   4–74

Background.—If acute rejection is not controlled in lung transplant recipients, they inevitably develop organ failure. Despite the use of cyclosporine and tacrolimus, azathioprine, and prednisone, 75% of lung transplant patients still develop acute rejection. These authors evaluated whether aerosolized cyclosporine (which delivers a high concentration of drug to the lung tissues) could improve acute cellular rejection when traditional immunosuppressive therapies were unsuccessful.

Methods.—Single-lung (n = 10) or double-lung (n = 8) transplant recipients with acute rejection (≥ grade 2 rejection) were enrolled. These 18 patients were treated with aerosolized cyclosporine (300 mg/day) in addition to standard triple-drug immunosuppressive regimens. Results of therapy were measured by transbronchial biopsy 4 weeks after the start of aerosolized cyclosporine and at regular intervals thereafter. The historical control group consisted of 23 lung transplant recipients with acute refractory rejection who were treated before the advent of aerosolized cyclosporine.

Findings.—Of the 18 patients, 2 could not tolerate the aerosolized cyclosporine because of airway hyperresponsiveness and were dropped from the study. Of the remaining 16 patients, in 14 (88%) aerosolized cyclosporine maximally or completely resolved the histologic inflammation associated with acute rejection. In the other 2, pulmonary function improved, but histologic changes after aerosolized cyclosporine were null or minimal. Histologic rejection improved with treatment time. In fact, in 5 of the patients in whom removal of aerosolized cyclosporine was attempted, 4 redeveloped cellular rejection. Compared with controls, patients receiving aerosolized cyclosporine had significant improvements in forced vital capacity and forced expiratory volume. Renal function was not significantly changed by the addition of aerosolized cyclosporine to the baseline triple-drug immunosuppressive regimen.

Conclusions.—In 14 of 18 lung transplant recipients with acute rejection refractory to traditional immunosuppressive therapies, the addition of aerosolized cyclosporine successfully improved both histologic and clinical measures of rejection. The main limitation to its use was airway irritation. Although further study is needed, the increased effectiveness of aerosolized cyclosporine in delivering the drug to target tissues may enable a reduction in the doses of oral immunosuppressive drugs, which could reduce the risk of systemic toxicity.

▶ Despite the use of prednisone, azathioprine, cyclosporine, or tacrolimus, acute rejection affects as many as 75% of patients after lung transplantation. Although increased steroid or cytotoxic therapy is used, it is not always effective. Persistent acute rejection is the preeminent risk for chronic rejection or death in the first year after transplantation.[1] These investigators explored the feasibility and outcome of aerosolized cyclosporine in lung transplant recipients with acute rejection. Although it is not a randomized, placebo-controlled, blinded study, the results are quite encouraging. Sixteen patients with acute rejection ($\geq$ A2) were selected to receive 300 mg of cyclosporine per day as a single treatment through a jet nebulizer after the drug was dissolved in propylene glycol. Patients were premedicated with 5 ml of 2% lidocaine delivered by nebulizer. Therapy was continued on a 3 times per week schedule, once the patient was discharged.

Of the 16 patients, only 2 were unable to tolerate the therapy secondary to cough and mucosal irritation. In patients receiving oral tacrolimus, cyclosporine levels ranged from 140 to 419 ng/mL 60 minutes after treatment. Trough levels 24 hours later ranged from 0 to 37 ng/mL. There were no changes in renal or hepatic function observed with the addition of inhaled cyclosporine. Recognizing that aerosol deposition will not be uniform, aerosolized cyclosporine significantly reduced the incidence of acute histologic rejection nearly fourfold. If confirmed by a randomized study, this could be a significant addition to the regimen for treatment of refractory acute rejection.

M.R. Silver, M.D.

Reference

1. Kesten S, Maidenberg A, Winto T, et al: Treatment of presumed and proven acute rejection following six months of lung transplant survival. *Am J Respir Crit Care Med* 152:1321–1324, 1995.

5 Trauma and Burns

Trauma

Incremental Benefit of Individual American College of Surgeons Trauma Triage Criteria

Henry MC, Hollander JE, Alicandro JM, et al (State Univ of New York, Stony Brook)
Acad Emerg Med 3:992–1000, 1996   5–1

Purpose.—The American College of Surgeons (ACS) trauma triage criteria are intended to identify patients who need specialized trauma care in spite of appearing initially well. However, the addition of mechanism criteria to physiologic and anatomic criteria may lead motor vehicle crash (MVC) victims without serious injuries to be triaged to trauma centers. This study examined the incremental benefit of individual ACS trauma triage criteria to the prediction of severe injuries in MVC victims.

Methods.—The prospective, cross-sectional study included 1,545 MVC victims transported to 1 of 12 hospitals in a suburban/rural county. Structured instruments were used to collect data on demographics and individual ACS criteria. Information on patient disposition was collected from the ED. Study outcomes included admission, operative interventions (OR), major nonorthopedic operative interventions or death (Maj-OR), and injury severity score (ISS). Receiver operating characteristic curve analysis was performed to optimize the sensitivity and specificity of out-of-hospital triage decision rules.

Results.—Thirteen percent of the MVC victims were admitted, 6% had OR, 1% had Maj-OR, and 3% had an ISS of 16 or greater. The physiologic and anatomic criteria were the most useful in predicting all outcomes. Specificity was considerably reduced by certain additional criteria—such as crash speed, vehicle deformity, and axle displacement—without improving sensitivity. The optimal ROC curve for Maj-OR—with a sensitivity of 85% and specificity of 87%—was determined by systolic blood pressure of less than 90 mm Hg, Glasgow Coma Scale score less than 13, respiratory rate less than 10 or greater than 29, death of a same-car occupant, penetrating injury, and an opposite-side compartment intrusion of 24 inches or greater. Factors predicting an ISS of 16 or greater—with a sensitivity of 86% and specificity of 70%—were GCS score of less than 13, respiratory rate of less than 10 or greater than 29, penetrating injury, 2 proximal long bone fractures, flail chest, opposite-side compartment intrusion of 24 inches or greater, patient ejection, rollover, and age less than 5 or greater than 55 years.

Conclusions.—In the evaluation of MVC victims, physiologic and anatomic criteria can be used to predict high levels of hospital resource utilization and severe injury. The addition of mechanism criteria may lower specificity with little or no improvement in sensitivity. Crash speed and extent of vehicle deformity are of particularly little predictive value.

▶ This is a rather large study of over 1,500 trauma patients, 13% of whom were admitted. The results of this study showed the superiority of physiological and anatomical criteria in determining acuity and outcome. The crash information seemed to provide little value, with the exception of the death of a same car occupant and ≥ 24-inch opposite-side compartment intrusion. In general, scoring systems do need to be tested on separate populations. This type of study does serve an important role in evaluating prognostic models in critically ill patients.

J.E. Calvin, Jr., M.D.

J.E. Parrillo, M.D.

Posttraumatic Multiple-organ Dysfunction Syndrome: Role of Mediators in Systemic Inflammation and Subsequent Organ Failure
Pastores SM, Thakkar A, Gennis P, et al (Montefiore Med Ctr, Bronx, NY; Bronx Municipal Hosp Ctr, NY; Albert Einstein College of Medicine, Bronx, NY)
Acad Emerg Med 3:611–622, 1996   5–2

Objective.—Despite the best emergency department (ED) treatment, some trauma victims die days or weeks later from multiple-organ dysfunction syndrome (MODS). Because strategies in preventing and treating MODS may one day begin in the ED, emergency physicians need to become familiar with the biology, pathophysiology, and clinical features of MODS.

Clinical Overview of MODS in Trauma Patients.—Deaths from trauma occur immediately, within hours, or days or weeks later as a result of MODS and/or sepsis. Sepsis is an example of systemic inflammatory response syndrome (SIRS), of which MODS is a complication. Trauma can lead to primary MODS as a result of the insult, or to secondary MODS as a result of SIRS.

Pathogenesis and Pathophysiology of Postinjury MODS.—MODS can develop with or without the presence of infection as a result of massive injury that produces SIRS. This SIRS evolves into MODS, or a lesser injury that leads to a lesser grade SIRS and a delayed infection precipitating late MODS.

Other Modes of Injury.—Excessive production of cytokines TNF-α, IL-1, IL-6, IL-8, and IFN-γ, resulting from injury, are associated with development of MODS. Reactive oxygen-derived metabolites are free radicals that can damage cells, cell membranes, nucleic acids, proteins, and enzymes. Eicosanoids, oxidation products of arachidonic acids, can lead to the production of inflammatory prostaglandins. Platelet activating factor (PAF) can enhance the damaging effects of cytokines. Enhanced production of nitric oxide during hemorrhagic shock decreases blood pressure.

Patterns of Mediator Release in Trauma.—Indications are that measurement of cytokine levels in tissue compartments may relate more to biologic activity than measurement of circulating concentrations.

Antimediator Therapies for SIRS/MODS.—Advances include anticytokine, antineutrophil, and antioxidant therapies; and eicosanoid synthesis inhibitors and receptor antagonists, therapies against PAF, NOS inhibitors, and immunomodulatory therapies.

Conclusion.—Advances in understanding and moderating or modulating cellular and molecular mechanisms at work in the development of MODS may lead to new and earlier therapeutic interventions to prevent and treat MODS.

▶ This article is a nice review of some of the current beliefs surrounding the pro-inflammatory mediators that are felt to be, at least in part, responsible for the development of multiple organ dysfunction/failure that complicates trauma and other serious injuries. There is also a brief review of some of the therapeutic strategies that have been evaluated as potential therapies for this uncontrolled inflammatory response. Current opinion is now suggesting that there is likely a disturbance in the normal balance between the pro-inflammatory and the compensatory anti-inflammatory response that eventually results in the complications of trauma and SIRS, namely, recurrent sepsis and multiple organ dysfunction/failure.[1] Proof of this hypothesis is needed, and we hope further refinements in our knowledge and understanding of this complex physiologic process will be coming in the next several years.

R.A. Balk, M.D.

Reference

1. Bone RC, Grodzin CJ, Balk RA: Sepsis: A new hypothesis for pathogenesis of the disease process. *Chest* 112:235–243, 1997.

Normal Values of SvO$_2$ as Therapeutic Goal in Patients With Multiple Injuries
Kremžar B, Špec-Marn A, Kompan L, et al (Univ Med Centre, Zalöska, Slovenia)
Intensive Care Med 23:65–70, 1997   5–3

Introduction.—The traditional treatment for patients with multiple injuries has included above normal levels of oxygen delivery. The effect of maintaining normal levels of venous oxygen saturation (SvO$_2$) on the survival of 40 patients with multiple injuries was evaluated to determine whether this approach is more relevant to survival than maintaining above-normal levels of oxygen transport.

Methods.—Patients were assigned to 1 of 2 groups. Normal SvO_2 was maintained in 23 patients by manipulation of oxygen transport variables (group A). Oxygen delivery was increased if SvO_2 diminished or the dobutamine test was positive. In group B (17 patients), oxygen delivery (DO_2) was maintained at above-normal levels by aggressive use of fluids and dobutamine. The oxygen transport–related variables and lactate concentrations were recorded every 12 hours in the first 5 days after injury for all patients.

Results.—Survival was significantly better and multiple organ failure was significantly lower in group A than group B. The average group A DO_2 was significantly lower than that of group B at day 2 and thereafter. To maintain normal SvO_2 and aerobic metabolism in group A, patients required average values of DO_2 of 605–688 mL/min/m². Ten group A patients needed dobutamine 2.5–5 µg/kg/min. In group B, the average DO_2 was 622 mL/min/m₂ on day 1, increasing to 835 mL/min/m₂ by day 5 after injury.

Conclusion.—Optimal oxygen uptake is better achieved by maintaining normal SvO_2 values and increasing DO_2 only when needed, compared with maintaining above-normal DO_2. The former approach may be more relevant than the latter approach for survival of patients with multiple injuries. It is important that the optimal DO_2 be defined for each patient.

▶ This nonrandomized, retrospective control study contributes no new information to the debate regarding above normal oxygen delivery. Although this debate will undoubtedly continue for years to come, rather convincing evidence has come forth in the last 3 years that casts a dubious shadow on this concept. Perhaps selected patients may benefit, but some recent evidence suggests that forcing supernormal levels of oxygen delivery may negatively impact outcome in some patient populations.

B.A. Shapiro, M.D.

Missed Injuries in a Rural Area Trauma Center

Robertson R, Mattox R, Collins T, et al (Univ of Arkansas, Little Rock)
Am J Surg 172:564–568, 1996

5–4

Background.—In rural areas, victims of trauma are often seen in multiple hospitals before reaching a trauma center. Studied were missed injuries in patients treated in rural community hospitals before trauma center care, and in patients injured in urban areas and taken directly to a trauma center.

Methods.—Data were obtained on 3,996 patients treated at level 1 trauma centers between January 1993 and June 1995. Missed injuries were defined as those not detected in the first 24 hours after trauma.

Findings.—A total of 70 missed injuries were identified in 56 patients. Compared with patients in whom injuries were not missed, those with missed injuries had experienced more blunt trauma, were injured more severely, had longer stays in ICUs and in the hospital, and a lower mortality. Sixty percent of the missed injuries occurred in patients who had been transferred.

Conclusions.—The risk for missed injuries is greatest in transferred patients with blunt injuries. Delayed transports and the previous performance of examinations may contribute to missed injuries. All patients with trauma must be assessed thoroughly and repeatedly. In addition, diagnostic studies must be reviewed for adequacy.

▶ Patients are commonly transferred from 1 center to an another because of a lack of medical facilities or subspecialities or for financial reasons. The authors did the study to identify injuries that were not found within 24 hours of the trauma and compared them with those of the typical patient with trauma. They found that unidentified injuries occurred 70 times in 56 of the total 3,996 patients. Sixty percent of the missed injuries were in transferred patients. The take-home messages from this study include ensuring good communication between the referring and receiving physicians, obtaining original studies whenever possible instead of just reports, and requiring the receiving physician to obtain a thorough history and perform a physical examination on all patients.

J. Samuel, M.D.

Burns

Bioactive Substance Accumulation and Septic Complications in a Burn Trauma Patient: Effect of Perioperative Blood Transfusion?
Nielsen HJ, Reimert CM, Dybkjur E, et al (Natl Univ, Hvidovre Univ, Denmark; Copenhagen)
Burns 23:59–63, 1997   5–5

Introduction.—The risk of postoperative infectious complications is increased with perioperative transfusion of homologous blood. Posttransfusion morbidity and mortality may be related to acute and delayed adverse transfusion reactions to whole blood, leukocyte-depleted blood, and platelet and plasma products. The development of adverse effects may be related to blood storage time. It is still unknown what the potential clinical effects of bioactive substances in blood transfusion products are. The clinical effects of accumulation of various substances in a burn trauma patient, in relation to the content of the substances in the transfused products, were evaluated during transplantation.

Methods.—A 2-step transplantation operation was performed on a patient with 40% second- and third-degree burn trauma. Before, during, and after the operation, samples for analysis of histamine, eosinophil cationic protein, eosinophil protein X, neutrophil myeloperoxidase, and interleukin-6 were drawn. Samples were also drawn from transfused red cells,

infection. This is not the preferred approach for most settings, but it may be effective if the outbreak does not respond to less intrusive measures.

▶ A rapid outbreak of methicillin-resistant MRSA in a university hospital burn unit. Using pulsed-field gel electrophoresis, the infection control team was able to identify the likely reservoir of the outbreak, which, not surprisingly, turned out to be a house officer and a nurse. Measures to control outbreaks of MRSA in the intensive care unit continue to be a source of debate among epidemiologists. This article presents a review of the recommendations that physician directors and nurse coordinators will want to become familiar with.

C. Franklin, M.D.

Burn Resuscitation: Crystalloid Versus Colloid Versus Hypertonic Saline Hyperoncotic Colloid in Sheep
Guha SC, Kinsky MP, Button B, et al (Univ of Texas, Galveston)
Crit Care Med 24:1849–1857, 1996   5–7

Background.—The value of early colloid use in burn victims has not been definitively established. It was hypothesized that initial and early use of a colloid or hyperosmotic colloid decreases fluid requirements and edema.

Methods.—Eighteen female sheep were studied in the blinded, controlled study. The sheep were scalded and treated by 1 of the following 3 regimens: (1) lactated Ringer's solution, (2) hetastarch, and (3) hypertonic saline dextran. Ten mL per kg was infused 30 minutes after injury, at a rate sufficient enough to restore and maintain the baseline oxygen delivery values.

Findings.—Scalding caused an initial 30% decline in cardiac output, a 20% decrease in mean arterial pressure, and a 10% to 15% increase in hematocrit. All the solutions restored and maintained baseline oxygen delivery within 1 hour, but hetastarch and hypertonic saline dextran decreased the net fluid volume by 48% and 74%, respectively, over 8 hours, compared with lactated Ringer's solution. Treatment did not affect burn wound edema. Hypertonic saline dextran decreased edema in nonburned skin, compared with lactated Ringer's solution and hypertonic saline dextran. The hetastarch and hypertonic saline dextran groups had significantly higher plasma colloid osmotic pressures. The lactated Ringer's solution and hetastarch groups had a continuous decline in plasma sodium concentrations from baseline values over 8 hours. Plasma sodium levels were increased at 4 hours in the hypertonic saline dextran group, but normalized within 8 hours.

Conclusions.—Initial resuscitation of large body surface area burn injury with a colloid can markedly decrease net volume loading. Further reductions can be achieved by using hypertonic saline colloid. Hyponatremia occurred in the isotonic crystalloid- and colloid-treated sheep, but not in sheep given hypertonic saline colloid.

▶ Short-term infusion of hypertonic dextran and hetastarch reduced the volume necessary for fluid resuscitation in burns without increasing wound edema. Further studies are needed to confirm this finding and to demonstrate the safety and efficacy of these solutions.

Y. Friedman, M.D.

Resuscitation of Thermally Injured Patients With Oxygen Transport Criteria as Goals of Therapy

Barton RG, Saffle JR, Morris SE, et al (Univ of Utah, Salt Lake City)
J Burn Care Rehabil 18:1–9, 1997   5–8

Purpose.—For patients with burns, the key to successful treatment is adequate resuscitation from burn shock. Burn resuscitation has generally been based on the end points of adequate blood pressure and urine output. In trauma and surgical patients, shock resuscitation is often based on oxygen transport criteria. This approach has been little used in burn patients. This preliminary study examines the oxygen transport characteristics of burn resuscitation.

Methods.—The study included 9 adult burn patients, 6 with inhalation injuries. The patients' mean age was 33 years, and their mean burn size was 45% of total body surface area. In each patient, oxygen transport criteria were used to guide resuscitation. Hemodynamic and oxygen transport parameters were measured hourly for 6 hours by the Fick method, using pulmonary artery balloon flotation catheters. Fluid resuscitation was initially calculated by the Parkland formula. In addition, fluid boluses were given to reach a pulmonary artery wedge pressure of 15 mm Hg, at which point dobutamine infusions of 5 µg/kg/min were started.

Results.—Resuscitation was associated with a rise in cardiac index (from 2.5 to 6.6 L/min/m^2) and a fall in systemic vascular resistance (from 1,534 to 584 dyne sec/cm^5). Oxygen delivery increased from 573 to 1,028 mL/min/m^2 and oxygen consumption from 132 to 172 mL/min/m^2. At oxygen delivery levels of less than 800 mL/min/m^2, oxygen consumption was dependent on oxygen delivery. Fluid resuscitation was significantly greater than predicted by the Parkland formula: approximately 23,000 mL vs. 14,000 mL over the initial 24 hours.

Conclusion.—As in patients with other causes of shock, volume loading and inotropic support restore depressed cardiovascular function in patients with burns. At least at oxygen delivery levels of less than 800 mL/kg/min, oxygen consumption in burn patients is dependent on oxygen delivery; it remains to be seen whether oxygen consumption can be made independent of oxygen delivery. More fluid is needed when oxygen transport criteria serve as the basis of resuscitation. The effects of this method of resuscitation on morbidity, survival, and other outcomes require further study.

▶ This study actually compares volume resuscitation according to a fixed calculation method (the Parkland formula) with volume resuscitation by hemodynamic measurements. Not surprisingly, the resuscitation was better with hemodynamic end points.

I have the impression that the authors were rather surprised that cardiac output increased with volume loading, even when pulmonary artery wedge pressure stayed relatively stable. They convincingly showed that empiric formulas for volume resuscitation in critically ill patients are not as effective as using hemodynamic end points. Welcome to the fold!

B.A Shapiro, M.D.

Predicting Mortality in Adult Burned Patients: Methodological Aspects of the Construction and Validation of a Composite Ratio Scale
Coste J, Wasserman D, Venot A (Hôpital Cochin, Paris)
J Clin Epidemiol 10:1125–1131, 1996   5–9

Background.—Approximately 15% of patients with severe burns die despite being provided aggressive and expensive medical care. A severity index, which would predict mortality risk, is needed for intelligent selection of treatment options based upon likely patient outcome. Previous attempts at developing predictive models of outcome for patients with severe burns have not maintained their predictive power when applied to populations other than those used for construction of the model. These models have also simply categorized patients into high- and low-risk groups rather than providing specific risk estimates for individual patients. The development of a continuous model of mortality risk in burn patients and the validation of the model in additional populations were described.

Methods.—Data pertaining to demography, injury, and outcome were collected prospectively for 708 victims of severe burns, aged 15 years or older, seeking treatment at the Cochin Hospital Burn Center in Paris between 1987 and 1992 (the training population). Similar data sets were collected, for validation of the statistical model, for burn victims treated at the same institution from 1993 to 1994, and for burn victims treated in all burn centers in France, except for Cochin from January to December, 1990.

Results.—The mortality rate among the training population was 8.5%. Survivors were younger than nonsurvivors (40.0 vs. 61.1 years), had a lower percentage of total body surface area burned (TBSA) (17.4% vs. 48.0%), and had a lower percentage of full-thickness body surface area burned (5.3% vs. 29.0%). Inhalation injury and patient sex did not differ between the 2 groups. The statistical model most predictive of mortality, for the training group ($R^2 = 0.95$) and validated by the 2 additional patient cohorts ($R^2 = 0.945$ and 0.954), involved a logistic transformation of a score, calculated as follows: 2 × (Age − 50) + TBSA, if the patient was

An outstanding resource for your nursing colleagues!

Yes! Begin my one-year subscription to *Heart and Lung®: The Journal of Acute and Critical Care* (6 issues).

Name ___________________________________

Institution _______________________________

Address __________________________________

City ____________________________ State _______

ZIP/PC __________ Country ________________

Specialty ________________________________
(Students, please list Institution)

Subscription prices (through 9/30/98)

		USA	Canada*	Int'l
Individuals	❑	$45.00	$69.55	$65.00
Institutions	❑	144.00	175.48	164.00
Students (full-time)	❑	24.00	47.08	44.00

Method of payment

Enclose payment (check or credit card number) and we'll send an extra issue FREE!

❑ **Check** (in U.S. dollars, drawn on a U.S. bank, and payable to *Heart and Lung®: The Journal of Acute and Critical Care*)

❑ VISA ❑ MasterCard ❑ Discover

❑ AmEx ❑ Bill me Exp. date__________

Card #_____________________________________

Signature _________________________________

*Includes Canadian GST

Individual/student subscriptions must be in the name of, billed to, and paid for by the individual.

Canada/Int'l prices include airmail postage.
Prices subject to change without notice.

J002983YA

Reservation Card for the Year Book

Yes! I would like my own copy of *Year Book of Critical Care Medicine®* at the price of **$78.00** plus sales tax, postage, and handling. Please begin my subscription with the current edition according to the terms described below.* I understand that I will have 30 days to examine each annual edition.

Name ____________________________________

Address __________________________________

City ________________________________ State __________ ZIP ____________

Method of Payment

Check (in U.S. dollars, drawn on a U.S. bank, payable to *Year Book of Critical Care Medicine®*)

❑ VISA ❑ MasterCard ❑ Discover ❑ AmEx ❑ Bill me

Card number ____________________________ Exp. date: __________

Signature _________________________________

Prices are subject to change without notice.

PMC-009

---

*Your Year Book service guarantee:

When you subscribe to the *Year Book*, you will receive advance notice of future annual volumes about two months before publication. To receive the new edition, you need do nothing—we'll send you the new volume as soon as it is available. If you want to discontinue, the advance notice allows you time to notify us of your decision. If you are not completely satisfied, you have 30 days to return any *Year Book*.

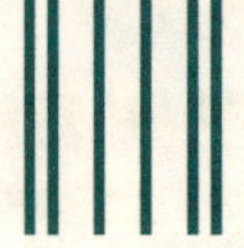

BUSINESS REPLY MAIL

FIRST-CLASS MAIL   PERMIT NO 135   ST LOUIS MO

POSTAGE WILL BE PAID BY ADDRESSEE

SUBSCRIPTION SERVICES
MOSBY–YEAR BOOK, INC.
11830 WESTLINE INDUSTRIAL DRIVE
ST. LOUIS   MO 63146-9988

BUSINESS REPLY MAIL

FIRST-CLASS MAIL   PERMIT NO 135   ST LOUIS MO

POSTAGE WILL BE PAID BY ADDRESSEE

M Mosby

PAT NEWMAN
11830 WESTLINE INDUSTRIAL DRIVE
PO BOX 46908
ST. LOUIS   MO 63146-9934

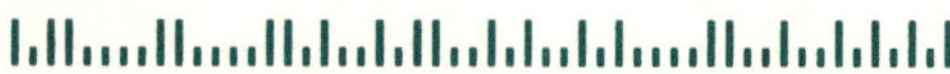

Want to speed up the process?

**To order the *Year Book*,
you also may call 1-800-426-4545**

**To subscribe to the journal today,
call toll-free in the U.S.:
1-800-453-4351
or fax 314-432-1158**

Outside the U.S., call: 314-453-4351

Visit us at:
www.mosby.com/Mosby/Periodicals

Mosby–Year Book, Inc.
Subscription Services
11830 Westline Industrial Drive
St. Louis, MO   63146 U.S.A.

M Mosby

older than 50 years. For patients younger than 50 years, the score was equal to TBSA. A nomogram for converting score to probability of death was constructed to allow ready and rapid use of the model.

Conclusions.—This composite measurement score is easily used and reproducible, has good predictive ability, and a high logistic ratio level, and has been validated using 2 patient populations in addition to that used in model construction. Persuading physicians to use this model, rather than more traditional indices, may be the most challenging task remaining.

▶ The simplicity of the data used in constructing the composite measurement scale (CMS) is very attractive. The CMS may be helpful as a guide to assessing severity, assuming the user applies the caveat of applying a general statistic to an individual patient. More extensive validation is needed before the scale is used on a widespread basis.

Y. Friedman, M.D.

Plasma Levels of Endothelin-1 and Thrombomodulin in Burn Patients
Nakae H, Endo S, Inada K, et al (Iwate Med Univ, Morioka, Japan; Iwate Life Science Inst, Morioka, Japan)
Burns 22:594–597, 1996   5–10

Background.—Endothelin-1 is a vasoconstrictive peptide that was detected as a secretion product of swine vascular endothelial cells and that has various other biological functions. Thrombomodulin is a protein found in vascular endothelial cell membranes. It is a thrombin receptor that has antithrombotic effects when activated. Vascular endothelial cells are stimulated by endotoxins and cytokines to produce endothelin-1 and thrombomodulin. Higher blood levels of endothelin-1 and thrombomodulin occur in patients with disseminated intravascular coagulation. Studies have previously reported a correlation between endotoxin, tumor necrosis factor-α (TNF-α), and the pathologic condition of patients with burn injuries. The relation of endothelin-1 and thrombomodulin to the severity of the burns and TNF-α is addressed.

Methods.—In 23 adult patients with burn injuries on 20% or more of their bodies, plasma levels of endothelin-1 and thrombomodulin were measured. The relation between these levels and the severity of the burns was examined. The relation of TNF-α to endothelin-1 and thrombomodulin was also examined.

Results.—A radioimmunoassay and an enzyme-linked immunosorbent showed that levels of endothelin-1 and thrombomodulin were significantly higher in patients who had sepsis than in those who did not (Figs 1 and 2). These levels were also significantly higher in patients who died than in those who survived. There was a significant correlation between maximum plasma endothelin-1 and maximum thrombomodulin and the Acute Physiology and Chronic Health Evaluation II score. Plasma levels of TNF-α

Methods.—Blood levels of TNF-α, IL-6, and IL-8 were determined immediately after the accidents in 24 adult patients with burn injuries. The relationship between these cytokines and infection and outcome was analyzed.

Results.—Almost no significant elevation of cytokine levels was seen in the early phase of the burn injury. Throughout the course of the injury, there were high levels of TNF-α, IL-6, and IL-8 in patients with burn injuries associated with sepsis and in patients who died.

Discussion.—In these patients with burn injuries, the levels of cytokines TNF-α, IL-6, and IL-8 reflected the severity of morbidity. This indicates that these cytokines form a complex network involved in the formation of the morbid condition.

▶ Yamada and co-workers measured the blood levels of several cytokines in patients with burn injuries immediately after the burn incidents and related blood levels of these cytokines to the morbid conditions that ensued. They found that, although cytokines could be measured after the initial burn, the levels of TNF-α, IL-6, and IL-8 were much higher in patients who had sepsis as compared with those who did not have sepsis. Thus, although showing that TNF-α, IL-6, and IL-8 reflect the severity of the burn injury when complicated by sepsis, the study does not deal with issues concerning treatment of these patients.

R.V. Rege, M.D.

Early Complications and Value of Initial Clinical and Paraclinical Observations in Victims of Smoke Inhalation Without Burns
Hantson P, Butera R, Clemessy J-L, et al (Université Paris VII; Service Médical d' Urgence de la Brigade des Sapeurs-Pompiers de Paris)
Chest 111:671–675, 1997   5–12

Background.—Smoke inhalation causes early respiratory injury and late complications, as well as secondary complications from infection. Toxic gases and soot deposits may directly injure upper and lower airways and lung parenchyma. Most studies of such complications from smoke inhalation have been of patients with extensive burns.

Methods.—In a retrospective study, the medical records of 64 patients admitted to the ICU with smoke inhalation were reviewed. Patients with cutaneous burns, multiple trauma, blast injury, or cardiac arrest were excluded. The mean patient age was 47 years.

Results.—Patients spent a mean of 5.8 days in the ICU. Two patients died from progressive respiratory failure. The mean stay in the ICU was longer for patients who had soot deposits in the oropharynx, dysphonia, or rhonchi at first examination; patients with a positive sputum bacteriologic analysis; and patients needing parenteral bronchodilator agents for more than 24 hours. Mechanical ventilation was required in 35 patients for a mean of 101.2 hours. Patients who initially had rhonchi, high carbon monoxide levels (but not cyanide levels), or a positive bacteriologic sample tended to require longer mechanical ventilation. A positive bacteriologic sample correlated with the presence of dysphonia or rhonchi and immediate intubation. No correlation was shown with chest radiographs.

Discussion.—In this retrospective study of patients subjected to smoke inhalation without burns, respiratory injury was common. Results of the initial examination revealed that patients with initial dysphonia or rhonchi will need longer mechanical ventilation or longer stays in the ICU, and this may be associated with a positive sputum bacteriologic analysis. Patients with altered mental status from carbon monoxide intoxication will have similar complications. Aspiration frequently results in lung injury in such patients.

▶ Smoke inhalation without skin burns presents a clinical challenge as to the timing of tracheal intubation and mechanical ventilation. This retrospective study essentially shows that when these patients are seen initially with dysphonia and/or ronchi, they require intubation. When initial sputum cultures are positive, there will probably be a more prolonged course of mechanical ventilation. No new information here, but a useful review of the clinical tenets of care for patients with smoke inhalation.

B.A. Shapiro, M.D.

The Value of Early Enteral Nutrition in the Prophylaxis of Stress Ulceration in the Severely Burned Patient
Raff T, Germann G, Hartmann B (Burn Centre, Ludwigshafen, Germany)
Burns 23:313–318, 1997   5–13

Objective.—Burn patients are at risk of gastroduodenal ulcers and gastrointestinal bleeding (GIB). Medical prophylaxis against these ulcers is considered mandatory for burn patients. The prophylactic value of enteral feeding is uncertain, however. The effects of medicinal stress ulcer prophylaxis were compared with those of early intragastric feeding for the prevention of GIB in burn patients.

Methods.—The analysis included 425 patients treated in a burn ICU during a 4-year period. During the first part of the experience, all patients received ulcer prophylaxis with cimetidine, 400 mg IV. Antacids were given through a nasogastric tube if the intragastric pH fell to less than 3.5. During the second part of the experience, early enteral nutrition was used as the only form of ulcer protection; no additional prophylaxis was given. Throughout the experience, patients were monitored for overt signs of upper GIB. The ability of the 2 approaches to prevent GIB was assessed.

Results.—About 8% of patients had upper GIB with medicinal prophylaxis, with serious GIB occurring in 2%. The overall incidence of upper GIB in the group receiving enteral nutrition was 3%, with a serious bleeding rate of less than 1%. The difference in overall GIB rate was significant. No patient in either group died as a direct result of upper GIB.

Conclusions.—In burn patients, early enteral nutrition effectively prevents upper GIB. They do not require cimetidine or other forms of medicinal prophylaxis. The cost-effectiveness and mechanism of early enteral feeding remain to be determined.

▶ The benefits of enteral nutrition support in the critically ill patient may take a number of forms. Some advocate that enteral nutrition will prevent malnutrition from occurring during the catabolic period of critical illness. Others claim that enteral nutrition will prevent the translocation of bacteria and endotoxin from the terminal ileum and colon, which may be instrumental in the development of multiple organ dysfunction or failure. This study assessed the use of enteral nutrition, in comparison with the use of cimetidine with or without antacid in the prevention of stress-related GI hemorrhage in patients with severe burns.

Burns are a well-known risk factor for the complication of stress-related GIB. In this study, none of the deaths were related to bleeding from gastric ulcers. The use of enteral nutrition was associated with a significantly reduced rate of overt GIB, in comparison with the use of cimetidine. There was also less sepsis and multiorgan failure in the patients with upper GIB enteral nutrition.

Unfortunately, the authors did not assess the incidence of nosocomial pneumonias related to the use of cimetidine and antacid, in comparison with enteral nutrition. However, at least from the standpoint of GIB, the use of enteral nutrition appears to have multiple benefits in patients with severe burns.

R.A. Balk, M.D.

6 Infectious Disease

Prevention of Central Venous Catheter–related Bloodstream Infection by Use of an Antiseptic-impregnated Catheter: A Randomized, Controlled Trial
Maki DG, Stolz SM, Wheeler S, et al (Univ of Wisconsin, Madison)
Ann Intern Med 127:257–266, 1997   6–1

Introduction.—Nearly all vascular catheter–related bloodstream infections are related to the use of noncuffed central venous catheters. Preventive strategies include potent cutaneous antiseptic agents, topical application of antimicrobial agents, and attachment of a subcutaneous silver-impregnated cuff. A new antiseptic venous catheter was evaluated in a randomized, controlled clinical trial.

Methods.—The study was conducted in a medical-surgical ICU. Patients scheduled to have a catheter placed were randomly assigned to receive a control catheter or an antiseptic catheter. Test and control catheters were identical (noncuffed, triple-lumen, 30.5-cm, and 16-G), except that the test catheter's external surface was impregnated with minute quantities of chlorhexidine gluconate (0.75 mg) and silver sulfadiazine (0.70 mg). All catheters were examined for colonization and catheter-related bloodstream infection at removal, and patient tolerance of the catheter was recorded. In the case of infection, all potential sources were cultured and findings confirmed by restriction-fragment DNA subtyping.

Complete data were obtained for 403 catheters (195 control and 208 antiseptic) in 158 patients. Most patients in each group were highly vulnerable to nosocomial infection because of their medical conditions and multiple invasive medical devices. Catheters remained in place for an average of 6 days in each group.

Findings.—Compared with control catheters, antiseptic catheters were less likely to be colonized at removal (relative risk, 0.56) and fivefold less likely to produce bloodstream infection (relative risk, 0.21). Eight patients in the control group, but none in the antiseptic group, had bloodstream infection caused by *Staphylococcus aureus,* gram-negative bacilli, enterococci, or *Candida* species. There was a highly significant difference in the cumulative risk for catheter-related bloodstream infection in the 2 groups (Fig 1). The antiseptic catheter was not associated with any adverse effects.

Conclusion.—The antiseptic catheter was well tolerated, prevented catheter colonization, and reduced the incidence of bloodstream infection.

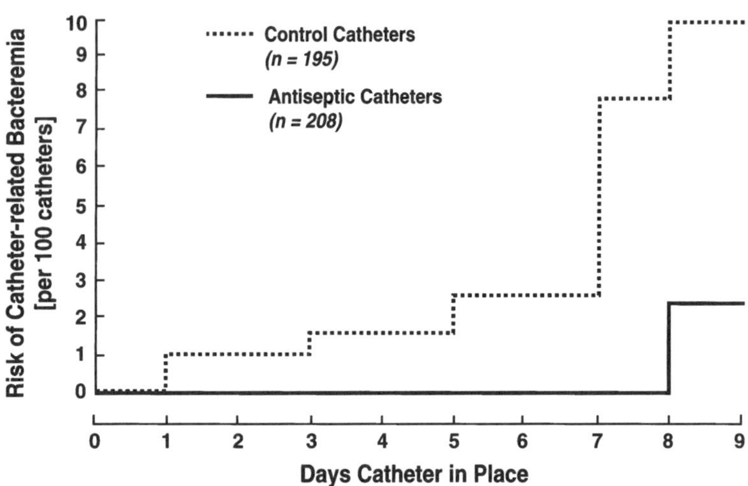

FIGURE 1.—Kaplan-Meier estimate of the cumulative risk for catheter-related bloodstream infection. The differences between groups are highly significant ($P = 0.01$, log-rank test). (Courtesy of Maki DG, Stolz SM, Wheeler S, et al: Prevention of central venous catheter–related bloodstream infection by use of an antiseptic-impregnated catheter: A randomized, controlled trial. *Ann Intern Med* 127:257–266, 1997.)

Because nosocomial bloodstream infections are associated with high mortality, prolonged hospitalization, and additional cost (approximately $29,000), the antiseptic catheter should also prove cost effective.

Central Venous Catheters Coated With Minocycline and Rifampin for the Prevention of Catheter-related Colonization and Bloodstream Infections: A Randomized, Double-blind Trial
Raad I, and The Texas Med Ctr Catheter Study Group (Univ of Texas, Houston)
Ann Intern Med 127:267–274, 1997   6–2

Introduction.—Central venous catheters are the leading cause of primary nosocomial bloodstream infection. Topical application of antiseptic and antibiotic agents at the insertion site can lower the risk for catheter colonization and infection, but a more effective strategy might be the coating of venous catheters with these agents. A multicenter clinical trial compared the incidence of catheter-related colonization and bloodstream infections with coated and noncoated central venous catheters.

Methods.—Study participants were 281 hospitalized patients at 5 university-based medical centers. The coated catheters were pretreated with tridodecylmethyl-ammonium chloride, then coated 18 hours later with minocycline and rifampin. Both coated and uncoated catheters were triple-lumen, polyurethane, 7F, and 20 cm long. All were inserted into the subclavian, internal jugular, or femoral vein, and were not exchanged over guidewires. Insertion sites were cleaned with an antiseptic agent at the time

TABLE 3.—Frequency and Microbiological Cause of Catheter Colonization and Bloodstream Infections

Variable	Uncoated Cultured Catheters ($n = 136$)	Coated Cultured Catheters (fv;2n = 130)	P Value
Catheter colonization, n (%)*	36 (26)	11 (8)	<0.001
Staphylococcus epidermidis	16 (12)	2 (2)	<0.001
Other coagulase-negative staphylococci	3 (2)	0	0.01
S. aureus	1 (1)	0	>0.2
Gram-negative bacilli	3 (2)	2 (2)	>0.2
Candida albicans	1 (1)	3 (2)	>0.2
C. tropicalis	0	1 (1)	>0.2
Polymicrobial	12 (9)	3 (2)	>0.02
Catheter-related bloodstream infections, n (%)†	7 (5)	0	<0.01
Infections confirmed by DNA typing, n (%)†	5 (4)	0	0.02
Infections/1000 catheter-days, n‡	7.34	0	<0.01
Infections confirmed by DNA typing/ 1000 catheter-days, n‡	5.16	0	0.03

*Catheter colonization was defined as the isolation of at least 15 colony-forming units of any organism by the roll-plate method or at least 10^3 colony-forming units by the sonication method. The Fisher exact test was used to compare the 2 groups. Relative risk for colonization for uncoated catheters was 3.13 (95% confidence interval, 1.66 to 5.88).

†Exact log-rank test was used; relative risks were undefined.

‡Binomial exact test was used.

(Courtesy of Raad I, and the Texas Med Ctr Catheter Study: Central venous catheters coated with minocycline and rifampin for the prevention of catheter-related colonization and bloodstream infections: A randomized, double-blind trial. *Ann Intern Med* 127:267–274, 1997.)

of insertion and at each dressing change. Sites were inspected every 72 hours. Catheter segments were cultured at the time of removal; skin samples from the insertion site were cultured at insertion and within 24 hours after catheter removal.

Results.—Patients in the 2 catheter groups were similar in age, sex, underlying diseases, degree of immunosuppression, therapeutic interventions, and risk factors for catheter infections. The incidence of colonization was significantly lower in coated catheters (8%) than in uncoated catheters (26%). Seven patients in the uncoated catheter group, but none in the coated catheter group, had catheter-related bloodstream infections (Table 3). Rates of these infections were 7.34 for uncoated vs. 0 for coated catheters (per 1,000 catheter-days). Coating central venous catheters with minocycline and rifampin was an independent protective factor against catheter-related colonization. These catheters caused no adverse effects, nor were they associated with antimicrobial resistance. Because of the high cost of treating colonization and bloodstream infections, the coated catheters could lead to significant savings.

Conclusion.—The venous catheters coated with minocycline and rifampin decreased the risk for colonization and infection without causing

sepsis was defined as sepsis abating following catheter removal per 1,000 catheter-days.

Results.—In the chlorhexidine group, the rate of significant catheter colonization and catheter-related sepsis was significantly lower. In the chlorhexidine group, the rate of central venous catheter colonization and central venous catheter-related sepsis per 1,000 catheter-related days were also significantly lower. In the chlorhexidine group, the rate of arterial catheter colonization per 1,000 catheter-days was also significant lower; however, the rate of arterial catheter-related sepsis per 1,000 catheter-days was similar for the antiseptic groups. In preventing gram-positive bacteria, the chlorhexidine solution was superior to the povidone iodine solution, but in preventing gram-negative infections, the chlorhexidine solution was nonsignificantly superior to the povidone iodine solution.

Conclusion.—For insertion-site care of short-term central venous and arterial catheters, the 4% alcohol-based solution of 0.25% chlorhexidine gluconate and 0.025% benzalkonium chloride was more effective than the 10% povidone iodine solution. The chlorhexidine gluconate solution was more effective with gram-positive bacteria than with gram-negative bacteria.

▶ This is a well-designed study with blinding of the laboratory personnel who processed all the cultures . The authors' conclusion of the superiority of a combination solution of chlorhexidine gluconate and benzalkonium chloride is well supported by the data. Their findings are quite relevant to all who care for central venous or arterial lines.

J.E. Calvin, Jr., M.D.

J.E. Parrillo, M.D.

Antimicrobial Resistance in Isolates From Inpatients and Outpatients in the United States: Increasing Importance of the Intensive Care Unit
Archibald L, Phillips L, Monnet D, et al (Natl Ctr for Infectious Disease, Atlanta, Ga; Emory Univ, Atlanta, Ga)
Clin Infect Dis 24:211–215, 1997   6–5

Background.—The emergence of antimicrobial-resistant pathogens has represented a significant challenge in the control of infectious diseases, particularly in a hospital setting. Although antimicrobial resistance is generally more prevalent in hospitals than in the community, the magnitude of the problem in the 2 populations, particularly among patients in the ICU, has not been clarified. A clear understanding of antimicrobial resistance in these populations is needed to prioritize and appropriately focus control measures in hospitals. Antimicrobial resistance was determined for bacterial isolates from both inpatients and outpatients from 8 American hospitals, in this study, to compare the prevalence of resistance between hospital- and community-acquired infections.

TABLE 1.—Resistance to Specific Antimicrobials in Isolates From Inpatients vs. Outpatients for Sentinel Antimicrobial-Pathogen Combinations

Antimicrobial/pathogen combination	No. of resistant isolates/total no. of isolates tested (%)		P value
	Inpatients	Outpatients	
Methicillin/coagulase-negative *Staphylococcus*	922/1,881 (49.0)	250/697 (35.9)	<.01
Methicillin/*Staphylococcus aureus*	861/2,633 (32.7)	233/1,594 (14.6)	<.01
Ceftazidime/*Enterobacter cloacae*	145/559 (26.0)	15/126 (11.9)	<.01
Imipenem/*Pseudomonas aeruginosa**	164/1,368 (12.0)	31/477 (6.5)	<.01
Ceftazidime/*P. aeruginosa*	147/1,889 (7.8)	26/63 (4.0)	<.01
Vancomycin/*Enterococcus* species	92/1,459 (6.3)	8/575 (1.4)	<.01
Ciprofloxacin/*Escherichia coli*	16/3,189 (0.5)	28/3,997 (0.7)	NS
Ceftazidime/*E. coli*	5/2,348 (0.2)	9/1,887 (0.5)	NS

*Two hospitals not included.
Abbreviation: NS, not significant.

(Courtesy of Archibald L, Phillips L, Monnet D, et al: Antimicrobial resistance in isolates from inpatients and outpatients in the United States: Increasing importance of the intensive care unit. *Clin Infect Dis* 24:211–215, 1997. Published by the University of Chicago. © 1997 by The University of Chicago. All rights reserved.)

Methods.—Resistance patterns were determined for bacteria isolated from patients at 8 hospitals in the United States between 1994 and 1995. Comparisons were made among patient populations using 8 antimicrobial–pathogen combinations (Table 1), based on their clinical relevance.

Results.—The prevalence of antimicrobial resistance was significantly greater in inpatients than it was in outpatients for all antimicrobial–pathogen combinations, except ceftazidime–*Escherichia coli* and ciprofloxacin–*E. coli* (Table 1). When the inpatient population was subdivided, the percentage of isolates resistant to antimicrobials was significantly greater in ICU patients than it was in other inpatients for each antimicrobial–pathogen combination initially identified as more prevalent in the hospital, with the exception of imipenem/*Pseudomonas aeruginosa*. There was a stepwise decrease in resistance rates, from ICU patients, to non-ICU patients, to outpatients, for all six antimicrobial/pathogen combinations.

Conclusions.—The rate of antimicrobial resistance in nosocomial pathogens appears to be significantly greater for inpatients than it is for outpatients, and greater in ICU patients than in non-ICU inpatients. These data lend further support to the presumption that emphasis should continue to be placed on the hospital, particularly the ICU, in efforts to control antimicrobial resistance in pathogens.

▶ Many clinicians are concerned about increasing antibiotic resistance to available antimicrobial agents. Emergence of *Streptococcus pneumoniae* penicillin resistance, *Enterococcus* species vancomycin resistance, and recent reports of vancomycin-resistant *Staphylococcus aureus* affect all physicians, regardless of their specialty or practice location. This report analyzes data from the National Nosocomial Infections Surveillance system, which is the only national information source of hospital-acquired infections and their patterns of resistance. The authors document that antimicrobial resistance is a problem in all locations, but that it is much more prevalent in ICUs. With the exception of *Escherichia coli* resistance to ciprofloxacin and ceftazidime, inpatient units were much more likely to have imipenem- or ceftazidime-resistant *Pseudomonas aeruginosa;* methicillin-resistant, coagulase-negative, gram-positive cocci or *S. aureus;* vancomycin-resistant *Enterococcus* species; or ceftazidime-resistant *Enterobacter cloacae.* Furthermore, resistance for most of these organisms was more common in ICUs than in general hospital beds. Interestingly, the percentage of resistance for methicillin-resistant *E. cloacae* was comparable between outpatients and general medical wards.

If these data can be generalized to other hospitals, then the emergence of resistance seems to be the greatest problem in the ICU. Strategies such as restricted formulary, protocol for empiric therapy as well as proven infections, and patient cohorting will be more likely to have a microbiological impact if targeted at ICU patients and physicians.

M.R. Silver, M.D.

Nosocomial Bacteremia in Critically Ill Patients: A Multicenter Study Evaluating Epidemiology and Prognosis
Vallés J, for the Spanish Collaborative Group for Infections in Intensive Care Units of Sociedad Española de Medicina Intensiva y Unidades Coronarias (SEMIUC) (Hosp de Sabadell, Barcelona; et al)
Clin Infect Dis 24:387–395, 1997   6–6

Background.—Nosocomial infections occur most often in ICUs, and they are associated with a high mortality rate. What factors specifically influence this mortality rate? These authors analyzed clinical, microbiological, and therapeutic variables to determine their impact on hospital-acquired infections in ICU patients.

Methods.—From 30 multidisciplinary center ICUs, 481 patients with 590 episodes of true bacteremia were studied (infection rate 3.6 per 100 admissions). Only those whose bacteremia occurred 72 hours or less after hospital admission were included to ensure that the infection was indeed acquired in the hospital. Univariate and multivariate analyses were performed to determine the relative contributions of various factors to the clinical course of these patients.

Findings.—Of the 481 patients, 200 died in the ICU (41.6% mortality rate), although death was directly related to the bacteremia in only 112 of the 590 episodes (19%). The most common causes of bacteremia were intravascular catheter infections (37.1%), lower respiratory tract infections (17.5%), and intra-abdominal infections (6.1%). Almost half of the infections were caused by gram-positive microorganisms, with about one third caused by gram-negative bacilli. The following factors were significantly associated with crude mortality in these patients: acute renal failure, an Acute Physiology and Chronic Health Evaluation (APACHE) II score of 15 or greater at diagnosis, chronic liver failure, mechanical ventilation, multiple organ failure, respiratory distress syndrome, and septic shock.

The following variables were independent predictors of directly related mortality: acute renal failure, gram-negative or candidal bacteremia, multiple organ failure, respiratory distress syndrome, septic shock, severe sepsis, and a source of infection other than the intravascular catheter.

Conclusions.—Bacterial sepsis in ICU patients with nosocomial infection is more often caused by gram-positive bacteria than by gram-negative ones. Typically, these bacteremias result from intravascular catheters and lower respiratory tract infections. Thus, bacteremia in the ICU could be reduced with close attention to intravascular catheters and nosocomial pneumonia. Furthermore, crude mortality was associated not only with the systemic response but also with the severity of the patient's underlying condition. Thus, in addition to the selection of an appropriate antibiotic, therapies directed at septic shock and its associated complications are important modifiable factors in these patients.

▶ Nosocomial bacterermias are a significant problem for ICU patients. The incidence of nosocomial infections in hospitalized patients is between 5% and 10%, with a disproportionate share of those occurring in ICU patients.[1] In this report of 590 nosocomial bacteremias in ICU patients, the incidence of bacteremia was 3.6 episodes per 100 admissions. The following factors increased mortality among patients with bacteremias: parenteral nutrition, mechanical ventilation, dialysis, previous surgery, previous shock, previous antibiotic therapy. Unfortunately, most ICU patients have several of these characteristics. Of the 481 first episodes of bacteremia, 36% (175 of 481) were definitely catheter related. There were another 32 cases (approximately 7%) of bacteremias with gram-positive cocci. Catheter colonization was not significant enough to be classified as definitely catheter related. Gram-positive cocci accounted for 41.9% of the isolates.

Three articles examining catheter related bacteremias recently appeared in the same journal.[2–4] In 2 studies,[2, 3] noncuffed catheters coated with either chlorhexidine-silver sulfadiazine or minocycline and rifampin reduced catheter colonization from 24% to 26% to 8% to 13.5%. Catheter-associated bacteremia was reduced fivefold to sevenfold in these studies. The other study[4] examined salvage rates in dual lumen dialysis catheters associated with bacteremia. In this study, antibiotic therapy without catheter removal was successful only 32% of the time. However, there were no significant complications associated with attempted catheter salvage.

In summary, ICU bacteremias are a result of indwelling central venous catheters nearly 50% of the time. Antibiotic-impregnated uncuffed catheters reduce the likelihood of bacteremia developing. Although these catheters are more expensive, given the frequency of catheter-related bacteremias, these catheters may actually be cost-effective.

M.R. Silver, M.D.

References

1. Jarvis WR, Edwards JR, Culver DH, et al: Nosocomial infection rates in adult and pediatric intensive care units in the United States: National Nosocomial Infection Surveillance System. *Am J Med* 91:185S–191S, 1991.
2. Maki DG, Stolz SM, Wheller S, et al: Prevention of central venous catheter-related bloodstream infection by use of an antiseptic-impregnated catheter. *Ann Intern Med* 127:257–266, 1997.
3. Raad I, Darouiche R, Dupuis J, et al: *Ann Intern Med* 127:267–274, 1997.
4. Marr KA, Sexton DJ, Conlon PJ, et al: Catheter-related bacteremia and outcome of attempted catheter salvage in patients undergoing hemodialysis. *Ann Intern Med* 127:275–280, 1997.

Nocardial Infections in Bone Marrow Transplant Recipients

Chouciño C, Goodman SA, Greer JP, et al (Vanderbilt Univ, Nashville, Tenn; Nashville Veterans Administration Hosp, Tenn)
Clin Infect Dis 23:1012–1019, 1996

6–7

Introduction.—In patients whose immune systems are compromised by lymphoreticular neoplasms, AIDS, autoimmune disorders, and immunosuppression associated with transplantation, *Nocardia* species—aerobic actinomycetes often found in decaying organic matter and natural soil—may cause opportunistic infections. Whereas the risk of nocardial disease in recipients of solid organ transplant is well known, after bone marrow transplantations, there have been only 4 patients reported. Six patients who had nocardial disease after bone marrow transplantation at 1 institution over a 14-year period were described.

Cases.—Each patient's records were examined for demographic, clinical, laboratory, and radiologic data. These were also compared with those of 4 patients found in a literature review. The patients ranged in age from 23 to 49 years. Underlying diseases included chronic myelogenous leukemia, acute myelogenous leukemia, non-Hodgkin's lymphoma, and aplastic anemia. Symptoms at presentation included headache, dry cough, fever, purulent sputum, abdominal pain, and toe swelling. Nine patients received allogeneic bone marrow transplants, and 1 was autologous. Immunosuppressive medications were given to all 10 patients; acute or chronic graft-vs.-host disease was associated with all but 1 allogeneic bone marrow transplant. Despite receiving prophylaxis with trimethoprim-sulfamethoxazole on an intermittent basis 2 to 3 times a week, 3 patients had nocardiosis.

Results.—Among autologous bone marrow transplant recipients, the rate of nocardial infection at this institution was 0.2%, and among allogeneic bone marrow transplant recipients, the rate was 1.7%. Death was more often caused by complications of graft-vs.-host disease and associated invasive infection with *Aspergillus* species than with nocardial infection. In this group, 70% of patients died.

Conclusion.—Nocardial infection is associated with a high rate of invasive fungal infection and is an important, although infrequent, complication of bone marrow transplantation. Infection cannot be reliably protected against with trimethoprim-sulfamethoxazole.

▶ This article reports on cases of nocardial infections in patients receiving bone marrow transplantation and reviews 4 cases from the literature. The fact that there have been only 4 reported cases of nocardial infection in bone marrow transplant recipients in the past 30 years, but this 1 center has had 6 cases in 14 years, makes one think that there is something unique about this center. This institution is providing the world's experience with an otherwise rare problem.

L.C. Casey, M.D., Ph.D.

Cerebrospinal Fluid Concentrations of Leukotriene B$_4$ in Bacterial Meningitis

Santer R, Sievers E, Schaub J (Univ of Kiel, Germany)
Acta Paediatr 85:902–905, 1996   6–8

Background.—Research has shown that interleukin (IL) 1β, tumor necrosis factor (TNF) ᾽α, and other mediators play a key role in the pathophysiology of bacterial meningitis. However, no one has reported on leukotriene B$_4$ (LTB$_4$) levels in cerebrospinal fluid (CSF). The presence of this potent polymorphonuclear leukocyte (PMN) mediator in the CSF of patients with bacterial meningitis was investigated.

Methods and Findings.—Nonpleocytic CSF from 5 children and CSF from 8 children with aseptic meningitis were analyzed. Concentrations of LTB$_4$ were less than the detection limit (less than 0.2 ng mL^{-1}) in these samples. In the 0–20 ng mL^{-1} range, the recovery rate of LTB$_4$, added to nonpleocytotic CSF, exceeded 90%. Seven CSF specimens with PMN counts exceeding 1000/mL were also analyzed. In 6 of these samples, LTB$_4$ was detectable at levels ranging from 0.35 to 3.3 ng mL^{-1}. Concentrations of LTB$_4$ and PMN were significantly correlated.

Conclusions.—Determining LTB$_4$ in CSF fluid apparantly does not provide useful diagnostic or clinical information in addition to that provided by neutrophil count. However, knowing such values may contribute to the understanding of the pathophysiology of bacterial meningitis. Further research in patients receiving and in those not receiving dexamethasone treatment is warranted.

▶ This article reports that LTB$_4$ is elevated in spinal fluid in patients with bacterial meningitis. Unfortunately, the levels of LTB$_4$ failed to provide any additional diagnostic or clinical information, compared with neutrophil count. If this work were to follow the path of sepsis and cytokines, clinical trials

Utilization and Diagnostic Yield of Blood Cultures in a Surgical Intensive Care Unit

Darby JM, Linden P, Pasculle W, et al (Univ of Pittsburgh, Pa)
Crit Care Med 25:989–994, 1997

6–11

Introduction.—Because of the associated high mortality rate, increased length of stay, and high costs, nosocomial bacteremias occurring in ICUs are of particular concern. The ICU case mix, the frequency of invasive device use, and length of stay are all factors that affect the rate of bacteremia. Because the true sensitivity of the blood culture test cannot be determined, the overall yield is relatively low, and the predictive value for true pathogens only approximates 50%, the value of blood cultures in patients suspected of bacteremia is questionable. In critically ill patients, the diagnostic yield of blood cultures has not been well studied. The use and diagnostic yield of blood cultures in a surgical ICU were determined. Factors potentially influencing their yield were examined.

Methods.—There were 206 patients who had a blood culture obtained during admission to a trauma/neurosurgical ICU in a 1-year period. Overall diagnostic yield was determined after blood culture isolates were categorized as pathogens or contaminants. Antimicrobial use data were also evaluated for all patients and their relationship to blood culture yield was analyzed.

Results.—In 4.6% of culture episodes, blood cultures were positive for pathogens, whereas in 5.5% of culture episodes, contaminants were isolated (Table 1). In 21 patients, a total of 23 true bacteremias were identified, producing an overall rate of bacteremia of 3.6 per 100 admissions. At the time of blood culture in 65.3% of all culture episodes, concurrent antibiotics were being used. When cultures were obtained when patients were receiving antibiotics, the yield for pathogens was significantly lower (2.2%) when compared with culture episodes obtained when patients were

TABLE 1.—Overall Culture Results

	Patients (N)	Culture Sets (N)	Culture Episodes (N)
Total	206	1106	635
Positive	52	83	64
	(25.2)	(7.5)	(10.1)
Pathogen	21	44	29
	(10.2)	(4.0)	(4.6)
Contaminants	31	39	35
	(15.0)	(3.5)	(5.5)
Contamination rate (%)	59.6	46.9	54.7

Note: Numbers in parentheses indicate percentages.
(Courtesy of Darby JM, Linden P, Pasculle W, et al: Utilization and diagnostic yield of blood cultures in a surgical intensive care unit. *Crit Care Med* 25(6):989–994, 1997.)

not receiving antibiotics (6.4%). In approximately 32% of all culturing episodes, single-set blood culture episodes were obtained, producing an overall yield for pathogens of these culturing episodes lower (2.9%) than that of multiple-set culture episodes (5.3%).

Conclusion.—In comparison with other published studies, blood culture yield in this surgical ICU was relatively low. Blood culture yield may be negatively influenced by the concurrent use of systemic antibiotics and inappropriate or excessive culturing.

▶ This retrospective study seeks to describe the diagnostic yield of blood cultures and the factors influencing the yield. Nosocomial ICU bacteremias are associated with high mortality, increased length of stay, and increased cost.[1] As many as 50% of nosocomial bacteremias occur in the ICU, with an overall rate that is 10 to 20 times that of non–ICU-hospitalized patients. In this study, 32% of the 645 patients admitted in 1 year to a 10–bed trauma/neurosurgical unit had at least 1 set of blood cultures drawn. Using a 24-hour time frame to define the blood culturing episode, 10% of blood culture episodes were positive. Of these, 5.5% were contaminants, whereas only 4.5% were true bacteremias. The most common causes for true bacteremia were catheter infection (9/21) and pneumonia (4/21).

Not surprisingly, the concurrent use of antibiotics was associated with a threefold reduction in the likelihood of obtaining a positive blood culture. The yields were lower than the contamination rates and higher than those reported in other studies. This study reinforces the generally held belief that (1) the yield of a blood culture is significantly lower when the patient is already receiving antibiotics; (2) multiple sets of blood cultures are more likely to have positive yields; and (3) excessive culturing may reduce blood culture yields.

M.R. Silver, M.D.

Reference

1. Pittet D, Tarara D, Wenzel RP: Nosocomial bloodstream infection in critically ill patients: Extra length of stay, extra costs, and attributable mortality. *JAMA* 271:1598–1601, 1994.

Significance of the Isolation of *Candida* Species From Respiratory Samples in Critically Ill, Non-neutropenic Patients: An Immediate Post-mortem Histologic Study
El-Ebiary M, Torres A, Fàbregas N, et al (Universitat de Barcelona)
Am J Respir Crit Care Med 156:583–590, 1997   6–12

Objective.—The diagnosis of pulmonary candidiasis is difficult because the significance of isolation of *Candida* species from the lungs of immunocompetent patients is unclear. In immunocompetent mechanically ventilated patients who died in the ICU, the incidence and significance of the isolation of *Candida* species in quantitative cultures of different respiratory sampling techniques were assessed prospectively, comparing them with the histology and microbiology of immediate postmortem pulmonary biopsy specimens.

Methods.—Endotracheal aspirates (EAs), protected specimen brush (PSB), bronchoalveolar (BAL) lavage, blind biopsies (an average of 14 per patient), and bilateral bronchoscopically guided biopsies (2 per patient) were obtained immediately after death from 25 patients. Lung specimens were examined histopathologically and cultured for *Candida* species.

Results.—*Candida* species were isolated from biopsy samples of 10 patients, 9 from PSB, 5 from EAs, 6 from BAL, 13 from blind lung biopsies, and 12 from guided lung biopsies. Two patients received a diagnosis of *Candida* pneumonia. Of the 470 microorganisms isolated from 280 of the 375 lung biopsy specimens, 40 (9%) were *Candida* species. *Candida* species. represented 14% of organisms isolated from PSB, 12% of organisms isolated from EAs, and 9% of organisms isolated from BAL cultures. All sampling techniques showed significant agreement with each other.

Conclusions.—Whereas *Candida* was found in specimens throughout the lung, its presence was not necessarily an indicator of the presence of *Candida* pneumonia. *Candida* species were found in 40% of mechanically ventilated, nonneutropenic patients who died.

▶ *Candida* is frequently isolated from sputum samples from patients in the ICU. This study found that only 8% of the positive cultures were associated with actual *Candida* pneumonia. Thus, like bacterial cultures of sputum, fungal cultures also frequently result in overtreatment of patients using "toxic" antibiotics for the treatment of pneumonias that aren't present (No-monia).

L.C. Casey, M.D., Ph.D.

Candidemia in Non-neutropenic Critically Ill Patients: Analysis of Prognostic Factors and Assessment of Systemic Antifungal Therapy
Nolla-Salas J, Sitges-Serra A, León-Gil C, et al (Unidad de Cuidados Intensivos, Barcelona; Autonomous Univ of Barcelona; Hosp de Ntra Sra de Valme, Selvilla, Spain; et al)
Intensive Care Med 23:23–30, 1997   6–13

Objective.—Nosocomial *Candida* infections account for 8% to 15% of all hospital-acquired blood infections and result in a mortality rate of 33% to more than 50%. Few studies have examined treatment and outcome in critically ill, nonneutropenic patients with candidemia. In a prospective multicenter study, the incidence of candidemia in a large sample of critically ill patients was determined, clinical and microbiologic features were assessed, risk factors for mortality were defined, and the results of systemic antifungal therapy were evaluated.

Methods.—During a 15-month period, candidemia was diagnosed in 46 patients (19 women), aged 18–89 years, in medical/surgical ICUs in 28

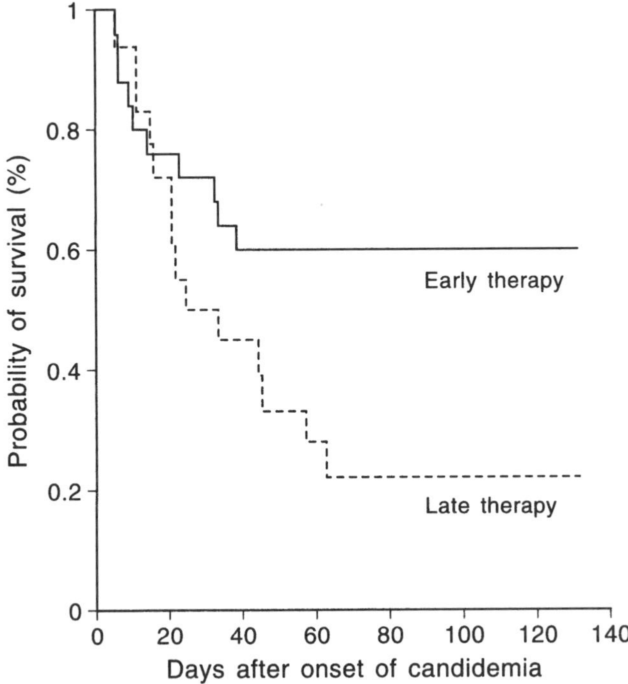

FIGURE 2.—Kaplan-Meier estimated probability of survival after first blood culture positive for *Candida* according to the time that elapsed between the episode of candidemia and the start of antifungal therapy ("early": < 2 days vs. "late": > 2 days). (Courtesy of Nolla-Salas J, Sitges-Serra A, León-Gil C, et al: Candidemia in non-neutropenic critically ill patients: Analysis of pronostic factors and assessment of systemic antifungal therapy. *Intensive Care Med* 23:23–30. Copyright 1997, Springer-Verlag.)

hospitals in Spain. Predisposing factors, species isolated, length of ICU stay, early (initiated within 48 hours of first positive blood culture) or late therapy, and outcome were recorded. A Kaplan-Meier survival analysis was performed. Severity of illness was scored on the Acute Physiology and Chronic Health Evaluation (APACHE II) scale.

Results.—The incidence of candidemia was 1 per 500 ICU admissions. The median number of risk factors was 8, and all patients had more than 1 risk factor. Of the 47 organisms identified, *Candida albicans* represented 60% of isolates and C. *parapsilosis* 17%. Fluconazole was administered to 27 (58.7%) patients, amphotericin B to 10 (21.7%), sequential antifungal therapy to 6 (13%), and nothing to 3 (6.5%). The clinical cure and eradications rates for fluconazole-treated patients (74% and 78%, respectively) were not significantly different from those for amphotericin B–treated patients (40% and 60%, respectively). Overall mortality was 56.5% and mortality attributable to candidemia was 21.7%. Univariate analysis showed that an APACHE II score of less than 21 at disease onset, early antifungal therapy (Fig 2), and short hospital stay significantly improved survival. No variables significantly affected outcome according to multivariate analysis.

Conclusions.—The incidence of candidemia in ICUs is low. Survival is higher in patients with an APACHE II score of less than 21 at disease onset, when early antifungal therapy is administered, and when the hospital stay is short. Larger studies need to be conducted to determine the effects and duration of therapy on candidemia.

▶ Although the incidence of candidemia in nonneutropenic patients is low (1 per 500 ICU admissions), this study found that there was a an overall mortality of 56% and an attributable mortality of 22%. Early treatment might decrease the mortality.

L.C. Casey, M.D., Ph.D.

The Fluconazole Era: Management of Hematogenously Disseminated Candidiasis in the Nonneutropenic Patient
Kramer KM, Skaar DJ, Ackerman BH (Philadelphia College of Pharmacy and Science)
Pharmacotherapy 17:538–548, 1997   6–14

Introduction.—For critically ill patients without neutropenia, hematogenously disseminated candidiasis caused by nosocomial fungal infection is a life-threatening complication. During the 1980s, the rate of nosocomial fungal infections in the United States doubled, the most frequently isolated pathogen being *Candida albicans.* In the past, the only available agent for the treatment of these infections was amphotericin B, which is associated with toxic effects and infusion-related reactions. Fluconazole, a much less toxic drug, has been studied as an alternative for the treatment of candidemia and hematogenously disseminated candidiasis. One factor making it difficult to interpret these studies is that candidal infections may range in severity from transient candidemia to life-threatening, hematogenously disseminated candidiasis. The evidence on fluconazole as therapy for hematogenously disseminated candidiasis is reviewed.

Fluconazole for Candidiasis.—Fluconazole has proved highly effective in the treatment of cryptococcal meningitis and oropharyngeal pharyngitis in immunocompromised patients. However, questions remain about its use in proved or presumed hematogenously disseminated candidiasis. In open, uncontrolled trials in various patient populations, fluconazole showed good cure rates at daily doses of < 400 mg/day (Table 1). Data from the largest randomized, controlled trial performed to date suggest that fluconazole is as effective as amphotericin B for the treatment of candidemia in nonneutropenic patients. However, these data are most applicable to patients with catheter-associated candidemia in which *C. albicans* or *Candida tropicalis* is isolated. For other types of patients, there is no solid evidence to support the use of fluconazole over amphotericin B. Fluconazole may be appropriate for patients with catheter-associated candidemia, with *C. albicans* or *C. tropicalis* as the likely pathogen. If no clinical response occurs within 48 hr, however, amphotericin B should be given.

TABLE 1.—Uncontrolled Trials of Fluconazole for Serious Fungal Infections

No. of Patients	Patients with Candidal Infection	Patients with Candidemia	Immuno-compromised Patients*	Antifungal Dose (mg/day)	Mean Treatment Duration Days (range)	Cure Rate Candidal Infection (%)
17	11	0	8	50	33 (8–194)	73[36]
125	64	18	NR	50–100†	NR (7–61)	88[37]
26	25	5	0	200–400	15 (5–26)	85[38]
6	6	6	1	100–200	20 (12–38)	100[39]
40	38	12	17	200	15 (2–38)	65‡,[40]
60	60	60	37	5 mg/kg, 30 pts	16 (7–38)	43[41]
				10 mg/kg, 30 pts	19 (7–79)	63[41]

*Patients with AIDS, hematologic malignancy, organ transplant, or receiving corticosteroid therapy or other immuno-suppressive therapy.

†Other antifungal drugs used in 13% of patients.

‡Patients with *C. albicans* only (n = 36).

Abbreviation: NR, not reported.

(Courtesy of Kramer KM, Skaar DJ, Ackerman BH: The fluconazole era: Management of hematogenously disseminated candidiasis in the nonneutropenic patient. *Pharmacotherapy* 17:538–548, 1997.)

For patients with candidemia or hematogenously disseminated candidiasis associated with another portal of entry, or in institutions with fluconazole-resistant fungi such as *Candida krusei* and *Candida glabrata*, amphotericin B should continue to be the initial agent of choice. Fluconazole may be used in these patients if unacceptable and unmanageable toxic effects develop.

Summary.—The evidence on fluconazole to replace amphotericin B as a treatment for hematogenously disseminated candidiasis is reviewed. Fluconazole is effective for catheter-associated candidemia in critically ill patients when the likely pathogen is *C. albicans*; for other patients, amphotericin B continues to be the first-line agent.

▶ This is an excellent, readable review of the management of serious candidal infections. The article includes a discussion of the increasing incidence of *Candida* as a pathogen, as well as a brief review of the 2 major antifungal agents, fluconazole, and amphotericin B. The final section of the article discusses the recent studies comparing the 2 agents in the treatment of candidiasis. The authors are cautious in their recommendation of fluconazole for nonneutropenic patients with candidemia. They are in favor of substituting fluconazole for amphotericin in patients with catheter-associated candidemia when *C. albicans* or *C. tropicalis* is isolated. In other seriously ill patients, they still recommend amphotericin as first-line therapy. While some authorities may disagree, their conclusions are not unreasonable. For those who have not kept up with the most recent developments in antifungal therapy in the ICU, this is a good article to begin with.

C. Franklin, M.D.

Conclusion.—Although the fatality rate was high in these patients with severe stroke, one third were still alive 1 year after admission. Early death appears to be influenced by baseline variables, but treatment in the NICU with early intubation and mechanical ventilation can reduce the fatality rate. Among survivors in this series, 59.5% had only slight or no long-term disability.

▶ Outcomes research is an important part of our current medical environment. The authors have attempted to define predictors of outcome in patients suffering severe stroke. This study helps to further define what factors can be used as an indicator of survival at 2 months following stroke. Such information is very important in helping to guide family counseling and patient-care plans.

W.T. Peruzzi, M.D.

Abnormal Heart Rate Variability as a Manifestation of Autonomic Dysfunction in Hemispheric Brain Infarction

Korpelainen JT, Sotaniemi KA, Huikuri HV, et al (Univ of Oulu, Finland)
Stroke 27:2059–2063, 1996   7–2

Introduction.—In patients with coronary artery disease, abnormal heart rate variability carries an increased risk of unfavorable ventricular arrhythmias and sudden arrhythmic death. In patients with acute stroke, evidence of abnormal heart rate variability may appear on short-term ECG recordings. However, the meaning of heart rate variability in stroke patients is unknown. The clinical significance and prognostic value of heart rate variability in patients with ischemic stroke were prospectively studied.

Methods.—Twenty-four-hour ECG recordings were obtained in 31 consecutive patients with hemispheric brain infarction, and in the same number of age- and sex-matched healthy controls. Time domain and frequency domain measures of heart rate variability were analyzed. The findings were used to assess the effects of brain infarction on autonomic cardiac regulation, and to determine the clinical and prognostic significance of heart rate variability.

Results.—In the stroke patients, all measures of heart rate variability were lower than in controls, including standard deviation of RR intervals, total power, very-low-frequency power, low-frequency power, and high-frequency power. The difference was apparent both in the acute phase and after 1 and 6 months. The more severe the poststroke neurologic deficit and disability, the greater the impairment of heart rate variability. No relevant spectral components were detected in 5 patients with large brain infarctions causing increased intracranial pressure.

Conclusions.—Abnormalities of heart rate variability, apparently resulting from damage to the cardiovascular autonomic regulatory system, are seen in patients with hemispheric brain infarction. The autonomic damage appears to be long-lasting, as found in heart rate abnormalities up to 6 months after the stroke. Abnormal heart rate variability in the acute phase after stroke may be an unfavorable prognostic factor.

▶ Abnormalities in heart rate variability have been described in patients sustaining an acute myocardial infarction, and is particularly important when left ventricular function is abnormal. The authors in this study suggest abnormal heart rate variability may be of prognostic importance in hemispheric stroke. More patients are necessary, possibly including patients with smaller strokes, to prove that hypothesis. It is unclear whether the mortality in this study is caused by the abnormal heart rate variability or whether abnormal heart rate variability is just a marker for the size of the stroke.

J.E. Calvin, Jr., M.D.

J.E. Parrillo, M.D.

Early Spontaneous Hyperperfusion After Stroke: A Marker of Favourable Tissue Outcome?

Marchal G, Furlan M, Beaudouin V, et al (INSERM U320, Caen, France; Univ of Caen, France)
Brain 119:409–419, 1996   7–3

Background.—Focal cerebral hyperperfusion is a common but poorly understood consequence of stroke. The deficit appears to be reversible if it can be demonstrated by imaging studies early after the onset of stroke. Little is known regarding the associations between hyperperfusion and stroke outcome. This study used positron emission tomography (PET) and CT to assess the relationships between early spontaneous hyperperfusion and tissue outcome, as well as the pathophysiologic basis of these relationships.

Methods.—In 30 consecutive patients with a symptomatic initial stroke in the territory of the middle cerebral artery (MCA), the investigators compared the acute-stage perfusion PET scans with the chronic-stage CT scans. All patients were apparently free of hemorrhage at the time of the admission CT scan. The patients were studied initially within 5 to 18 hours after stroke onset. About 1 month later, a plain CT scan, co-registered with PET, was obtained. Cerebral blood flow, cerebral blood volume, oxygen extraction fraction, and cerebral metabolic rate of oxygen consumption parametric images were obtained by PET and the oxygen-15 equilibrium method.

The acute perfusion images were used to identify 10 surviving patients with focal hyperperfusion in the appropriate MCA territory. The late CT scans were used to determine the topography and volume of both the hyperperfused and infarcted areas. The PET values from both areas in the acute and late phases were analyzed as well.

Findings.—Wide, patchy areas of hyperperfusion were identified in the cortical MCA territory. The hyperperfused areas were distinct from and larger than the small, deep-seated final infarcts. No MCA stem occlusion was demonstrated in any patient undergoing transcranial Doppler ultrasonography. During the acute phase, the areas of hyperperfusion showed increased acute-stage perfusion, blood volume, and oxygen consumption, with a significant reduction in oxygen extraction fraction. By the chronic phase, all of these values had normalized significantly. The final infarction showed no hyperperfusion in the acute stage. In the acute stage, the hyperperfused areas showed vasodilation and "luxury perfusion," which are signs of postcanalization hyperperfusion. Increased oxidative metabolism, which had previously been reported only in animals, was also revealed in these patients.

Conclusion.—In patients with MCA-territory stroke, extensive areas of hyperperfusion can be identified as distinct from the smaller area of the final infarction. The findings suggest that spontaneous, nonhemorrhagic hyperperfusion is a harmless and possibly even beneficial phenomenon, particularly if associated with increased cerebral metabolic rate of oxygen consumption. The findings could have implications for therapeutic trials of acute stroke, where more readily available perfusion imaging techniques could be used to demonstrate hyperperfusion.

▶ The appropriate treatment that maximizes the chance for recovery from stroke and minimizes the risk to the patient is still not known, despite an increasing number of observations. This well-done study goes a long way in determining whether the hyperperfusion seen after an embolic stroke is causally associated with the resultant neurologic injury. In this study, it was determined that the hyperperfusion observed is not related to the cerebral area of injury and, in fact, may be a marker for improved prognosis. These results need to be confirmed in further human studies, which could result in significant clinical implications for future patients.

E. Gluck, M.D.

Drugs and Brain Death
Kennedy MC, Moran JL, Fearnside M, et al (St Vincents Hosp, Sydney, Australia; Queen Elizabeth Hosp, Adelaide, Australia; Westmead Hosp, Sydney, Australia; et al)
Med J Aust 165:394–398, 1996   7–4

Introduction.—In Australia, brain death is defined as irreversible cessation of all function of the brain and is present when there is irreversible loss of consciousness and irreversible loss of brain stem reflex responses and respiratory center function, or irreversible cessation of intracranial blood flow. These definitions describe the lack of clinically observable brain function and not the absence of activity at an organ or cellular level. The Harvard Guidelines and all subsequent guidelines and protocols state that brain death can only be diagnosed in the absence of any drug effect on the brain. The Australian Society of Clinical and Experimental Pharmacologists and Toxicologists held a multidisciplinary symposium on this topic in 1995, using a hypothetical case report of an apparent brain death in which CNS function might be masked by drug effects. The complicated decisions related to withdrawal of treatment and life support were described.

> *Hypothetical Case Report.*—Male, 20, was found unconscious with severe injuries and in cardiac arrest after leaving a party where drugs were reported to have been consumed. He was successfully resuscitated. His pupils were equal, small, and reacted to light; he had generalized flaccidity, and an extensor-plantar response to painful stimuli. Toxicology reports showed the presence of morphine, phenytoin (which the patient was taking for epilepsy), and possibly benzodiazepines. At 40 hours after admission, his condition deteriorated. Pupils were at midposition and no longer reactive to light, and his lower limbs exhibited only spinal reflexes. The withdrawal of life support was considered.

Recommendations for Patient Management.—Accepting a single screen result at face value for this patient is wrong. The attending physicians should request more information from the laboratory. They should ask whether the presence of benzodiazepine has been confirmed by the assay method used and whether further confirmation is possible; what other drugs could be present that had not, or could not, be detected by the method used; and whether the staff could vouch for the certainty of the assays. If the laboratory is unable to answer these questions, a reference laboratory with properly educated staff should be used.

Physicians are legally justified in removing life support from patients considered brain dead by standard medical criteria. They are at legal risk if they ignore any drug-related factors. Ethically, physicians should err on the side of continuing life support.

Conclusion.—At 40 hours after hospital admission, in the hypothetical case report presented, further analytic data regarding plasma phenytoin level, further drug screen results, and perhaps further toxicological data are needed before informing relatives that the patient is brain dead or that life support can be withdrawn.

▶ This is an interesting colloquy on the diagnosis of brain death in Australia, with an emphasis on toxicologic analysis and how drug effects may mask CNS function. The discussants also analyze the legal and ethical implications of discontinuing life support in Australia. For those intersted in how these problems are approached in another country, this article, taken from an Autralasian multidisciplinary symposium, is worth reading.

C. Franklin, M.D.

Brain Death: MR and MR Angiography

Ishii K, Onuma T, Kinoshita T, et al (Sendai City Hosp, Japan)
AJNR 17:731–735, 1996   7–5

Introduction.—The method for diagnosing brain death must be free of error, verifiable, and accomplished easily and quickly. Described are MRI and MR angiography findings in 4 patients in whom brain death was diagnosed. The diagnostic role of these imaging techniques was discussed.

Methods.—In 4 patients in whom the diagnosis of brain death was based on neurologic and EEG findings, the cause of brain death was head injury in 2 patients, cerebral hypoxia resulting from asthma in 1 and subarachnoid hemorrhage in 1. Patients underwent MR angiograms and single photon emission CT (SPECT) immediately before or after MRI.

Results.—On neurologic examination, all patients were devoid of a cephalic or brain stem response, and none had evidence of spontaneous respiration. Flat EEGs were recorded for all 4 patients. All patients died within 4 days of the MR evaluations. No uptake of radioactivity in the cranial cavity was detected in any of the patients upon brain SPECT. These findings suggest brain death. The common MR findings in this cohort were diffuse brain swelling, especially gyral swelling, associated with diffuse prolongation of T1 and T2 signal in the cerebral gyri and cerebellar cortex, representing hypoxic/ischemic brain damage; downward displacement of the diencephalon and brain stem; and loss of flow void in the intracranial portions of both internal carotid arteries. Magnetic resonance angiograms detected no intracranial vessels above the level of the supraclinoid portion of the internal carotid arteries in 3 patients; the cervical portions of the vertebral arteries were observed in 1 patient.

Conclusion.—Magnetic resonance imaging and MR angiography can provide data suggestive of brain death. These tests are noninvasive and may be considered reliable in the diagnosis of brain death.

▶ The authors performed MRI and MR angiography on 4 patients with clinical brain death. They discuss the findings in these patients and the role MR resonance examination may have in the diagnosis of brain death. Although the exact place of MR has yet to be established, it is important to study noninvasive imaging techniques for their value in confirmation of the diagnosis.

C. Franklin, M.D.

Intravenous Angiography in Brain Death: Report of 140 Patients

Braun M, Ducrocq X, Huot J-C, et al (Saint Julien Univ Hosp, Nancy, France)
Neuroradiology 39:400–405, 1997   7–6

Introduction.—In some cases, testing to confirm the absence of cerebral perfusion is needed to fulfill the diagnosis of brain death. The definitive test of cerebral blood flow is angiography. An experience with IV digital subtraction angiography (DSA) for the diagnosis of brain death is presented.

Methods.—Intravenous DSA was performed in 140 adult patients with clinical evidence of brain death. All patients were studied within 1 to 12 hours of the clinical diagnosis. In most cases, contrast medium was injected through a 14 or 16 G needle cannulating a brachial vein. The value of IV DSA for the diagnosis of brain death was analyzed.

Results.—The patients were divided into 4 groups, based on the angiographic appearance of the vertebrobasilar system. In 115 patients, circulatory arrest at the V3–V4 vertebral level was demonstrated. Fifteen patients had stasis of contrast medium within the basilar or posterior cerebral arteries, with no signs of flow during the 60 second filming sequence. Nine patients had delayed, very slow vertebrobasilar blood flow with cessation of flow at different internal carotid levels. It took 25 to 35 seconds after contrast injection for partial but persistent posterior fossa blood flow to appear. All 5 patients had cessation of brainstem function, in addition to meeting all clinical criteria for brain death. One patient who had undergone craniotomy for acute subdural hematoma had a false-negative angiographic diagnosis of brain death.

Conclusions.—Intravenous DSA offers a simple and reliable approach to confirming the diagnosis of brain death. The findings should always be considered in the light of clinical signs and tests of brain stem function. Transcranial Doppler can define the appropriate timing of IV DSA in sedated patients with nondiagnostic electroencephalogram and evoked brain-stem responses.

▶ For intensivists who are involved in the diagnosis of brain death, it is important to keep abreast of new diagnostic modalities that help confirm cessation of higher brain function. In this study, the authors examined IV DSA. This technique is appealing because it is relatively convenient and reasonably safe both in terms of cardiovascular stability and organ preservation. The radiologists who performed this study endorse IV DSA as a reliable test of confirming brain death (in conjunction with clinical examinations). IV DSA should be evaluated for its precise role in diagnosing brain death in different situations. It has the potential to replace the electroencephalogram in certain settings and may solidify the brain death diagnosis in others. The limiting factor may be the exact time in which to perform the test. This is one aspect of IV DSA that should be studied in the future before it is practically recommended.

C. Franklin, M.D.

cept can be shown to be beneficial to the patient and the hospital under certain circumstances (a la percutaneous tracheostomy), I cannot develop a rationale for applying this to the placement of Burr holes. Because any critical care program that deals with head trauma will have a neurosurgeon available at all times, it would seem imprudent to me to allow less experienced personnel to perform such a procedure. Finally, for the purpose of promoting this idea, the authors compare the associated morbidity with that of central venous line placement. This comparison has no validity and cannot be used to defend their hypothesis.

E. Gluck, M.D.

Significance of Intracranial Pressure Waveform Analysis After Head Injury

Czosnyka M, Guazzo E, Whitehouse M, et al (Univ of Cambridge, England)
Acta Neurochir (Wien) 138:531–542, 1996   7–9

Introduction.—Among patients with severe head injury, those with increased intracranial pressure (ICP) and reduced cerebral perfusion pressure (CPP) have worse outcomes. It has been suggested that the relationship of intracranial amplitude to mean pressure may have further prognostic significance. It is difficult to monitor simultaneously all of the phenomena that could affect outcomes. Using computer-supported bedside technology, the investigators sought to establish the time-dependent relationship between ICP pulse amplitude, mean ICP, and CPP.

Methods.—The study included 56 mechanically ventilated patients with head injury. All underwent continuous ICP monitoring with either a Camino transducer or subdural catheter. The patients had a mean Glasgow Coma Score of 6; the postresuscitation score was greater than 8 in 5 patients. Outcomes, classified according to Glasgow Outcome Score 12 months after the injury, were as follows: good recovery or moderate disability (30 patients), severe disability (13 patients), and persistent vegetative state or death (13 patients). Relationships among the amplitude of the ICP pulse wave and the mean values of ICP and CPP were analyzed. To avoid problems with distortion caused by the different frequency responses of the pressure transducers used, the fundamental harmonic of the pulse waveform (AMP) was used to assess ICP pulse wave amplitude.

Results.—In patients who died, the ICP pulse amplitude increased at the time the mean ICP increased to 25 mm Hg, decreasing thereafter. Patients in the moderate-to-good outcome categories did not have the upper breakpoint of the AMP-ICP relationship. Time-dependent changes in the correlation between amplitude and mean ICP were described in terms of the R-symbol of correlation between amplitude and pressure (RAP), a moving correlation coefficient between the fundamental harmonic of the ICP pulse wave and mean ICP. Patients who died or were left in a vegetative state had a significantly lower RAP than survivors. There were 7 deaths from uncontrolled intracranial hypertension; in these patients, the RAP either oscillated or decreased to 0 or below well before brain stem herniation occurred. A negative outcome was predicted by an ICP of greater than 20 mm Hg for longer than 6 hours plus a low correlation between amplitude and pressure, i.e., RAP of less than 0.5.

Conclusion.—The outcome of head injury is affected not only by mean CPP and ICP but also by the relationship between ICP amplitude and mean ICP. Patients with poor outcomes have not only high ICP and low mean CPP but also an impaired tolerance of intracranial hypertension, as reflected by a lower time-averaged RAP value. More experience with this type of analysis will be needed before subgroup analyses of different pathologies and therapeutic approaches can be performed.

▶ Measurement of ICP is still somewhat controversial. The precise interpretation of the pressure and associated waveform is still debated, as patients with elevated intracranial pressure have varied outcomes. The authors note that analysis of ICP waveform, in addition to measuring the absolute pressure, can help prognostication in patients with severe brain injury. A combination of prolonged elevation of the ICP and lack of correlation between pressure and amplitude was generally associated with very poor outcome. The sophisticated analysis used in this study will probably not be generally available to clinicians. Further studies need, first, to corroborate this information and then to package the technique in a more user-friendly application before bringing it to the bedside.

E. Gluck, M.D.

Clinical Grading and Outcome After Early Surgery in Aneurysmal Subarachnoid Hemorrhage

Hirai S, Ono J, Yamaura A (Chiba Univ, Japan)
Neurosurgery 39:441–447, 1996

7–10

Objective.—Treatment for ruptured intracranial aneurysms requires an evaluation of the severity of subarachnoid hemorrhage (SAH). This has generally been done using the Hunt and Hess or Hunt and Kosnik grading system. The World Federation of Neurological Surgeons (WFNS) system uses 2 factors to differentiate grades: consciousness level, as classified by the Glasgow Coma Scale (GCS), and focal neurologic deficits. The correlation between these grading systems was studied, including a new modification to strengthen correlations with the surgical results.

Methods.—The retrospective study included 304 patients with ruptured cerebral aneurysms on the anterior circle of Willis. Before undergoing surgery, each patient was assessed by the Hunt and Kosnik scale, the WFNS scale, and the GCS. Surgery was performed within 72 hours after symptom onset in all patients. Postoperatively, all patients underwent hyperdynamic therapy, the results of which were evaluated by the Glasgow Outcome Scale. Correlations between the various grading systems were assessed, together with the outcomes of early surgery.

Results.—Most patients were in grade II or III in the Hunt and Kosnick system vs. grade I or II in the WFNS system. On the GCS, most patients had scores of 13 or greater. Outcomes for patients with Hunt and Kosnick grades of II and III were significantly different from those with grades of III and IV. On the WFNS scale, the only significant difference was for patients with grades of I and II (Fig 1). On the GCS, there were significant differences in outcome between patients with scores of 13 vs. 14 (Fig 2). Patients who were oriented had better outcomes than those who were confused. Outcome was unrelated to eye opening or the presence of focal deficit.

Conclusion.—Results of the correlation of various clinical grading systems with outcome in patients undergoing early surgery for aneurysmal

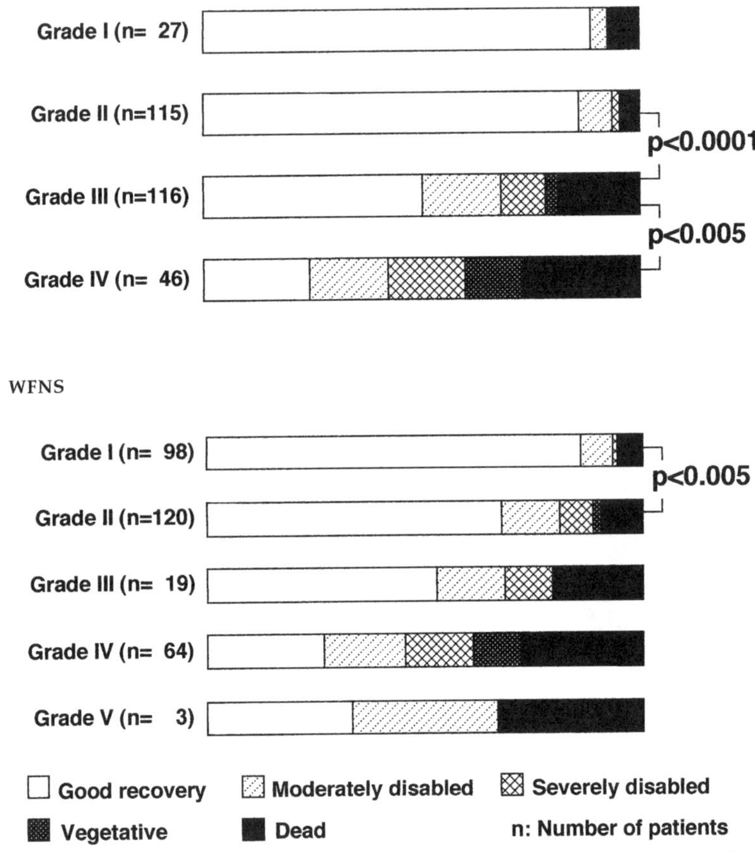

FIGURE 1.—Hunt and Kosnik and World Federation of Neurological Surgeons (WFNS) gradings and outcome at 6 months after initial subarachnoid hemorrhage. In the Hunt and Kosnik system, the patient outcome was significantly different between grades II and III (*P* less than 0.0001) and between grades III and IV (*P* less than 0.005). In the WFNS system, there were no significant differences among the adjacent grades except between grades I and II (*P* less than 0.005). (Courtesy of Hirai S, Ono J, Yamaura A: Clinical grading and outcome after early surgery in aneurysmal subarachnoid hemorrhage. *Neurosurgery* 39:441–447, 1996.)

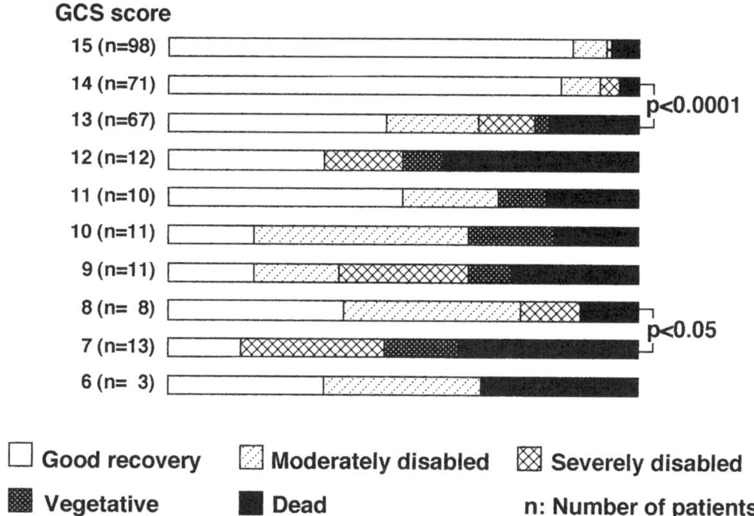

FIGURE 2.—The Glasgow Coma Scale (GCS) and outcome at 6 months after initial subarachnoid hemorrhage. Significant differences were observed at 2 borders, between scores of 13 and 14 (*P* less than 0.0001) and between scores of 7 and 8 (*P* less than 0.05). (Courtesy of Hirai S, Ono J, Yamaura A: Clinical grading and outcome after early surgery in aneurysmal subarachnoid hemorrhage. *Neurosurgery* 39:441–447, 1996.)

SAH suggest that separate recording of 3 responses on the GCS should be performed to achieve an objective grade. Even if the total score is the same, patients with confused verbal responses should receive a lower grade than those who are oriented. Further study, including that of SAH patients in poorer condition, is needed to establish a comprehensive grading system for SAH, as well as the optimal treatment.

▶ This study, performed in Japan, recommends the adoption of a different grading system for SAH. The authors base the need for a modification of the prevailing systems on the observation that patients with a GCS of 13 or 14 have very different outcomes depending on which areas of the GCS are more adversely affected; i.e., a patient could achieve a score of 13 in several different ways, some of which have poorer outcomes than others.

Because the scope of interventions may be based on the initial evaluation, it becomes of paramount importance to be able to accurately predict which patients have a reasonable expectation of recovery. However, a major shortcoming of the study is that the data were collected over a 7-year period. During this time, many changes have evolved in the treatment of SAH, which could confound interpretation of these data. The authors do demonstrate that with this modification they are able to more accurately separate out patients with different prognoses, even when these patients have a similar GCS.

E. Gluck, M.D.

Predicting Outcome in Poor-grade Patients With Subarachnoid Hemorrhage: A Retrospective Review of 159 Aggressively Managed Cases

Le Roux PD, Elliot JP, Newell DW, et al (Univ of Washington, Seattle)
J Neurosurg 85:39–49, 1996   7–11

Background.—Twenty percent to 40% of patients admitted with subarachnoid hemorrhage (SAH) are in poor clinical grade, i.e., Hunt and Hess grade IV or V. Most of these patients will die unless treated, yet many neurosurgeons are reluctant to operate. There are no clear criteria to decide which poor-grade patients do and do not receive treatments. Factors affecting the outcomes of patients with SAH of poor clinical grade were analyzed retrospectively.

Methods.—The investigators reviewed 10 years' experience in the management of 159 patients with Hunt and Hess grade IV or V SAH. There were 106 women and 53 men (median age 54 years). All were managed according to a standard policy emphasizing early aneurysm obliteration. All patients except those who lacked brain stem reflexes or function were considered for treatment. Six-month outcomes were assessed by the Glasgow Outcome Scale. Models predictive of outcome were developed by multivariate analysis.

Findings.—Six-month outcomes were favorable—i.e., good or moderately disabled on the Glasgow Outcome Scale—in 38% of patients: 54% in grade IV and 24% in grade V (Table 5). The initial hemorrhage and the occurrence of intractable intracranial pressure or cerebral infarction were the major factors affecting outcome (Table 6). The multivariate models developed for the study correctly predicted 77% to 82% of outcomes. However, basing treatment decisions on criteria assessed at admission might have resulted in treatment being withheld from 30% of patients who went on to have favorable outcomes.

Conclusion.—For patients with poor-grade SAH, aggressive management can still be of benefit. Decisions regarding treatment should not be based solely on the patient's neurologic condition at admission. Rather, all

TABLE 5.—Admission Clinical Grade and Outcome in 159 Poor-Grade
Patients With Subarachnoid Hemorrhage

Admission Clinical Grade‡	No. of Patients	Good	Moderately Disabled	Severly Disabled	Vegetative	Dead
			Outcome (%)†			
Grade IV	76	18.4	35.5	19.7	1.3	25.0
Grade V	83	4.8	19.3	10.8	4.8	60.2

Note: Clinical grade at admission was evaluated according to Hunt and Hess and was not corrected for systemic disease or vasospasm.
*Outcome was assessed at 6 months according to the Glasgow Outcome Scale.
†Grade V at admission correlated with a worse outcome ($\chi^2 = 15$, $P = 0.0001$).
(Courtesy of Le Roux PD, Elliot JP, Newell DW, et al: Predicting outcome in poor-grade patients with subarachnoid hemorrhage: A retrospective review of 159 aggressively managed cases. *J Neurosurg* 85:39–49, 1996.)

TABLE 6.—Cause of Death in 69 Poor-Grade Patients With
Subarachnoid Hemorrhage

Cause of Death	No. (%)*
initial hemorrhage	46 (28.9)
rebleed	8 (5.0)
vasospasm	1 (0.6)
increased intracranial pressure	1 (0.6)
stroke	1 (0.6)
myocardial infarction	2 (1.3)
respiratory failure	5 (3.1)
sepsis	2 (1.3)
undetermined	3 (1.9)

*Percent of entire series of 159 patients.
(Courtesy of Le Roux PD, Elliot JP, Newell DW, et al: Predicting outcome in poor-grade patients with subarachnoid hemorrhage: A retrospective review of 159 aggressively managed cases. *J Neurosurg* 85:39–49, 1996.)

patients should receive initial aggressive management, with subsequent decisions based on continued evaluation.

▶ This large, retrospective review sought to determine whether there were any factors predictive of poor outcomes after SAH. These authors found that predicting outcome based solely on clinical and diagnostic criteria commonly applied would have resulted in the withholding of treatment from many patients who could benefit from these interventions. This article and others like it serve to underscore the fact that, in many instances, prognostication has no meaning for an individual patient. Making decisions for a single patient based on prior group characteristics is foolish. The type of intervention to be ultimately made must be based on close observation of individual patients and their response to treatment.

E. Gluck M.D.

Reducing the Risk of Rebleeding Before Early Aneurysm Surgery: A Possible Role for Antifibrinolytic Therapy

Leipzig TJ, Redelman K, Horner TG (Indianapolis Neurosurgical Group, Ind)
J Neurosurg 86:220–225, 1997   7–12

Background.—Approximately 3,000 patients die annually in North America from rebleeding of a ruptured cerebral aneurysm. The aim of neurosurgical treatment of these aneurysms is to prevent rebleeding. Recently, there has been interest in early surgical treatment to eliminate the risk of recurrent subarachnoid hemorrhaging, but because most patients cannot be prepared for surgery within several hours of the hemorrhage, these patients are still at risk for early rebleeding. Other studies have reported that antifibrinolytic therapy decreased the risk of rebleeding but increased the rate of ischemic strokes and hydrocephalus with long-term use of these agents. Antifibrinolytic treatment before early surgical treatment may reduce the risk of recurrent subarachnoid hemorrhaging without increasing morbidity.

Methods.—The safety and efficacy of preoperative high-dose antifibrinolytic therapy with epsilon-aminocaproic acid (EACA) to lower the risk of rebleeding was evaluated in 307 patients with subarachnoid hemorrhages from ruptured saccular intracranial aneurysms. All patients were admitted within 3 days of the hemorrhage. Patients' aneurysms were classified as Hunt and Hess grades I, II, or III.

Results.—Recurrent bleeding occurred in only 1.3% of patients. This compares favorably with the recurrent hemorrhage rate of 5.7% reported by the International Cooperative Study on the Timing of Aneurysm Surgery for the early surgery group. The rate of hydrocephalus or symptomatic vasospasms was not unduly high in patients given preoperative EACA. Temporary CSF drainage was needed in 11.4% of patients. Overall, 8.8% of patients needed a ventriculoperitoneal shunt. Patients who required a shunt were a mean of 10 years older than the general study population. Symptomatic vasospasms occurred in 23% of patients, and strokes occurred in 8.1% of patients.

Discussion.—These findings indicate that a short course of high-dose EACA is safe in patients with subarachnoid hemorrhaging from ruptured saccular intracranial aneurysms and may help lower the risk of recurrent hemorrhaging in patients with good-grade aneurysms before early surgery. A randomized, controlled evaluation of short-term, high-dose EACA before early surgical intervention is planned.

▶ Because of previous studies that have shown that antifibrinolytic therapy decreases the rate of rebleeding in patients with aneurysmal subarachnoid hemorrhaging, the authors studied a population of 307 candidates to see whether antifibrinolytic therapy could decrease early rebleeding rates before surgery was performed. In past studies, antifibrinolytic therapy was given on a long-term basis and resulted in increased rates of ischemic strokes and hydrocephalus. It was believed that these complications would not occur on a short-term basis, so the authors combined the administration of antifibrinolytic therapy with early operative management of the aneurysm. The results in their study are compared with historical data. The reported rate of rebleeding of 1.3% is much lower than previously reported rates of 6%. In addition, the rates of ischemic strokes compared favorably with other reports, indicating that antifibrinolytic therapy did not increase the incidence of these complications. The study was not a randomized, controlled study; however, because of these results, the authors are planning to perform one in the future. If, in fact, this combined therapy can reduce the rate of rebleeding, the morbidity and mortality of this disorder would be greatly decreased.

R.V. Rege, M.D.

Operative Treatment of Spontaneous Spinal Epidural Hematomas: A Study of the Factors Determining Postoperative Outcome
Groen RJM, van Alphen HAM (Slotervaart Municipal Gen Hosp, Amsterdam; Free Univ, Amsterdam)
Neurosurgery 39:494–509, 1996   7–13

Purpose.—Spontaneous spinal epidural hematoma (SSEH) is a rare condition typically associated with acute, severe back pain and rapidly evolving nerve root and/or spinal cord compression. Prompt surgery is usually required, but studies of operative treatment for this condition have been difficult to interpret. A review of the literature on SSEH was performed to elucidate the factors influencing postoperative outcomes.

Methods.—The analysis included 330 cases of SSEH from the literature, as well as 3 from the authors' experience. The patients were 196 males and 137 females (age range, 1 to 90 years). Data were collected on patient age; sex; medical history; mortality; hematoma size, position, and vertebral level; preoperative neurologic condition; time to surgery; and postoperative results. Postoperative neurologic condition was classified as unchanged, incomplete sensory and/or motor recovery, and complete recovery.

Findings.—All hematomas were either removed surgically or identified at autopsy. Postoperative outcome was unaffected by patient age or sex or by the position of the hematoma. Ten patients died either immediately before or after surgery. The neurologic condition after surgery was unchanged in 15% of patients; there was partial recovery in 44% of patients and complete recovery in 34%. Hematomas located at the cervical or cervicothoracic level carried higher mortality rates, particularly if the patient had cardiovascular disease or was taking anticoagulants. Outcomes were better for patients who had incomplete sensorimotor deficit preoperatively. For patients with complete sensorimotor loss, the results were better when surgical decompression was performed within 36 hours or less. For patients with incomplete sensorimotor deficit, decompression within 48 hours was associated with better recovery.

Conclusion.—In patients with SSEH, the major factors affecting recovery are the extent of the preoperative neurologic deficit and the time to surgery. Although cervical location is related to mortality, the level of the hematoma does not influence the results of surgical decompression. This suggests that the major cause of neurologic deficit is not vascular obstruction but rather local compression.

▶ This article presents a retrospective review of the published world experience with SSEHs. It suggests that the initial neurologic deficit and the interval until surgery are important factors in the ultimate recovery of the patient.

E. Gluck, M.D.

Neurologic Complications in Critically Ill Patients

Wijdicks EFM (Mayo Clinic and Mayo Found, Rochester, Minn)
Anesth Analg 83:411–419, 1996

7–14

Background.—This review describes common neurologic complications of serious illnesses often seen in the ICU.

Coma.—Coma is usually detected in the ICU when illness subsides, but the patient does not awaken. Accumulation of previously administered sedative drugs is associated with altered consciousness. An anoxic-ischemic insult from an episode of hypoxemia or hypotension may produce a diffuse encephalopathy. When coma is associated with sepsis, the outcome is poor. Cholesterol embolization may be an underreported cause of coma. Acute renal failure leading to acute uremic encephalopathy is a common cause of coma in the ICU. Ischemic strokes in multiple arterial territories or microemboli also are associated with failure to awaken. Resuscitation for cardiac or respiratory arrest can result in postanoxic-ischemic encephalopathy. Transplant patients, particularly those receiving heart or liver transplants, are at higher risk for coma than other ICU patients. Failure to awaken after liver transplant may be caused by brain edema, neurotoxicity to cyclosporine, seizure, and central pontine myelinolysis. Central pontine myelinolysis can be confirmed by MRI. Intracranial hematomas are not common but they can occur in ICU patients. There are multiple causes of coma in ICU patients. The cause of coma is usually obvious after a review of the medical record. Computed tomography scanning and cerebrospinal fluid analysis should be performed when patients fail to awaken.

Generalized Muscle Weakness.—There are 3 categories of muscle weakness: (1) axonal neuropathy, usually associated with sepsis; (2) acute steroid myopathy, which can be associated with the use of neuromuscular junction blockers; and (3) prolonged muscle weakness after neuromuscular junction blockers, which may be a toxic myopathy. Polyneuropathy is the most common cause of generalized muscle weakness in ICU patients and is often associated with sepsis. Other factors associated with polyneuropathy include age, extended ICU stay, hypoalbuminemia, and hyperglycemia. Clinical features include normal cranial nerve findings, distal limb weakness, areflexia, muscle wasting, and diminished pinprick in a stocking–glove pattern. Outcome is usually good, with progressive resolution over several months. Use of neuromuscular blocking drugs, such as pancuronium and vecuronium, also is associated with generalized muscle weakness. Patients with renal failure, metabolic acidosis, or hypermagnesemia are more likely to accumulate blocker metabolites. Outcome is good for this type of neuropathy. Acute necrotic myopathy can occur when a neuromuscular blocker is given intravenously in combination with large steroid doses. A myopathy has been described in lung transplant patients, in which there is a loss of myosin. There is no evidence of sepsis and no neuromuscular blocking agents were used. Normal creatine kinase levels are present. The cause of this myopathy remains unknown. Rhabdomyolysis can cause muscle weakness and is usually associated with trauma, ischemia, and sepsis.

Seizure.—Generalized tonic–clonic seizure is not common in the ICU. Seizures are associated with drug toxicity, drug withdrawal, and alcohol withdrawal. Metabolic disorders increase the risk of seizure. Most ICU seizures occur in those patients with postoperative hyponatremia. Seizures in transplant patients can indicate immunosuppressive drug toxicity. The incidence of seizures is increased by administration of cyclosporine, OKT3, and FK 506 administration.

Conclusions.—Critically ill patients are at increased risk of neurologic complications, which can have an unfavorable effect on outcome. The patient management plan must be reassessed when neurologic complications occur. This review describes neurologic complications frequently encountered in the ICU.

▶ This well-written and organized article describes the common neurologic complications seen in the intensive care unit. It renders precise information on reasonable diagnostic and treatment strategies for each complication. The information contained here should be part of the basic curriculum for intensivists. After reviewing this article, we have placed it in our reading syllabus for the critical care fellows and medical house staff.

E. Gluck, M.D.

Polyneuropathies in Critically Ill Patients: A Prospective Evaluation
Berek K, Margreiter J, Willeit J, et al (Universitätsklinik für Neurologie, Innsbruck, Austria; Univ Hosp, Innsbruck, Austria)
Intensive Care Med 22:849–855, 1996   7–15

Objective.—"Critically ill polyneuropathy" (CIP) is a relatively recently described phenomenon consisting of primary axonal degeneration of motor and sensory fibers without inflammatory changes and normal CSF. Many different causes have been proposed, but the condition seems to be associated with sepsis and multiple organ failure. A prospective study of CIP in patients with sepsis or systemic inflammatory response syndrome (SIRS) combined with multiple organ failure (MOF) was reported.

Methods.—The study included 22 adult patients with sepsis or SIRS combined with MOF. All patients met strict inclusion and exclusion criteria, the latter including any other disease that might have given rise to polyneuropathy. The patients were not treated with steroids or neuromuscular blocking agents. In the ICU, each patient underwent a thorough clinical neurologic examination and electrophysiologic studies, including electromyography/nerve conduction velocity measurements. These studies were repeated after 2 or 3 months. The data were analyzed to assess the incidence, severity, and course of polyneuropathies in this group of patients.

Results.—Nine of the patients (41%) had clinical signs of polyneuropathy when investigated in the ICU. The major clinical signs were motor weakness and reduced or absent tendon reflexes; varying degrees of sensory loss were also present but were more difficult to confirm. At follow-up, 7 of these patients still had clinical evidence of neuropathy. Electrophysiologic signs of polyneuropathy were detected in 18 patients (82%) in the ICU. In most patients, the tests showed axonal polyneuropathy with preserved conduction velocities, reduced compound muscle and sensory action potentials, and pathologic spontaneous activity with fibrillation potentials and positive sharp waves. At follow-up, 11 patients still had signs of polyneuropathy. Weaning problems were encountered in 8 patients who survived, as well as in 7 of 7 who died from MOF.

Conclusion.—This study finds a very high frequency of polyneuropathy among patients with sepsis or SIRS combined with MOF. This polyneuropathy is better detected by electrophysiologic studies than by clinical neurologic examination. The study rules out various drugs—such as steroids and neuromuscular blocking agents—in the etiology of CIP.

▶ The authors must be congratulated for completing this well-designed study under very difficult conditions. Whatever criticisms may be justified, this study has been better executed than most others in the literature that address the problem of polyneuropathies in the ICU. A brief historical review is warranted to emphasize the importance of this study.

The observation that severe polyneuropathy occurs in critically ill patients is not new. This so-called CIP gained significant clinical attention when the possibility was raised that certain neuromuscular blocking agents may be causing the disease state. Indeed, the debate over CIP began to focus on such questions as: Can the problem be avoided by using specific neuromuscular blocking agents? and Does the degree and/or time of paralysis influence the incidence and severity? This focus led to numerous clinical guidelines for avoiding CIP that included specific neuromuscular blocking agent (NMBA) protocols, monitoring of paralysis by twitch monitor, daily "drug holidays," etc. Recent studies have suggested that CIP is a common event in patients with sepsis and MODS, but the clinical manifestations of the pathology are often subtle and seldom dramatic.

This study convincingly demonstrates that CIP is common in patients with sepsis or SIRS and MODS. More convincing is the fact that the study excluded patients with suspected causes for CIP such as pre-existing neurologic disease or pre-existing disease that might possibly be responsible for CIP. Further, none of the remaining 22 patients received steroids or NMBAs. Nine of these 22 patients showed evidence of CIP by conduction studies, and all of the survivors were difficult to wean from the ventilator.

These data irrefutably demonstrate that CIP is a common event among critically ill patients. It is clear that NMBAs do not cause the pathology; however, the degree and length of paralysis may be significant in influencing the clinical severity of the pathology. The data convince me that CIP must be considered in patients who prove difficult to wean from the ventilator when lung and cardiovascular reserves appear adequate, regardless of NMBA usage.

B.A. Shapiro, M.D.

Critical Illness Polyneuropathy in Multiple Organ Dysfunction Syndrome and Weaning From the Ventilator
Leijten FSS, De Weerd AW, Poortvliet DCJ, et al (Westeinde Hosp, The Hague, The Netherlands)
Intensive Care Med 22:856–861, 1996   7–16

Background.—Patients with multiple organ dysfunction syndrome may also have acute polyneuropathy. Such "critical illness polyneuropathy" (CIP) has been associated with problems in weaning from ventilation. It was hypothesized that CIP is related to the degree and number of organ dysfunctions as well as weaning difficulty.

Methods.—Thirty-eight patients younger than 75 years were included in the prospective study. All patients had been receiving mechanical ventilation for more than 7 days and had no previous signs of or risk factors for polyneuropathy. A dynamic scoring system was used to quantify organ dysfunctions on a scale from 0 to 12. Electromyography was done during mechanical ventilation to identify patients with and without CIP.

Findings.—Eighteen patients were found to have CIP, which was associated with an increased organ dysfunction score and number of organs involved, especially cardiovascular, renal, and hematopoietic failure. Patients with CIP had received mechanical ventilation for a longer time, but this was not clearly because of more difficult weaning. Two of 4 patients weaned normally had CIP.

Conclusions.—Axonal polyneuropathy is associated with the severity of multiple organ dysfunction syndrome. However, its presence does not necessarily mean that weaning from mechanical ventilation will be difficult.

▶ Neurologic dysfunction is a significant part of multiple organ system failure. This study sheds some light on the degree of peripheral nerve involvement that occurs with multiple organ dysfunction syndrome. This is important information because the peripheral nervous system is frequently overlooked when dealing with such critically ill patients.

W.T. Peruzzi, M.D.

Administration of Methylprednisolone for 24 or 48 Hours or Tirilazad Mesylate for 48 Hours in the Treatment of Acute Spinal Cord Injury: Results of the Third National Acute Spinal Cord Injury Randomized Controlled Trial
Bracken MB, for the National Acute Spinal Cord Injury Study (Yale Univ, New Haven, Conn)
JAMA 277:1597–1604, 1997   7–17

Purpose.—The National Acute Spinal Cord Injury Study (NASCIS) 2 found that high-dose methylprednisolone administered for 24 hours improved neurologic outcomes after acute spinal cord injury. This treatment is likely to work by suppressing lipid peroxidation and hydrolysis, which destroy neuronal and microvascular membranes. These processes extend beyond the 24-hour period after an injury. Another trial evaluated the use of a 48-hour maintenance dose of methylprednisolone. It also examined the use of the lipid peroxidation inhibitor tirilazad mesylate compared with high-dose methylprednisolone, in the hope of reducing complications.

Methods.—The randomized, double-blind, clinical trial included 499 patients with acute spinal cord injuries treated at 16 North American NASCIS centers. All patients were treated within 8 hours after injury. Treatment began with an IV bolus infusion of methylprednisolone, 30 mg/kg. The patients were then randomized into 3 groups. Those in the 24-hour group received a methylprednisolone infusion of 5.4 mg/kg/hr for 24 hours. Those in the 48-hour group received methylprednisolone at the same dose rate for 48 hours. Those in the tirilazad group received tirilazad mesylate in one 2.5 mg/kg bolus infusion every 6 hours for 48 hours. The 3 groups were compared for motor function changes from baseline at 6 weeks and at 6 months after injury. They were also evaluated for changes in the Functional Independence Measure (FIM) at 6 weeks and at 6 months.

Results.—Motor recovery at 6 weeks and at 6 months was significantly better in the 48-hour methylprednisolone group than the 24-hour methylprednisolone group. At both times, these differences were significant for patients who started treatment at 3 to 8 hours after injury. For patients starting treatment within this time, the 48-hour methylprednisolone infusion significantly increased the chances of improving by 1 full neurologic grade at 6 months and increased the chances of improvement in the Functional Independence Measure at 6 months. These patients also had more severe sepsis and pneumonia than the other 2 groups. However, other complications and mortality rates were similar among groups. Outcomes for patients in the tirilazad group were comparable with those in the 24-hour methylprednisolone group.

Conclusion.—Patients with spinal cord injuries in whom treatment is started within 3 hours of injury should receive high-dose methylprednisolone for 24 hours. For those starting treatment within 3 to 8 hours of injury, methylprednisolone treatment should be extended to 48 hours. The study finds no rationale for the use of tirilazad, although further study with different dosing regimens may be indicated.

▶ It is well documented that methylprednisilone administered soon after spinal cord injury improves neurologic outcome. Debate concerning how long the therapy should be administered has been vigorous, but could only be settled by a well-designed, prospective multicenter study. Congratulations to the NASCIS centers for producing a definitive investigation. If you still wonder what is meant by "outcomes studies," you should read this article.

B.A. Shapiro, M.D.

Acute Myopathy of Intensive Care: Clinical, Electromyographic, and Pathological Aspects

Lacomis D, Giuliani MJ, Cott AV, et al (Univ of Pittsburgh, Pa)
Ann Neurol 40:645–654, 1996   7–18

Background.—Critically ill patients given IV corticosteroids and neuro-muscular junction-blocking agents may have acute myopathy of intensive care. The full clinicopathologic spectrum of this disorder is unclear. The clinical, electrodiagnostic, and histopathologic characteristics of 1 group of patients in whom acute myopathy of intensive care developed after organ transplantation or during treatment of severe pulmonary disorders and sepsis were reported.

Methods and Findings.—Fourteen patients were included in the study. High-dose IV corticosteroids were administered, usually in conjunction with relatively low-to-moderate doses of neuromuscular junction-blocking agents. After the latter drugs were discontinued, most patients had diffuse, flaccid weakness with failure to wean from mechanical ventilation. Findings on electromyograms were consistent with a necrotizing myopathy. The histopathologic study of muscles showed myopathy with a loss of thick filaments in 79%, mild myopathic changes in 14%, and atrophy of type 1 and 2 fibers in 7%. Thick filament loss was detected in muscle

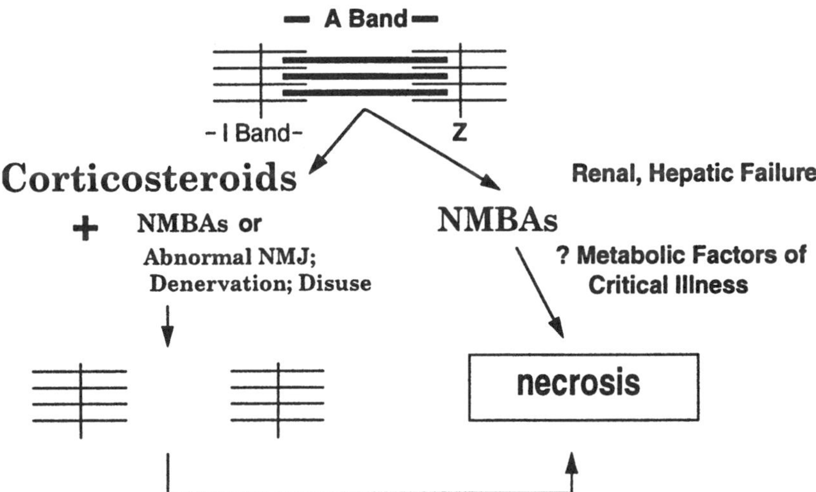

FIGURE 4.—A theoretical model of acute myopathy of intensive care. Loss of A bands and thick filaments occurs after exposure to high-dose IV corticosteroids, but neuromuscular junction-blocking agents (NMBAs), denervation, other causes of a motor end-plate disturbance, or disuse are necessary to trigger the process. Overt myofiber necrosis (with disorganization of all myofilaments) can also result from this combination of factors. The NMBAs and metabolic disturbances associated with critical illness may also induce a necrotizing myopathy without selective loss of thick filaments. So-called NMBA toxicity, including prolonged neuromuscular junction (NMJ) blockade, may be intensified in the setting of renal or hepatic failure. Z indicates Z line. (Reprinted from Lacomis D, Giuliani MJ, Cott AV, et al: Acute myopathy of intensive care: Clinical, electromyographic, and pathological aspects. *Annals of Neurology* 40(4):645–654, 1996 by permission of Little, Brown and Company, Inc.)

biopsy specimens acquired a mean of 30 days after IV corticosteroid therapy but not in those obtained earlier (Fig 4).

Conclusions.—Acute myopathy of intensive care may develop in critically ill patients, including transplant recipients, after exposure to IV corticosteroids and neuromuscular junction-blocking agents, even when exposure to the latter is minimal. Selective loss of thick filaments is common in this disorder, particularly if the muscle biopsy specimen is obtained 2 or more weeks after IV corticosteroid exposure.

▶ This study sheds more light on the pathophysiologic process involved with the myopathy associated with concurrent neuromuscular blockade and steroid administration. Further information regarding the pathophysiologic characteristics of this disease entity may assist in therapy or prevention of this disease entity. This also provides better definition of the disease picture, which should be of assistance if the diagnosis is in question.

W.T. Peruzzi, M.D.

8 Other Concerns

Pediatric Critical Care and Obstetrics and Gynecology

Poor Discriminatory Performance of the Pediatric Risk of Mortality (PRISM) Score in a South African Intensive Care Unit

Wells M, Riera-Fanego JF, Luyt DK, et al (Baragwasath Hosp, Johannesburg, South Africa; Univ of the Witwatersrand, Johannesburg, South Africa)
Crit Care Med 24:1507–1513, 1996   8–1

Introduction.—The Pediatric Risk of Mortality (PRISM) score has been validated in the United States and Europe, but its ability to predict mor-

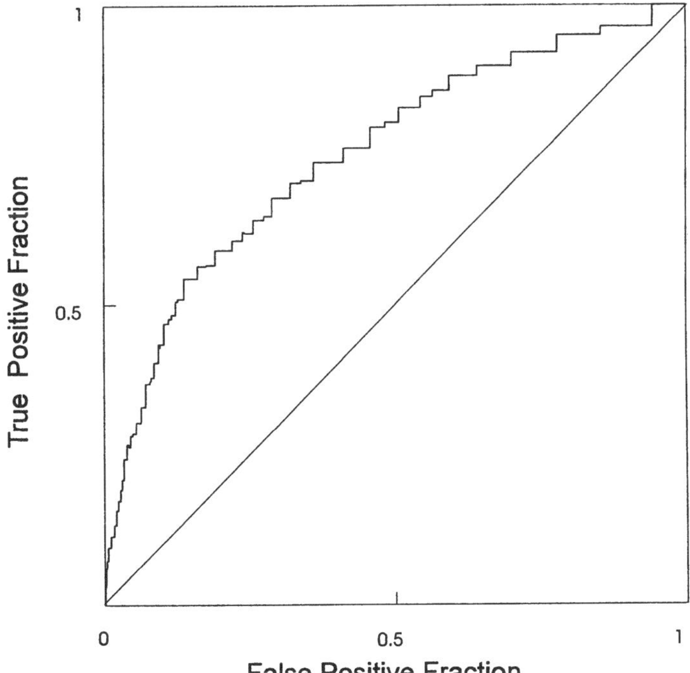

FIGURE 4.—The receiver operating characteristic curve for the study population, at cutpoint intervals of 1%. The area under the curve is 0.73 ± 0.01 (SEM). (Courtesy of Wells M, Riera-Fanego JF, Luyt DK, et al: Poor discriminatory performance of the Pediatric Risk of Mortality (PRISM) score in a South African intensive care unit. *Crit Care Med* 24(9):1507–1513, 1996.)

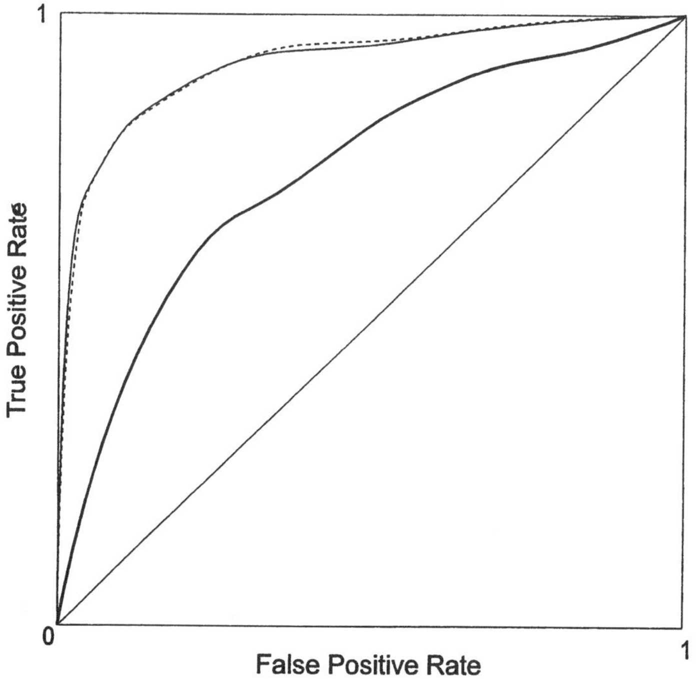

FIGURE 5.—A comparison between the receiver operating characteristic curves of the original pediatric risk of mortality population (*upper solid line*, A_2 = 0.92 ± 0.02 [SEM]), another European population (*dotted line*, Dutch study, A_2 = 0.92 ± 0.02 [SEM]), and the current study population (*lower solid line*, A_2 = 0.73 ± 0.01 [SEM]). *Solid diagonal line* represents the area under the curve (A_2) of 50% which for receiver operating characteristics means pure chance correlation. (Courtesy of Wells M, Riera-Fanego JF, Luyt DK, et al: Poor discriminatory performance of the Pediatric Risk of Mortality (PRISM) score in a South African intensive care unit. *Crit Care Med* 24(9):1507–1513, 1996.)

tality has not been evaluated in a less affluent society. Scoring systems should usually be used only in populations similar to the reference model from which the prediction model was created. The applicability of the PRISM score was prospectively evaluated at Baragwanath Hospital in South Africa.

Methods.—Between January 1989 to June 1994, 1,528 consecutive pediatric patients were examined. Data were gathered regarding demographic and clinical data, PRISM scores, and Therapeutic Intervention Scoring System scores. The prediction of actual mortality by PRISM scoring was assessed by the Hosmer and Lemeshow goodness-of-fit test. Receiver operating characteristic (ROC) curves were developed and compared with curves for United States and European pediatric ICU populations. Individual ROC curves were created for surgical and nonsurgical patients, age categories, and diagnostic categories.

Results.—Compared with European and United States ICU populations, South African patients were younger, stayed longer in ICU, and were more severely ill, with higher admission PRISM scores and overall mortality rates. Most South African patients were given respiratory and septic diagnoses. There were very few surgical patients. The PRISM scoring system failed to accurately predict mortality over a wide range of expected mortality rates and the ROC showed a poor predictive power, with an area under the curve significantly below that for the PRISM reference population (Figs 4 and 5). For all age groups and diagnostic categories, the PRISM score showed equally poor discriminatory function.

Conclusion.—The PRISM score should be recalibrated or recalculated for the patient population in South Africa because of the high discrepancy and poor discriminatory function observed. It may be that part of the inaccuracy results from different demographic characteristics of the ICU population and a different pattern of diseases. The PRISM scoring system is probably not population dependent.

▶ One of the ongoing concerns in the development of critical illness scoring systems is whether the system will have broad applicability in different patient populations. One recurring question has been whether systems developed and validated in Europe and North America will work in other parts of the world, where significant socioeconomic factors figure into patient outcome. The PRISM scoring system did not perform as well as expected in the South African pediatric ICU studied here. If other studies demonstrate similar results, it may indicate the need for a complete rethinking of how and when we use scoring systems.

C. Franklin, M.D.

Extracorporeal Life Support for the Treatment of Viral Pneumonia: Collective Experience From the ELSO Registry
Meyer TA, Warner BW (Children's Hosp Med Ctr, Cincinnati, Ohio)
J Pediatr Surg 32:232–236, 1997   8–2

Background.—Viral pneumonia is the most common indication for extracorporeal life support (ECLS) in children. ECLS has been used in patients with a range of viral infections. There are no studies on the outcome of patients according to viral type.

Methods.—Data were collected from the Extracorporeal Life Support Organization registry on the national experience of pediatric and neonatal patients with viral pneumonia and ECLS. A review identified 127 patients with positive cultures or serology for viral infection. These patients were classified according to viral type: respiratory syncytial virus (RSV), herpes simplex virus (HSV), adenovirus, cytomegalovirus (CMV), and "other," which included varicella, influenza, parainfluenza, and enterovirus. Outcomes were compared according to viral type and survival.

Results.—Patients differed in age and weight according to type of virus. Patients with RSV, HSV, CMV, and adenovirus were younger than patients with other viral infections. The groups had similar pre-ECLS PaO_2 mean airway pressure, oxygenation index, mode, or duration of ECLS. Overall survival of patients with viral pneumonia was 57%, but survival in pa-

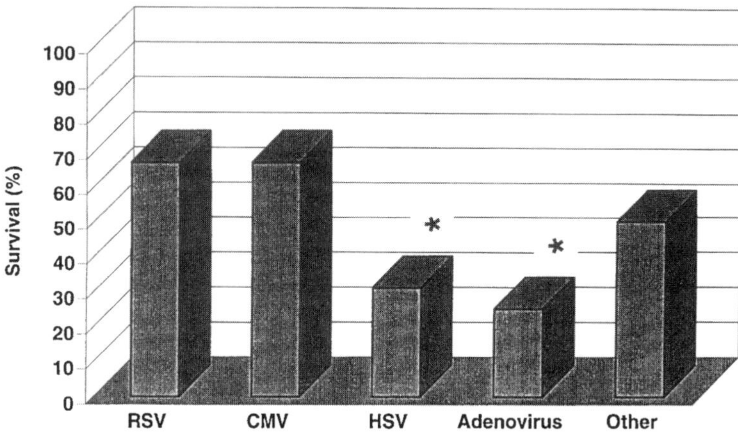

FIGURE 1.—Percent survival of ECLS patients according to their type of viral pneumonia. The group termed "other" consists of patients with varicella, influenza, parainfluenza, and enterovirus. *$P < 0.05$ vs. RSV group. (Courtesy of Meyer TA, Warner BW: Extracorporeal life support for the treatment of viral pneumonia: Collective experience from the ELSO registry. *J Pediatr Surg* 32:232–236, 1997.)

tients with RSV or CMV was 67%. Survival was significantly lower in patients with HSV or adenovirus compared to patients with RSV (Fig 1). Patients with RSV had fewer cardiovascular complications than patients with several of the other viruses. In contrast to survivors, nonsurvivors exhibited a higher last pre-ECLS mean airway pressure and a higher rate of elevated creatinine and renal failure requiring dialysis.

Discussion.—ECLS is important in the management of pediatric and neonatal patients with viral pneumonia. The survival of these patients varies according to viral type. The treatment of these patients seems to be improving.

▶ The use of ECLS to treat severe respiratory failure in neonates and pediatric patients is not infrequent. There is, in fact, a registry of ECLS that has data on 1789 patients. This database was used to answer questions about viral pneumonia which is said to be the most common diagnosis for which ECLS is used in the neonatal and pediatric populations. The charts of 127 patients with culture or serologically proven viral pneumonia were retrospectively reviewed for this study. In this review, only a small percentage of the patients from the registry were found to satisfy the entry requirements. The majority of the confirmed infections were attributed to RSV. An increased mortality rate for HSV and adenovirus infections were noted in comparison to RSV and CMV infections. The reduced survival with HSV infection is surprising in light of antiviral therapy for this infection.

Registry data are helpful to answer many questions regarding the use of ECLS. Standardization of indications, methodology, and end points are necessary for this registry to be able to answer the important future questions that will influence patient care and determine the value of this complicated procedure for pediatric patient care. This becomes more important as additional techniques for patient management become available, techniques such as high frequency oscillation, liquid ventilation, and inhaled nitric oxide, to name but a few.

R.A. Balk, M.D.

ECMO in Evolution: The Impact of Changing Patient Demographics and Alternative Therapies on ECMO
Wilson JM, Bower LK, Thompson JE, et al (Children's Hosp, Boston)
J Pediatr Surg 31:1116–1123, 1996   8–3

Background.—The incidence of neonatal extracorporeal membrane oxygenation (ECMO) is declining nationally, presumably because of the use of alternative technologies. The current study determined changes over time in ECMO use at one center.

Methods.—Data on 455 patients receiving ECMO during a 12-year period were analyzed. The 370 neonates included in the study were categorized according to diagnostic group.

Findings.—During the study period, the total number of patients receiving ECMO per year declined, which was attributed to a decrease in the total number of neonates (except for those with congenital diaphragmatic hernia [CDH]) treated. The complexity of each ECMO run increased over time, evidenced by marked increases in mean ECMO duration per patient and an increase in the incidence of patient complications on ECMO. Overall, survival decreased significantly. The patient mix shifted from more straightforward neonatal cases to more complex pediatric and cardiac cases because of improvements in pre-ECMO management of neonates. However, there was also a worsening in the severity of the condition in each diagnostic group.

Conclusions.—If these trends continue, ECMO will be increasingly used for pediatric, cardiac, and CDH patients. Existing ECMO centers must be prepared to develop programs that support such patients, in addition to neonates. The difficulty of transporting these unstable patients and the likelihood that the number of active ECMO centers will decline may necessitate ECMO centers to develop long distance transport capabilities.

▶ As new approaches to prevent and treat the respiratory distress syndrome of newborns, and new therapeutic and support approaches to acute lung injury in children are developed, there may be less need to turn to therapies such as ECMO. That is exactly what the authors of this study postulated and found at their center. Whether this is true at all centers depends on the criteria used to select patients for ECMO therapy and the array of other modalities available for use at the center. It was interesting to note that the patients referred for ECMO were now sicker and had a longer time on this support, as well as a poorer outcome. It would be interesting to ask these same questions of the ECMO registry to see if this is true at all or a majority of centers. I also would be curious to ascertain the explanation as to which therapy or change in management has resulted in this shift away from ECMO use.

R.A. Balk, M.D.

Effects of High-frequency Oscillatory Ventilation on Circulation in Neonates With Pulmonary Interstitial Emphysema or RDS
Nelle M, Zilow EP, Linderkamp O (Univ of Heidelberg, Germany)
Intensive Care Med 23:671–676, 1997   8–4

Introduction.—Rising transpulmonary pressure during mechanical ventilation can interfere with cardiovascular function. The effects of high-frequency oscillatory ventilation (HFOV) on cardiovascular function are unclear. The effects of HFOV on circulatory parameters were studied in newborns with respiratory failure.

Methods.—The prospective study included 18 critically ill infants with respiratory failure resulting from surfactant deficiency (RDS) or pulmonary interstitial emphysema (PIE). Mean postnatal age was 47 hours. In the 8 infants with RDS, mean gestational age was 27 weeks and mean birth weight, 1,620 g. The 10 patients with PIE had a mean gestational age of 28 weeks and birth weight of 1,740 g. All were studied before and 2 hours after the start of HFOV with a piston oscillator. Doppler US was used to measure changes in left ventricular output and blood flow velocities in the anterior cerebral artery, internal carotid artery, and celiac artery.

Results.—In both the RDS and PIE groups, mean airway pressure was the same during HFOV as during intermittent mandatory ventilation. Many of the circulatory parameters studied changed significantly during HFOV. In patients with RDS, HFOV was associated with an increase in the ratio of partial pressure of oxygen in arterial blood to fractional inspired oxygen (PaO_2/FIO_2). At the same time, the partial pressure of carbon dioxide in arterial blood decreased from 49 to 35 mm Hg. For patients with PIE, PaO_2/FIO_2 increased from 63 to 72 mm Hg, whereas $PaCO_2$ decreased from 63 to 40 mm Hg. The PIE group had a significant reduction in heart rate during HFOV, from 135 to 115 min^{-1}; a significant increase in systolic blood pressure, from 43 to 51 mm Hg; and a significant increase in left ventricular output, from 210 to 245 mL/kg. None of these parameters changed significantly in the RDS group, and neither group had changes in shortening fraction or systemic resistance. The PIE group showed 45% to 65% increases in mean blood flow velocity in the internal carotid, anterior cerebral artery, and celiac artery; these changes did not occur in the RDS group.

Conclusions.—In neonates with respiratory failure caused by RDS or PIE, rescue therapy with HFOV improves oxygenation, CO_2 elimination, and circulation. Patients with PIE have the greater improvement in systemic, cerebral, and intestinal circulation, perhaps because of their higher pulmonary compliance.

▶ This prospective clinical study evaluated the effects of HFOV on ventilation, oxygenation, and hemodynamics in neonates with RDS or PIE. The study confirmed that HFOV improves both ventilation and oxygenation in this population. This study also showed that when mean airway pressures are maintained at those levels used at conventional ventilation, hemodynamics are also improved with HFOV. The important points to consider in reviewing this article include the neonates being hemodynamically stable with no significant compromise before the initiation of HFOV and also that the mean airway pressures were maintained at the same levels as was used for conventional ventilation. The questions one must ask involve whether or not the neonates would have responded in a similar way if they had a marginal hemodynamic status or if they required higher mean airway pressures. High-frequency oscillatory ventilation most certainly can improve oxygenation and ventilation in infants with critical lung disease, but the hemodynamic consequences of this ventilation most probably relate to the need for higher mean airway pressure and/or the state of the infant's hemodynamic compromise before the initiation of this therapy.

S.D. Barnes, M.D.

Noninvasive Monitoring of Carbon Dioxide During Respiratory Failure in Toddlers and Infants: End-Tidal Versus Transcutaneous Carbon Dioxide

Tobias JD, Meyer DJ (Univ of Missouri, Columbia)
Anesth Analg 85:55–58, 1997   8–5

Background.—Noninvasive CO_2 monitoring provides a useful measure of the adequacy of ventilation. End-tidal (ET) CO_2 monitoring is an accurate technique, but prone to sampling changes and affected by alterations in the patient's ventilation-perfusion status. Because of these and other problems, $ETCO_2$ is generally a poor approach to estimating $PaCO_2$ in the pediatric ICU setting. End-tidal CO_2 monitoring was compared with another noninvasive measure of $PaCO_2$, transcutaneous CO_2 ($TCCO_2$) monitoring.

Methods.—Twenty-five mechanically ventilated infants and toddlers with respiratory failure were studied. All were younger than 4 years of age. Each patient underwent simultaneous monitoring with $ETCO_2$ and $TCCO_2$. The monitoring values were then compared with the measurement of $PaCO_2$ on arterial blood gas analysis. A total of 100 sets of $PaCO_2$, $ETCO_2$, and $TCCO_2$ values were compared.

Findings.—The mean difference between $ETCO_2$ and $PaCO_2$ values was 6.8 mm Hg, and the mean difference between $TCCO_2$ and $PaCO_2$ values was 2.3 mm Hg. In 96% of comparisons, the absolute difference between the 2 noninvasive measurements was 4 mm Hg or less. In 38% of cases, the difference between $ETCO_2$ and $PaCO_2$ was 4 mm Hg or less. On Bland-Altman analysis, the comparison between $TCCO_2$ and $PaCO_2$ showed a bias of -0.68 and a precision of ±2.35. On comparison of TCCO$_2$ and PaCO$_2$, bias was -6.68 and precision ±5.01.

Conclusions.—For noninvasive monitoring of PaCO$_2$ in infants and toddlers with respiratory failure, TCCO$_2$ is more accurate than ETCO$_2$. With either technique, periodic calibration with PaCO$_2$ is recommended. The 2 invasive monitors should be used in a complementary fashion—if 1 is inaccurate, the other should be tried. End-tidal monitoring CO$_2$ provides information on endotracheal tube position that is not available with TCCO$_2$.

▶ This is a prospective clinical study comparing the accuracy of 2 noninvasive monitors of arterial CO$_2$, end-tidal and transcutaneous. The study was performed in mechanically ventilated infants and toddlers with respiratory failure. The study showed that TCCO$_2$ was more accurate, i.e., most closely approximated the PaCO$_2$, better than ETCO$_2$ in this population. The authors describe problems with both of these noninvasive monitoring techniques, including the inaccuracy associated with CO$_2$ monitoring using ETCO$_2$ in diseases of ventilation-perfusion mismatch. They note problems involved in TCCO$_2$ monitoring, mainly the risk of burns and need for diligent and well-trained personnel. It was also pointed out well in the article that the ETCO$_2$ may be used for reasons other than tracking the arterial CO$_2$, such as documenting intratracheal position of the endotracheal tube and thus serving as an additional safety monitor. Taking everything into consideration, one must agree that the TCCO$_2$ monitor in the right hands is the more accurate of the available noninvasive CO$_2$ monitors in this population. In the current noninvasive environment, we must continue to develop and critically evaluate techniques for noninvasive monitoring of ventilation and oxygenation.

S.D. Barnes, M.D.

Fluconazole *vs.* Amphotericin B for the Treatment of Neonatal Fungal Septicemia: A Prospective Randomized Trial
Driessen M, Ellis JB, Cooper PA, et al (Med Univ of South Africa; Univ of the Witwatersrand, South Africa)
Pediatr Infect Dis J 15:1107–1112, 1996   8–6

Introduction.—Disseminated fungal infections are particularly devastating in newborn infants. Anecdotal and preliminary reports suggest that fluconazole can be used successfully in neonates with fungal septicemia, with effective antifungal activity and mild side effects. A prospective, randomized study compared outcome in neonates treated with fluconazole or amphotericin B.

Methods.—Two centers participated in the study, each enrolling 12 infants with proven fungal septicemia. Half at each center were randomized to fluconazole and half to amphotericin B. Fluconazole was given orally or IV at an initial dose of 10 mg/kg, then 5 mg/kg once daily. Amphotericin B was administered as an IV infusion, 1 mg/kg/day. Therapy continued until all cultures were negative for 1 week and there was no clinical and/or laboratory evidence of infection.

Results.—One infant was not a proven case of disseminated fungal infection, leaving 12 on fluconazole and 11 on amphotericin B eligible for analysis. The 2 groups were comparable in birth weight, age at enrollment, and disease profiles. A comparison of the last values obtained during treatment showed no significant differences between the 2 groups for hematologic and renal functions, but total bilirubin, alkaline phosphatase, and direct bilirubin levels were higher in the amphotericin B group. The fluconazole group showed a significant increase in platelet count. Two weeks after treatment was stopped the 2 groups had comparable hematologic, renal, or hepatic function tests. The total number of days of IV antifungal therapy was 57 for the fluconazole group and 162 for the amphotericin group, a significant difference. Central catheters were needed for 3 infants given amphotericin B, but not for any treated with fluconazole. Fatality was 33% with fluconazole and 45% with amphotericin B treatment.

Conclusion.—The current treatment for disseminated infection, amphotericin B alone or with 5-fluorocytosine, can cause devastating toxicity in newborns. In this group of infants both oral and IV fluconazole were as effective as amphotericin B. Fluconazole was less toxic and more convenient to use, and with reduced hospital stays, it may be more cost-effective.

▶ It appears fluconazole has great advantages (oral administration, shorter duration of treatment, less need for central access, less toxicity) and equal efficacy when compared with amphotericin treatment of neonatal fungal septicemia

W. Hayden, M.D.

Meningococcal Disease: A Comparison of Eight Severity Scores in 125 Children

Derkx HHF, van den Hoek J, Redekop WK, et al (Univ of Amsterdam)
Intensive Care Med 22:1433–1441, 1996   8–7

Introduction.—A combined prospective and retrospective study examined the accuracy of 8 different prognostic scores in the prediction of fatal outcome in meningococcal disease. Most of these scoring systems were developed based on the analysis of small, heterogenous patient populations, and few have been validated in a separate data set.

Methods.—The study setting was a pediatric ICU providing tertiary care for severely ill patients younger than 18. Medical records were reviewed to identify all those admitted with meningococcal disease between April 1, 1986, and April 1, 1994. A standardized treatment protocol was employed during the study period. Antibiotic therapy consisted of ampicillin and chloramphenicol initially, changing to penicillin when *N. meningitidis* was cultured. Patients were categorized on the basis of clinical findings and

Gram-stain of blood, CSF, and/or skin biopsy. Prognostic scores calculated for all patients were the Stiehm, Niklasson, Leclerc, Garlund, and MOC scores, the Tesero, the Glasgow Meningococcal Septicemia Prognostic score (GMSPS), and the Tüysüz.

Results.—During the 8-year period, 125 children with culture-proven meningococcal disease were studied. The mean age of the group was 4 years 10 months. Thirty-four had meningitis, 33 had septic shock, and 58 had both. The overall case mortality rate from meningococcal disease was 20.8%. Rates were lower for meningococcal meningitis (5.9%) and meningitis with septic shock (13.8%) than for meningococcal septic shock (48.5%). Twenty-one of the 26 non-survivors died within 48 hours after admission. All 8 scoring systems discriminated above average between survivors and nonsurvivors, as expressed by the corresponding Receiver Operator Characteristic (ROC) curves. The area under the ROC curve ranged from 0.74 (Garlund) to 0.93 (GMSPS). Overall, the GMSPS performed significantly better than the other 7 prognostic scores. All patients whose GMSPS scores were less than or equal to 5 survived. When logistically transformed into a probability of mortality, the GMSPS exhibited above average calibrations. None of the scores correctly identified non-survivors.

Discussion.—The GMSPS, which uses clinical variables and 1 laboratory variable, can be scored quickly. However, one of the variables, the base deficit, introduces a delay. The low GMSPS values predictive of zero mortality could be used to exclude such patients from clinical trials of new treatment alternatives.

▶ The Glasgow Meningococcal Septicemia Prognostic Score (GMSPS) is easy to use, and compared to the other scoring systems, most accurately identified survivors of meningococcal disease. None of the scoring systems including the GMSPS were very good at predicting mortality. Worldwide, thousands die of this disease each year and this study provides some data which can be used to study mortality-comparable groups of patients.

W. Hayden, M.D.

Vancomycin Cerebrospinal Fluid Concentrations After Intravenous Administration in Premature Infants
Reiter PD, Doron MW (Univ of Colorado, Denver)
J Perinatol 16:331–335, 1996
8–8

Introduction.—Vancomycin has become the drug of choice to treat neonates with proven or presumed nosocomial staphylococcal infections. Newborns, especially premature infants, with such infections are at high risk for bacterial seeding of the CNS and development of meningitis. In a multiple-dose, open label case series, investigators sought to determine vancomycin cerebrospinal fluid (CSF) concentrations and penetration after IV administration in critically ill premature infants.

Methods.—Three infants with suspected or proved sepsis were studied. The infants were born at 26 to 31 weeks of gestation and weighed from 670 to 1265 gm. Vancomycin was administered by a 60-minute slow IV infusion at dosages of 20 mg/kg every 18 to 24 hours. Target peak and nadir serum concentrations were 20 to 40 µg/mL and 5 to 10 µg/mL. Calculated serum vancomycin concentrations were used to determine CSF vancomycin penetration.

Results.—Lumbar puncture results with calculated CSF vancomycin penetration are reported for 6 occasions ranging from antibiotic day 1 to antibiotic day 11. Concentrations of vancomycin in CSF ranged from 2.2 to 5.6 µg/mL; vancomycin CSF penetration ranged from 26% to 68%.

Discussion.—Overall, serum vancomycin pharmacokinetics were consistent with previously reported data. Cerebrospinal fluid penetration of the antibiotic after IV administration was much higher in these premature infants, however, than that reported in older infants and children. The higher CSF vancomycin concentrations may be accounted for by more permeable blood-brain barriers and slower vancomycin clearance. These findings should be encouraging to clinicians who choose vancomycin to treat CNS infections in critically ill premature infants.

▶ Although CSF vancomycin levels are higher in prematures than in others, the levels are still quite near the levels required for adequate killing and inhibition of sensitive organisms. Careful monitoring of patient status and blood levels of vancomycin are still indicated in meningitis patients. Cerebrospinal fluid levels of vancomycin should be considered when there is poor clinical response.

W. Hayden, M.D.

Prevalence of *Candida* Species in Hospital-acquired Urinary Tract Infections in a Neonatal Intensive Care Unit

Phillips JR, Karlowicz MG (Eastern Virginia Med School, Norfolk)
Pediatr Infect Dis J 16:190–194, 1997   8–9

Purpose.—Though previous reports have described hospital-acquired urinary tract infections (UTIs) in children, none have specifically examined UTIs in the neonatal ICU (NICU). It has been suggested that the prevalence of candidal UTI is increasing in the pediatric ICU setting. The prevalence and clinical features of candidal UTIs in the NICU were assessed retrospectively.

Methods.—Neonatal ICU records were reviewed to identify all hospital-acquired UTIs occurring over a 6½-year period. To meet the study definition of hospital-acquired, all infections had to have occurred in an infant at least 7 days of age and hospitalized since birth. The study definition of UTI was urine culture yielding a single organism with more than 1,000 colony-forming units/mL if taken by suprapubic aspiration or more than 10,000 colony-forming units/mL if taken by urethral catheterization.

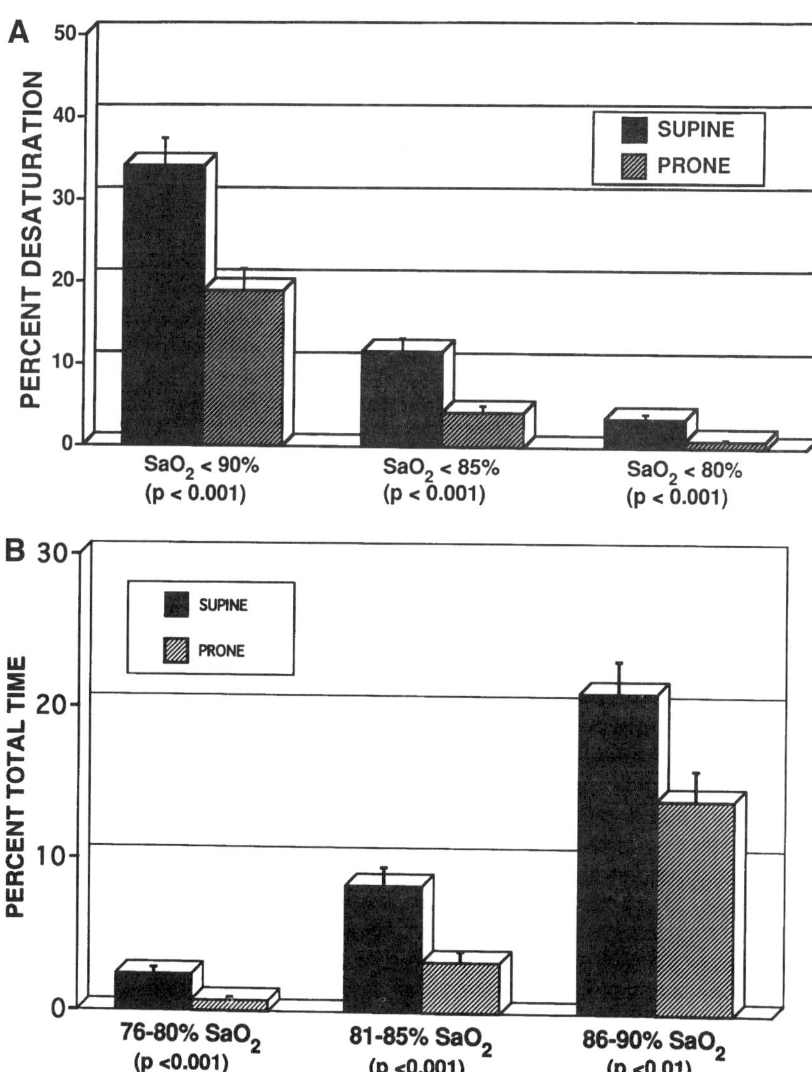

FIGURE.—**A,** Spontaneous hypoxemia (% desaturation) to levels of less than 90%, 85%, and 80% Sao_2 in 55 infants with CLD, weighing 1,000 g or less (mean ± SEM). Mean Sao_2 was 92% (*supine*) and 94.1% (*prone*), respectively. **B,** Ranges of Sao_2 (% total time) in 55 infants with CLD, weighing 1,000 g or less (mean ± SEM). (Courtesy of McEvoy C, Mendoza ME, Bowling S, et al: Prone positioning decreases episodes of hypoxemia in extremely low birth weight infants (1000 grams or less) with chronic lung disease. *J Pediatr* 130:305–309, 1997.)

have been no quantitative studies of the effect of position on oxygenation in extremely low birth weight (ELBW) infants with CLD. Results of a prospective crossover study comparing average oxygenation and episodes of hypoxemia in ELBW infants with CLD in the prone versus the supine position are presented.

Methods.—Fractional inspired oxygen concentration, pulse oximeter oxygen saturation, and transcutaneous oxygen tension were measured in 55 neonates with CLD in the prone and supine positions. Data obtained in both positions were compared statistically.

Results.—Pulse oximeter oxygen saturation increased significantly from 92% to 94.1% in the prone position (Figure). Prone positioning improved the oxygenation of infants on mechanical ventilation. Prone positioning significantly reduced the number of episodes of hypoxemia to oxygen saturation levels below 85% and 80%.

Conclusion.—Findings demonstrate that prone positioning improves oxygenation and reduces the number of episodes of hypoxemia in ELBW infants with CLD.

▶ Traditionally, the supine patient position has been more convenient for staff. Data such as these continue to accumulate, indicating that in certain instances in adult, pediatric, and neonatal medicine, the prone position may be physiologically advantageous. Keep in mind, however, that the supine position is being advocated by pediatricians to prevent sudden infant death syndrome (SIDS).

W. Hayden, M.D.

High Endothelin-1 in the Airways of Preterm Infants Is Associated With Less Severe Respiratory Distress During the Early Postnatal Period
Andersson S, Merritt TA, Orpana A, et al (Oregon Health Sciences Univ, Portland; Univ of Helsinki)
Pediatrics 99:545–547, 1997   8–12

Introduction.—A powerful natural vasoconstrictor, endothelin-1 (ET-1) also acts to constrict the tracheal smooth muscles. In the lung, it is found in both endothelial and epithelial cells. In vitro studies have found it to be a potent inducer of surfactant excretion from type II alveolar cells and to stimulate proliferation of airway epithelial cells. Airway levels of ET-1 in premature infants were analyzed in terms of the degree of respiratory distress.

Methods.—The study included 11 preterm infants (mean gestational age, 28 weeks) during their first week after birth. Analysis of ET-1 in tracheal aspirates was performed and compared with the existence of and the severity of the infants' respiratory distress syndrome.

Findings.—Respiratory distress syndrome was classified as severe in 3 infants, mild in 6, and absent in 2. The ET-1 concentration in tracheal aspirates varied widely, with a median value of 293 pg/mL. The mean log ET-1 during the first 7 days of life was negatively correlated with mean airway pressure and with fraction of inspired oxygen. The mean log ET-1 on the first day of life was positively correlated with the arteriolar-alveolar oxygenation ratio.

Conclusion.—In preterm infants, high concentrations of ET-1 in the airway are associated with less severe respiratory distress in the first week after birth. This peptide may play a key biological role in the lungs of preterm infants. Possible sources of ET-1 in the airway include plasma leakage, vascular endothelium, macrophages, and bronchial and glandular epithelium. Levels of ET-1 measured in tracheal aspirates from preterm infants are up to 1,000 times higher than in bronchoalveolar lavage fluid from adult patients with asthma.

▶ Neonatal cytokine biology progresses. ET-1 negatively correlates with mean airway pressure and fraction of inspired oxygen, 2 determinates of neonatal respiratory distress syndrome severity. The implications are unclear at this time.

W. Hayden, M.D.

Circulating Erythropoietin and Interleukin-6 Concentrations Increase in Critically Ill Children With Sepsis and Septic Shock

Krafte-Jacobs B, Bock GH (Children's Natl Med Ctr, Washington, DC; Fairfax Hosp, Falls Church, Va)
Crit Care Med 24:1455–1459, 1996   8–13

Objective.—In children with sepsis or septic shock, oxygen-carrying capacity can be increased by stimulating erythropoietin production. Interleukin-6 (IL-6) injections have been shown to stimulate erythropoiesis in rats. The relationship between plasma erythropoietin and interleukin-6 in children with sepsis or septic shock was examined by studying the modulatory effects of plasma from these patients on erythropoietin production in vitro using the Hep 3B cell line.

Methods.—Plasma samples were collected from 16 children, aged 0 to 18, with sepsis (n=9) or septic shock (n=7) and from 16 control patients. Plasma erythropoietin and IL-6 concentrations were determined. Hep 3B cells were cultured, and erythropoietin production was induced under hypoxic conditions. Recombinant human IL-6 in concentrations from 0.05 to 20 ng/mL was added to the cell cultures. Cell cultures with media containing 25% patient plasma were also incubated under a 12.5% oxygen concentration. Plasma IL-6, plasma erythropoietin, and hypoxia-induced erythropoietin production in Hep cells were measured. Plasma IL-6 and plasma erythropoietin values were compared using linear regression.

Results.—Compared with the control group, children with sepsis or septic shock had significantly higher plasma erythropoietin and IL-6 levels. Children with septic shock had higher plasma IL-6 levels than did children with sepsis whereas plasma erythropoietin levels were similar. IL-6 caused a dose-dependent increase in hypoxia-induced erythropoietin production. Erythropoietin production was significantly increased in Hep 3B cells incubated with control patients' plasma. Erythropoietin production in children with sepsis or septic shock was significantly correlated with their IL-6 concentrations.

Conclusion.—Plasma erythropoietin and IL-6 levels are increased in children with sepsis or septic shock. Addition of IL-6 results in a dose-response increase in hypoxia-induced erythropoietin production suggesting that IL-6 may be an important mediating factor in the up-regulation of erythropoietin.

▶ The observation of elevated levels of erythropoietin in the circulation of children with sepsis and septic shock leads to speculation concerning the significance of this finding. We typically associate elevated levels of erythropoietin with conditions of hypoxemia; however, the elevation in the setting of sepsis may signify that tissue or cellular hypoxia is occurring. On the other hand, it may turn out that erythropoietin is another of the family of acute phase reactants, and may parallel the elevations in IL-6 and other acute inflammatory mediators. The significance and implications of this observation requires further study and may shed light on the cellular/molecular aspects of the systemic inflammatory response.

R.A. Balk, M.D.

Inhaled Nitric Oxide in Neonatal and Pediatric Acute Respiratory Distress Syndrome: Dose Response, Prolonged Inhalation, and Weaning
Demirakça S, Dötsch J, Knothe C, et al (Justus Liebig Univ, Giessen, Germany; Philipps Univ, Marburg, Germany)
Crit Care Med 24:1913–1919, 1996   8–14

Objective.—Acute respiratory distress syndrome (ARDS) can occur in newborns, often with secondary persistent pulmonary hypertension. The pathophysiology of neonatal ARDS can lead to right ventricular failure with low cardiac output, with resultant multiple organ dysfunction. In this situation, treatment with selective pulmonary artery vasodilators could have significant benefits. The effects of long-term nitric oxide inhalation therapy were assessed in patients with pediatric and neonatal ARDS, including dosage, prolonged inhalation, and weaning from the nitric oxide.

Methods.—The study included 17 consecutive patients with severe ARDS. In keeping with the definition of the American-European consensus conference on ARDS, all patients had an acute onset, a partial pressure of arterial oxygen (PaO_2)/fraction of inspired oxygen of less than 200 mm Hg, radiographic infiltrates in both lungs suggesting the presence of lung edema, no signs of left atrial hypertension on echocardiography, and no chronic lung disease. All patients with neonatal ARDS had to be past a gestational age of 34 weeks and had to have some clear underlying diagnosis; this was to exclude patients with primary surfactant deficiency. There were 9 neonatal and 8 pediatric patients; neonatal patients were defined as those with a postconceptional age of less than 44 weeks. All

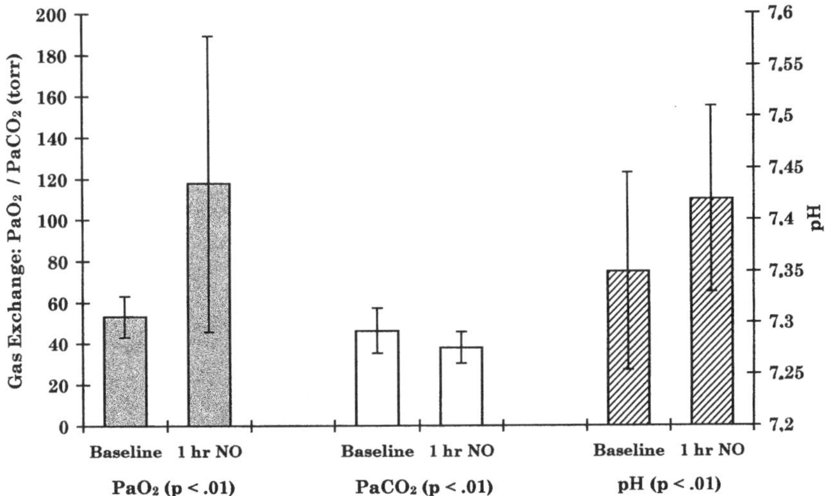

FIGURE 1.—Acute effects after the first hour of 20 ppm of inhaled nitric oxide on gas exchange (mean ± SD). No change in other therapies was made during this treatment period. To convert torr to kPa, multiply the value by 0.1333. *Abbreviations: NO*, nitric oxide; *PaO₂*, partial pressure of arterial oxygen; *PaCO₂*, partial pressure of arterial carbon dioxide. (Courtesy of Demirakça S, Dötsch J, Knothe C, et al: Inhlaed nitric oxide in neonatal and pediatric acute respiratory distress syndrome: Dose response, prolonged inhalation, and weaning. *Crit Care Med* 24(11):1913–1919, 1996.)

patients with neonatal ARDS had persistent pulmonary hypertension as shown by echocardiography. All patients received conventional therapy, including pressure-limited inverse ratio ventilation with positive end-expiratory pressure and permissive hypercapnia. They also received analgesia; sedation; muscle paralysis; and hemodynamic support, including optimization of IV fluid volume and catecholamine administration. The initial dose of nitric oxide inhalation therapy was 20 ppm for 1 hour. Nitric oxide was then withdrawn for 15 minutes, followed by dose-response testing at 1, 5, 10, 20, 40, and 80 ppm. Continuous nitric oxide inhalation was then given at the dose that produced the best PaO_2.

Outcomes.—The cause of ARDS was severe infection in 14 of the 17 patients. In all patients but 1, nitric oxide inhalation therapy produced substantial clinical improvement, After the first hour of therapy, mean PaO_2 increased from 53 to 118 mm Hg, whereas partial pressure of arterial carbon dioxide decreased from 46 to 38 mm Hg (Fig 1). The oxygenation index increased by 56%. The best effective dose of nitric oxide was 20 ppm for 7 of the 8 neonatal patients and 5 to 10 ppm for the pediatric patients. The patients received nitric oxide for a mean of 9 days. Sixteen patients survived, and only 1 of these was discharged with supplemental oxygen. The only death resulted from severe cardiovascular failure in a patient with congenital anomalies. In all patients, methemoglobin concentrations stayed within 3% or less of total hemoglobin.

Conclusion.—In patients with neonatal and pediatric ARDS, nitric oxide inhalation therapy appears to have important benefits in pulmonary gas exchange. It also stabilizes cardiocirculatory status. The best effective doses for both patient subgroups were reported; treatment should be continued to achieve an oxygenation index of 5 cm H$_2$O/mm Hg. The authors call for controlled trials to determine the effects of nitric oxide therapy on respiratory and neurologic outcomes and survival in patients with neonatal and pediatric ARDS.

▶ One unique aspect of this paper is the description of a disorder know as neonatal ARDS, which is characterized by (1) Gestational age greater than 34 weeks, (2) documented infection or meconium aspiration and (3) pulmonary hypertension by echocardiography.

W. Hayden, M.D.

Inhaled Nitric Oxide in Full-term and Nearly Full-term Infants With Hypoxic Respiratory Failure
Ehrenkranz RA, and The Neonatal Inhaled Nitric Oxide Study Group (Yale Univ, New Haven, Conn)
N Engl J Med 336:597–604, 1997   8–15

Background.—Persistent pulmonary hypertension is one of many causes of hypoxic respiratory failure in newborns. Conventional treatments have been unable to reduce mortality from this condition or to reduce the need for extracorporeal membrane oxygenation. Nitric oxide has been reported to be a selective pulmonary vasodilator, leading to treatment of neonates with pulmonary hypertension with inhaled nitric oxide. The ability of inhaled nitric oxide therapy to reduce mortality or avoid extracorporeal membrane oxygenation in newborns with hypoxic respiratory failure was investigated.

Methods.—The randomized, controlled, multicenter trial included 135 infants with hypoxic respiratory failure who were born at 34 or more weeks' gestation. All had an oxygenation index of at least 25. They were studied at age 14 days or less. The infants were randomized to receive either nitric oxide at a concentration of 20 ppm or 100% oxygen. If the patient responded, treatment was continued; if not, treatment was stopped for 15 minutes and then resumed at a maximal concentration of 80 ppm. If there was still no response, treatment was stopped. The main study hypothesis was that nitric oxide therapy would reduce the 120-day mortality rate or achieve a 40% relative reduction in the need for extracorporeal membrane oxygenation. Secondarily, changes in partial pressure of arterial oxygen (PaO$_2$), oxygenation index, and alveolar-arterial oxygen gradient were assessed. Blood methemoglobin was monitored as a safety measure.

Results.—The 2 treatment groups were similar in their baseline characteristics. The study was halted early on data review because the z value had crossed the boundary of statistical significance. By 120 days, 46% of nitric oxide–treated patients vs. 64% of control patients had either died or received extracorporeal membrane oxygenation. The mortality rates were

TABLE 5.—Results of the Subgroup Analysis

Variable	No. of Patients*	Percent with Improved Oxygenation†		Percent with Primary Outcome‡		Relative Risk (95% CI)§
		Control	Nitric Oxide	Control	Nitric Oxide	
Primary diagnosis						
Persistent pulmonary hypertension	41	14	61	73	32	0.43 (0.23–0.81)
Respiratory distress syndrome	25	8	60	47	50	1.07 (0.46–2.49)
Meconium aspiration	116	16	47	62	52	0.83 (0.61–1.15)
Pneumonia or sepsis	50	17	52	67	39	0.58 (0.33–1.00)
Pulmonary hypertension found by echocardiography						
Yes	176	15	54	65	47	0.72 (0.55–0.94)
No	50	14	44	50	39	0.79 (0.42–1.48)
Surfactant						
Yes	168	14	51	54	38	0.71 (0.51–0.99)
No	67	15	50	88	64	0.72 (0.55–0.95)
High-frequency ventilation						
Yes	130	14	57	66	46	0.70 (0.51–0.96)
No	105	16	43	61	45	0.74 (0.51–1.06)
Surfactant and high-frequency ventilation						
Both	88	13	59	57	37	0.64 (0.40–1.00)
Neither	25	14	40	93	64	0.69 (0.45–1.04)
Oxygenation index						
25.0–29.9	53	7	76	61	28	0.46 (0.24–0.88)
30.0–39.9	72	27	42	42	47	1.13 (0.67–1.91)
40.0–59.9	74	11	51	76	47	0.62 (0.43–0.89)
≥60.0	35	11	27	84	69	0.82 (0.56–1.18)

*Data on primary diagnosis are based on 232 patients; on pulmonary hypertension found by echocardiography, 226; and on oxygenation index, 234.

†Improved oxygenation was defined as a complete response (an increase of more than 20 mm Hg in the partial pressure of arterial oxygen) to the administration of 20 ppm nitric oxide or control gas at 30 minutes.

‡The primary study outcome was death by 120 days of age or the initiation of extracorporeal membrane oxygenation.

§Relative risks are shown for the occurrence of the primary study outcome in the nitric oxide group as compared with the control group.

Abbreviation: CI, confidence interval.

(Reprinted by permission of the *New England Journal of Medicine*, courtesy of Ehrenkranz RA, and The Neonatal Inhaled Nitric Oxide Study Group: Inhaled nitric oxide in full-term and nearly full-term infants with hypoxic respiratory failure. *N Engl J Med* 336:597–604, copyright 1997, Massachusetts Medical Society.)

similar between groups: 14% with nitric oxide and 17% with oxygen. However, 39% of patients in the nitric oxide group required extracorporeal membrane oxygenation, compared with 54% of the control group. The PaO_2 improved by 58 mm Hg in the nitric oxide group vs. 10 mm Hg in the control group. The nitric oxide group had a 14-point decrease in oxygenation index, compared with a 1-point increase in the control group. None of the patients required treatment discontinuation because of toxicity. None of the factors evaluated in post hoc subgroup analyses altered the results (Table 5).

Conclusion.—In critically ill newborns with hypoxic respiratory failure, nitric oxide inhalation therapy can significantly reduce the need for extracorporeal membrane oxygenation. The treatment has no apparent effect on mortality, however. Inhaled nitric oxide therapy is safe, well-tolerated, and fairly simple and is recommended for infants who do not improve with conventional therapy.

▶ The major conclusion of this study seems to me to be that if nitric oxide is added to the therapeutic options available for severe respiratory distress syndrome in neonates of more than 34 weeks' gestation, there will be less need for extracorporeal membrane oxygenation (ECMO) (20 fewer study children required ECMO in this study). Considering the huge investment (personnel, equipment, supplies, and medications) necessary for ECMO, nitric oxide has the advantage.

W. Hayden, M.D.

Noninvasive Capnometry Monitoring for Respiratory Status During Pediatric Seizures
Abramo TJ, Wiebe RA, Scott S, et al (Univ of Texas, Dallas)
Crit Care Med 25:1242–1246, 1997   8–16

Introduction.—In patients with seizure, impaired respiratory function during and after seizure activity is a major cause of mortality, which can be caused by diaphragmatic contractions that impede air movement, airway obstruction, or an imbalance between neurologic and mechanical respiratory drives. Hypoxemia and hypercapnia can result from these alterations. Blood gas analysis, an invasive procedure, is usually used to determine respiratory and acid base status in such patients. A noninvasive technique for monitoring expired partial pressure of carbon monoxide (PCO_2) is sidestream capnometry; it can be used with pulse oximetry to provide the clinician with a convenient method for continuously monitoring the adequacy of ventilation and oxygenation. In pediatric patients in the ictal and/or postictal state, the reliability and utility of a dual oral/nasal sidestream capnometry and pulse oximetry circuit were evaluated.

Methods.—Oral/nasal sidestream capnometry was used to obtain endtidal CO_2 for 166 patients, of whom 105 had active seizures and 61 were postictal. Every 5 minutes, pulse rates, oxygen saturation, and respiratory rates were recorded for 60 minutes. A capillary P_{CO_2} and clinical observation were compared to end-tidal CO_2 values.

Results.—The mean capillary P_{CO_2} reading was 43.4 ± 11.7 mm Hg, and the mean end-tidal CO_2 reading was 43.0 ± 11.8 mm Hg. There was a significant correlation between end-tidal CO_2 and capillary P_{CO_2}. There was established a relative average bias of 0.33 mm Hg with end-tidal CO_2 lower than capillary P_{CO_2} with 95% limits of agreement ± 4.2 mm Hg. Range of mean scores, age, and respiratory rates were not related to variability of difference scores. When compared with oxygen saturation, end-tidal CO_2 correlated better with respiratory rate changes.

Conclusion.—Using an oral/nasal cannula capnometry circuit, dependable end-tidal CO_2 values can be obtained in pediatric seizure patients. A reliable assessment of pulmonary status that can assist with decisions on providing ventilatory support is available to the clinician by continuous end-tidal CO_2 monitoring.

▶ The results of this study clearly suggest that oral/nasal capnometry is a reliable noninvasive monitor of physiologic ventilation (arterial P_{CO_2}) in pediatric patients after seizure. The remarkable difference in the reliability of this technique in the small children studied compared with adults is the result of the excellent cardiac function in the pediatric patients. Because cardiac output is well maintained, the partial pressure of arterial carbon dioxide/ $PETCO_2$ gradient remains small.

This study shows that in children under 6 years of age who are both postictal and have received antiseizure medication, an oral/nasal capnometer device will reliably trend the arterial P_{CO_2}. It is essential that these data not be applied to adult patients.

B.A. Shapiro, M.D.

Blunt Abdominal Trauma in Children: Risks of Nonoperative Treatment
Sjövall A, Hirsch K (Karolinska/S:t Görans Hosp, Stockholm)
J Pediatr Surg 32:1169–1174, 1997   8–17

Background.—Several reports have examined the safety of nonoperative management of blunt abdominal trauma in children. A major concern is delayed treatment of gastrointestinal canal perforation because it is very difficult to diagnose this type of injury. Late bleeding from spleen or liver injuries; bile duct injuries; septic complications from liver hematomas; and pancreatic, hepatic, and splenic posttraumatic cysts have been described. In 1978, a protocol for nonoperative treatment of splenic injuries was initiated in the authors' department, and a similar protocol was applied to liver injuries during the next 2 years. A retrospective review was conducted to examine the complications of nonoperative management, how patients who needed operative treatment were identified, and whether any patients were subject to unnecessary risks or discomfort because of conservative treatment.

Methods.—The medical records of 203 children with injury to the spleen, liver, pancreas, or gastrointestinal tract were reviewed. All injuries occurred between 1979 and 1993. There were 137 boys and 66 girls, and the mean patient age was 9.0 years. Most injuries were from bicycle accidents, falls, and horse-riding accidents.

Results.—Of 145 patients with splenic injury, 7 had surgery. The splenic salvage rate was 100%. Of 29 patients with hepatic injury, 4 had laparotomy. One patient who received conservative treatment had rebleeding and underwent 2 laparotomies. Of 10 patients with pancreatic injury, 3 had surgery; 1 of these patients had surgery 4 weeks after the trauma occurred because of a pseudocyst. There were 19 patients with gastrointestinal tract injuries. Of 7 patients with intramural hematoma, 5 were treated nonoperatively. There were 12 patients with gastrointestinal perforations; 7 had immediate laparotomy. Three patients had surgery 24 hours after admission because of severe abdominal rigidity or pneumoperitoneum. A severe in-hospital delay occurred in a patient in whom the physical findings were believed to result from splenic and hepatic injuries, but laparotomy 36 hours after admission showed a jejunal rupture and necrosis of the transverse colon. There were no deaths.

Discussion.—Nonoperative management of blunt abdominal trauma in children is very successful in cases of splenic rupture. Conservative treatment of hepatic injury carries a higher risk. The treatment of pancreatic injury is controversial. It is difficult to diagnose perforations of the gastrointestinal tract, and it is important to keep this in mind when considering conservative treatment of abdominal trauma.

▶ This retrospective study has 2 very important messages for all who care for trauma patients. First, there is no substitute for frequent and thorough clinical abdominal examinations when conservative treatment is contemplated. When clinical signs cannot be explained by imaging findings, surgery must take place. Second, appropriate pain relief must be provided and should not significantly diminish the reliability of clinical abdominal examinations.

B.A. Shapiro, M.D.

Survival and Functional Outcome of Children Requiring Endotracheal Intubation During Therapy for Severe Traumatic Brain Injury
Thakker JC, Splaingard M, Zhu J, et al (Med College of Wisconsin, Milwaukee)
Crit Care Med 25:1396–1401, 1997   8–18

Objective.—Traumatic head injury is a common cause of trauma-related hospitalization and death in children. The authors' pediatric ICU uses an aggressive, multitherapy approach to the management of children with traumatic brain injury, including appropriate neurosurgery, intracranial pressure monitoring, acute hyperventilation, and other approaches. This strategy yields improved survival in patients with severe traumatic brain injury, although it has been suggested that morbidity is increased as well. Survival and outcome were assessed in children with traumatic brain injury sufficiently severe to require endotracheal intubation and mechanical ventilation.

Methods.—Over 5 years, 105 children with traumatic brain injury severe enough to require endotracheal intubation and mechanical ventilation were admitted. Seventy-four percent of the patients were boys, and 70% were white; the median age was 43 months. Treatment data included vital signs during the first 24 hours after admission, Pediatric Risk of Mortality (PRISM) score, Glasgow Coma Score, duration of mechanical ventilation, and length of pediatric ICU and hospital stay. Chart review and telephone follow-up were used to grade the patients' functional status as normal, independent, partially dependent, or dependent in terms of locomotion, self-care, and communication. Predictors of survival and functional outcome were evaluated.

Results.—The patients' median Glasgow Coma Score was 6, whereas the median PRISM score was 13. The mortality rate was 18%, with 17 deaths occurring in the pediatric ICU and 2 after discharge from the hospital. The functional outcome was rated as normal or independent for 37% of children, partially dependent for 40%, and dependent for 7%. The median follow-up was 25 months and included 78 survivors. Of patients available for follow-up, 66% were rated as normal or independent, 8% were rated as partially dependent in at least 1 functional area, and 1% were rated as dependent in all functional areas.

Factors associated with death and a dependent functional outcome included younger age, lower Glasgow Coma Score, and a higher admission PRISM score. Forty-one percent of patients with a Glasgow Coma Score of 5 or less survived with normal or independent functional outcomes. In contrast, normal or independent outcomes were reached by only 21% of patients with PRISM scores of 20 or greater. Patients with a Glasgow Coma Score of 5 or less and a PRISM score of 20 or greater were 10 times more likely to have a bad outcome than patients with a Glasgow Coma Score of 5 or less and a PRISM score of less than 20.

Discussion.—This study shows a 72% survival rate among children with severe traumatic brain injury. For patients who survive, functional status continues to improve in the few years after discharge. A low Glasgow Coma Score is a risk factor for death or poor functional outcome. However, even if the Glasgow Coma Score is 5 or less, survival with good function is possible. Combining the PRISM score and Glasgow Coma Score adds to the ability to predict survival and functional outcome.

▶ Although the results of a retrospective, observational cohort study are always suspect, this study shows that severely brain-injured children who survive to hospital discharge continue to improve functionally over the next 2 years.

B.A. Shapiro, M.D.

Femoral Venous Access Is Safe in Burned Children: An Analysis of 224 Catheters

Goldstein AM, Weber JM, Sheridan RL (Harvard Med School, Boston)
J Pediatr 130:442–446, 1997   8–19

Objective.—Septic and mechanical complications are associated with the use of central venous catheters particularly in pediatric burn patients. One institution had reported that life-threatening mechanical complications can be avoided by using femoral vein access. The safety of femoral venous cannulation in pediatric burn patients, the risk of catheter-related sepsis when placed through burned skin, the relation between risk of sepsis and number of days a catheter is left in place or the duration of use of a given site, and the relation between risk of sepsis and use of catheters placed over a guide wire were investigated.

Methods.—Between January 1992 and December 1995, data on 224 catheter placements in 86 children, aged 1 to 19, with an average burn size of 38.4% was collected prospectively.

Results.—Catheters were in place for an average of 5.7 days, an average of 8.3 sites were used, and each patient had 1 to 18 catheters placed. Five factors influenced catheter-related sepsis (Table 2). Three patients had mechanical complications.

Conclusion.—Femoral venous access in pediatric burn patients is safe and carries a low incidence of mechanical complications and infection.

▶ A large prospective study strongly suggesting that femoral vein cannulation has no direct correlation with sepsis in burned children. Incidence of sepsis correlated with the severity of the major insult requiring admission and therapy (skin burn). If femoral cannulation is safe in this population, it certainly deserves examination in the adult population.

B.A Shapiro, M.D.

TABLE 2.—Factors Affecting the Incidence of Catheter-Related Sepsis

	Sepsis	No sepsis
Patient age (yr)	2.9 ± 4.0	5.5 ± 5.1*
Burn size (%BSA)	58.0 ± 32.5	36.1 ± 20.9†‡
Catheters placed (No.)	2.9 ± 2.5	2.3 ± 1.9
Days that catheter was in place (No.)	5.7 ± 2.2	5.7 ± 3.0
Consecutive days that site was used (No.)	8.3 ± 4.4	8.1 ± 5.6

Catheter-related sepsis as defined by Shriners Burn Institute criteria. Values expressed as mean plus or minus SD.
*Data did not achieve statistical significance by unpaired *t* test, except where otherwise specified.
†Burn size includes only patients with acute thermal burns, not those with exfoliating skin disorders.
‡*P* less than 0.01.
(Courtesy of Goldstein AM, Weber JM, Sheridan RL: Femoral venous access is safe in burned children: An analysis of 224 catheters. *J Pediatr* 130:442–446, 1997.)

Controlled Prospective Randomized Comparison of High-Frequency Jet Ventilation and Conventional Ventilation in Neonates With Respiratory Failure and Persistent Pulmonary Hypertension

Engle WA, Yoder MC, Andreoli SP, et al (Indiana Univ, Indianapolis)
J Perinatol 17:3–9, 1997   8–20

Objective.—Whereas uncontrolled studies have demonstrated that high-frequency ventilation can be used as a rescue method in neonates with respiratory failure when conventional ventilation fails, other studies were not able to find improved survival. The safety and efficacy of high-frequency jet ventilation in neonates with persistent pulmonary hypertension was compared with that of conventional ventilation in a prospective, randomized, controlled study.

Methods.—Eleven neonates in a level-3 intensive care unit were treated with high-frequency jet ventilation and 13 with conventional ventilation. Patients who failed either treatment were given extracorporal membrane oxygenation (ECMO). Survival analysis was used to compare time to ECMO or death for both groups.

Results.—Whereas the oxygenation index and alveolar-arterial oxygen gradient increased significantly in the high-frequency ventilator group, these parameters were essentially unchanged in the conventional ventilator group. Peak inspiratory pressure increased significantly from 37.7 to 44.4 cm H_2O in the conventional ventilator group. Both groups had similar survival rates without ECMO. Morbidity rates, incidence of chronic lung disease, number of patients requiring ECMO, number of pneumothoraces, and duration of ventilation, oxygen administration, hospitalization, ECMO, and causes of death were similar in both groups.

Conclusion.—High-frequency ventilation increased the oxygenation index and the alveolar-arterial oxygen gradient without increasing the peak inspiratory pressure or morbidity. Efficacy of the technique in the absence of ECMO and its effect on mortality should be evaluated in a multicenter cohort trial.

▶ This study required a great deal of time and energy to accomplish, and the authors are to be congratulated for their efforts. However, there are too many variables in this study to justify the conclusions. For example, there were 8 neonatologists involved in the care of these 24 patients, and each applied their own endpoints and therapies. The only conclusion I can make from the data is that the high-frequency jet ventilation in combination with conventional ventilation was as safe as the conventional ventilation alone. In my opinion, from the data presented there can be no conclusions about efficacy.

B.A Shapiro, M.D.

Analysis of Costs in a Pediatric ICU

García S, Ruza F, Alvarado F, et al (Hosp Infantil "La Paz," Madrid)
Intensive Care Med 23:218–225, 1997   8–21

Objective.—Despite the high costs of intensive care, there have been few studies analyzing these costs and their components in terms of resource utilization and consumption. Such cost analyses provide important information for economic evaluation of strategies for effective patient treatment using studies on cost-effectiveness and cost-utility. The costs of running a pediatric ICU are analyzed, including patterns of cost variation in different patient groups.

Methods.—The prospective, observational study was performed in the multidisciplinary 12-bed pediatric ICU of a tertiary university hospital. During the 17-month study period, 495 patients were admitted, 64% being medial and 36% surgical patients. Their mean length of ICU stay was 7 days. Calculation of fixed costs per patient per day included the services of physicians, nurses, and other personnel; structural depreciation; maintenance; consumption; and disposable materials. Variable costs were calculated for each patient, including the costs of routine procedures and costs for drugs, blood products, various tests and imaging procedures, and other procedures. For each patient, Physiologic Stability Index (PSI) was assessed at admission. The study sought to determine the actual costs of pediatric intensive care and its components, focusing on the variable costs of caring for different patient groups and the elements of those costs.

Results.—Mean fixed costs were $608 per patient per day, which accounted for 72% of total patient costs. Personnel costs made up 86% of fixed costs, including 58% for nurses and auxiliary staff. The remaining 28% of costs were variable costs, with a mean value of $218 per patient per day. Daily variable costs were $542 for nonsurvivors versus $179 for survivors. For nonsurvivors there were also higher costs related to nonsurvivors' longer stay in the ICU.

Variable daily costs increased from $155 for patients with a PSI score of less than 4 points, to $210 for those with a PSI of 5 to 9 points, to $324 for those with a PSI of 10–14 points, to $480 for those with a PSI of more than 15 points. This relationship was not apparent for all resources, however. Costs for treatments and biochemical and hematologic tests increased with PSI score. Costs for antibiotics, parenteral nutrition, blood products, and bacteriologic tests peaked in patients with PSI scores of up to 14 points. Radiology costs were not significantly affected by PSI score.

Conclusions.—Personnel costs account for 62% of total costs in the ICU, this study suggests. Variable costs are 3 times higher for nonsurvivors than for survivors; ICU stays are longer for survivors as well. Patients with an elevated PSI score on the first day of admission have increased variable costs. More severe illnesses are associated with increased costs for treatment techniques but not with increased costs for antibiotics, parenteral nutrition, bacteriologic testing, or radiology. Having unified cost calculation criteria would be helpful for performing comparative studies of different groups of patients, thus permitting economic assessment of different treatment strategies.

▶ This is a prospective observational study evaluating the cost of administering care to critical pediatric patients. This study was performed in a pediatric ICU in Madrid, Spain. The findings are not surprising in that they support that the sickest and therefore the nonsurvivors require the greatest expense devoted to their medical care. It is also not surprising that the greatest proportion of the cost is represented in personnel expense. Even though this study was performed in Spain, I suspect that the findings apply to pediatric intensive care settings in other parts of the world. One can only hope that with advances in medical care utilizing new technologies, the length of stay would decrease and survival would increase. The fear obviously is that with advanced technologies the sick patient will have longer and more involved lengths of stay which in fact will increase the expense of their care.

S.D. Barnes, M.D.

Outcome and Acute Care Hospital Costs After Warm Water Near Drowning in Children

Christensen DW, Jansen P, Perkin RM (Loma Linda Univ, Calif)
Pediatrics 99:715–721, 1997   8–22

Purpose.—Drowning continues to be a major cause of preventable death in children. Attempts have been made to classify pediatric near-drowning patients into prognostic groups using data available in the emergency department (ED). However, since these scoring systems cannot identify all patients who will survive intact, most EDs aggressively resuscitate all drowning victims. The characteristics and outcomes of pediatric near-drowning victims were analyzed in an attempt to reliably identify survivors early in their course.

Methods.—The retrospective study included 274 children admitted to a children's hospital for near-drowning over a 9½-year period. Nearly two thirds of the patients were boys; the median age was 24 months. Each child's outcome was classified as good, denoting near-normal function, or poor, i.e., dead or in a vegetative state. The factors best able to predict outcome were identified by discriminant analysis and used to create a clinical classification system. Acute care hospital costs for the 2 outcome groups were calculated as well.

Results.—Though the discriminant analysis classification had an accuracy of 95%, it predicted death in 6 patients who survived intact. No combination of variables was capable of distinguishing all intact survivors from the patients with poor outcomes. Accuracy was 93% with the clinical classification method, which predicted death for 5 patients who survived intact. Some patients went through a prolonged vegetative state before experiencing a complete recovery. Fourteen percent of patients survived in a vegetative state; they accounted for 53% of total acute care hospital costs. Though two thirds of patients were intact survivors, they accounted for only one third of total hospital costs.

Conclusions.—It is not possible to predict the outcome of pediatric near-drowning victims in the ED. This means that aggressive resuscitation is indicated for all such patients. Later decisions about withdrawal of life support should consider factors including the likelihood of survival, level of certainty, and parental and societal issues. Patients who survive in a vegetative state are very expensive to care for. Reducing spending on these patients could produce significant cost savings; however, it would also result in the loss of some intact survivors.

▶ This study involves a retrospective review of patients admitted following near drowning in an effort to predict who would likely fail to survive and also to get an idea of the expense involved in the care of such patients. It is not surprising that the patients who are determined to be persistently vegetative are the most expensive to care for whereas intact survivors are the least expensive. It is also not surprising that the majority of costs were spent on patients with poor outcomes. The efforts made to predict which patients would survive and which would not were not successful. The important point to be taken from this paper is that outcome cannot be reliably predicted in the emergency department, and aggressive resuscitation of near-drowning victims should take place with decisions to withdraw life-support made at a later time in the course of the patient's care when the state of cerebral function can be established.

S.D. Barnes, M.D.

A Comparison of Severity of Illness Scoring Systems for Critically Ill Obstetric Patients

El-Solh AA, Grant BJB (State Univ of New York, Buffalo; Buffalo Gen Hosp, NY; Dept of Veterans Affairs Med Ctr, Buffalo, NY)
Chest 110:1299–1304, 1996   8–23

Introduction.—Various predictive scoring systems have been proposed for use in clinical decision making. However, there are questions about how these systems apply to specific patient groups. Three different illness severity scoring systems were compared for their predictive ability on critically ill obstetric patients.

Methods.—The retrospective study included 93 critically ill obstetric patients and a control group of 96 nonobstetric critically ill patients. The patients, all between 17 and 41 years old, were drawn from a series of 12,740 consecutive ICU admissions. The 3 scoring systems compared for their predictive ability were the acute physiology and chronic health evaluation (APACHE II), the simplified acute physiology score (SAPS II), and the mortality probability models.

Methods.—Forty patients scheduled for potentially curative surgery for colorectal or gastric adenocarcinoma were studied prospectively. Twenty participants drank 1 L of a control enteral formula daily for the 7 days preceding surgery and were supplemented with the same formula by jejunal infusion for 7 days after surgery. The remaining patients received the enteral formula enriched with RNA, omega-3 fatty acids, and arginine on the same schedule. Immune function was estimated by the phagocytic activity of polymorphonuclear cells and the intensity of their respiratory burst. Plasma concentrations of C-reactive protein (CRP) were measured as an indicator of inflammatory response. Measured indicators of gut function included intestinal mucosa oxygen metabolism, intestinal micro-perfusion, and plasma concentration of the intestinal isoenzyme of alka-line phosphatase.

Results.—The phagocytic ability of polymorphonuclear cells decreased significantly in the control group, but not the treatment group, during the first 4 days after surgery. The intensity of the respiratory burst of poly-morphonuclear cells was greater in patients receiving enriched formula than in the control group on days 1 and 8 after surgery, but not on day 4. The CRP levels increased beginning 1 day after surgery in both groups; however, the magnitude of the increase was significantly less in patients receiving enriched formula than in controls. Intestinal microperfusion and intestinal mucosa oxygen metabolism were significantly greater in the enriched group than in controls, and plasma concentrations of the intes-tinal isoenzyme of alkaline phosphatase were 85%, 57%, and 63% lower in the enriched group than in the control group on postsurgical days 1, 4, and 8, respectively.

Conclusions.—Perioperative enteric supplementation, using an enriched formula, significantly modulated the expected postsurgical immunosup-pression and inflammation, and improved gut function in this patient cohort. Further research, involving larger patient cohorts, is required to confirm the modulatory effects of enriched enteric formulas administered during the perioperative period.

▶ Further evidence of the concept called "immunonutrition," i.e., enhanc-ing immune function through enteral feedings. The number of patients involved in the study was small, and the outcome variables did not involve survival, but the study is worth reading for those interested in this esoteric and poorly understood area of critical care.

C. Franklin, M.D.

Randomized, Double-blind Study of Intravenous Human Albumin in Hypoalbuminemic Patients Receiving Total Parenteral Nutrition

Rubin H, Carlson S, DeMeo M, et al (Northwestern Univ, Chicago)
Crit Care Med 25:249–252, 1997   8–26

Purpose.—Whether because of increased catabolism, decreased synthesis, or both, serum albumin increases in patients who have acute illness or have undergone major surgery. In hospitalized patients, serum albumin is a useful predictor of mortality. However, it is uncertain whether serum albumin is a useful marker of nutrition. Most previous studies have shown no reduction in morbidity with the administration of human serum albumin to patients receiving total parenteral nutrition (TPN). The effects of IV albumin administration were investigated in hospitalized patients with hypoalbuminemia.

Methods.—The randomized, blind, placebo-controlled trial included 31 patients with a serum albumin concentration of less than 2.5 g/dL who were receiving at least 6 days of TPN. All were adults and free of metastatic cancer, cirrhosis, and nephrotic syndrome. Each patient received 6 or more days of therapy with either albumin or placebo. All were monitored through discharge or death. Albumin kinetics were evaluated as well.

Results.—The 2 groups were comparable in terms of hospital days on TPN and days on their assigned drug. Death occurred within 30 days for 1 patient in the placebo group and 2 in the albumin group. Sepsis and bacteremia occurred in 1 and 3 patients, respectively. Pneumonia occurred in 4 patients in the placebo group and in 7 in the albumin group. None of these differences were significant. All patients in the albumin group had an increase in serum albumin, including 1 patient who received albumin for only 6 days. The mean increase in serum albumin was 1.42 g/dL in the albumin group, versus 0.29 in the placebo group. Albumin metabolism increased from 17.4–20.5 g/day. Overall, the results suggested that albumin was causing more harm than good, and the study was discontinued.

Conclusions.—Giving IV albumin to hospitalized patients with hypoalbuminemia does not appear to have any benefit, despite the fact that serum albumin increases during such treatment. Given the high cost of human serum albumin, the researchers recommend a reduction in its use for patients receiving TPN.

▶ This study is really too small to draw any strong conclusions about the routine use of intravenous albumin. However, there was really no evidence of a clinically important trend.

J.E. Calvin, Jr., M.D.
J.E. Parrillo, M.D.

Skeletal Muscle Glutathione Is Depleted in Critically Ill Patients

Hammarqvist F, Luo J-L, Cotgreave IA, et al (St Göran's Hosp, Stockholm; Hiddinge Univ, Stockholm; Karolinska Inst, Stockholm)
Crit Care Med 25:78–84, 1997

8–27

Objective.—In critically ill patients, the formation of oxygen free radicals and peroxides is increased. These reactive oxygen species can be detoxified by the endogenous scavenger glutathione, which, thus, counteracts oxidative injury. The muscle protein catabolic state observed in critically ill patients could affect the level of glutathione in their skeletal muscle. Reduced and total glutathione levels in the skeletal muscle of critically ill patients were assessed, including their relationship to the free amino acid pattern in muscle tissue.

Methods.—The prospective study included 11 mechanically ventilated, critically ill patients who had been in the ICU for at least 4 days. Each underwent measurement of reduced and total glutathione concentrations in skeletal muscle, in plasma, and in whole blood. Free amino acid concentrations in muscle were also measured. The same measurements were made in a group of metabolically healthy age- and sex-matched controls.

Results.—The reduced glutathione level in the critically ill patients was 57% that of controls; total glutathione was 62% of the control value. The ratio of reduced to total glutathione was 0.80 in critically ill patients vs. 0.91 in controls. Glutamine concentration in the ICU group was 72% of the control value. Glutamine was significantly correlated with total muscle glutathione and with the ratio of reduced and total glutathione in skeletal muscle. This suggested a relationship between glutathione redox status and tissue glutamine status.

Conclusion.—Critically ill patients have disturbances of muscle glutathione metabolism. The findings suggest a condition of oxidative stress, with reduced glutathione concentrations in muscle and a lowered ratio of reduced to total glutathione. The result may be impaired muscle defense against oxygen free radicals and changes in amino acid transport. These changes could play a role in the imbalance between protein synthesis and protein degradation observed in protein catabolism of critical illness.

▶ Although a great deal of attention has been paid to the role of cytokines in critical illness, less attention has been devoted to the role of oxygen free radicals. This study showed depletion of total and reduced glutathione levels in critically ill patients. Further study is needed to determine the prognostic value of this reduction and the possible benefit of amino acid replacement or oxygen radical scavengers.

Y. Friedman, M.D.

BLEED: A Classification Tool to Predict Outcomes in Patients With Acute Upper and Lower Gastrointestinal Hemorrhage
Kollef MH, O'Brien JD, Zuckerman GR, et al (Washington Univ, St Louis)
Crit Care Med 25:1125–1132, 1997   8–28

Background.—Acute gastrointestinal (GI) bleeding is a major cause of hospital and ICU admissions. It has been suggested that most patients with this diagnosis can be managed on the intermediate care unit or hospital ward, avoiding ICU admission. However, there has been no validated risk classification schema to predict outcomes for patients with acute GI hemorrhage. A previously described outcome predicting tool—the BLEED criteria—was validated for predictive accuracy in patients with acute upper or lower GI hemorrhage.

Methods.—The study included 465 patients with acute upper or lower GI hemorrhage admitted from the emergency department to 2 teaching hospitals. The emergency physicians made the decision as to whether patients should be admitted to the ICU or hospital ward. This decision was made without the use of the BLEED criteria: ongoing bleeding, low systolic blood pressure, elevated prothrombin time, erratic mental status, and unstable co-morbid disease. Patients meeting these criteria at their initial emergency department assessment were considered high risk. All others were considered low risk. The patients' courses were analyzed for the occurrence of in-hospital complications: recurrent GI bleeding, surgery to control bleeding, or hospital mortality.

Results.—Two hundred nine patients were classified as high risk and 256 as low-risk. The rate of in-hospital complications was greater for patients in the high-risk group, with relative risks of 2.47 at 1 hospital and 8.94 at the other. High-risk patients were more likely to have additional organ system derangements, need more units of transfused packed red blood cells, and have longer hospital stays. Patients at 1 of the hospitals were more likely to be admitted to the ICU than patients at the other hospital; relative risks of ICU admission were 4.21 for low-risk patients and 1.58 for high-risk patients. This practice difference had no apparent effect on patient outcome, however.

Conclusion.—Used in the initial emergency department diagnosis of patients with acute upper and lower GI bleeding, the BLEED criteria can accurately classify patients as to risk of hospital complications. This classification should produce more objective estimates of expected outcomes, thus leading to improvements in the delivery and evaluation of medical care for a common problem. The BLEED classification may prove useful in the development of clinical practice guidelines for acute GI bleeding.

▶ An interesting approach. It deserves further investigation.

B.A. Shapiro, M.D.

Improved Oxygenation After Discontinuing Neuromuscular Blockade

Wilson DF, Jiao J-H (Univ of Virginia, Charlottesville)
Intensive Care Med 23:214–217, 1997   8–29

Introduction.—Although there are guidelines for choice of agent and monitoring for neuromuscular blockade (NMB) during mechanical ventilation for respiratory failure, there are none for when it should be used. Short-term use of NMB may have harmful effects on lung volume and ventilation/perfusion matching. The effects of longer-term use are unknown. This retrospective study examined the effects of prolonged NMB in children with respiratory failure.

Methods.—The study included 68 pediatric ICU patients receiving at least 3 days of mechanical ventilation for pulmonary parenchymal disease. Of these, 28 received NMB at the start of mechanical ventilation and had at least 72 hours of continuous NMB. They were compared with patients not receiving prolonged NMB in terms of diagnoses, pediatric risk of mortality score, indications for and duration of mechanical ventilation and neuromuscular blockade, and blood gas values with corresponding ventilatory measures. In addition, cohort groups of infants with respiratory syncytial virus (RSV) disease who did and did not receive prolonged NMB were compared.

Results.—When NMB was stopped, there was significant improvement in oxygenation and reduction of mean airway pressures, with no change in peak inspiratory pressure. There were no signs of such improvement in the 48 hours before NMB was stopped. Among children with RSV disease, duration of mechanical ventilation was 14 days for those with prolonged NMB vs. 7 days for those without. This was despite the lack of difference in demographic characteristics, illness severity, or impairment of oxygenation.

Conclusion.—In children with respiratory failure receiving mechanical ventilation, cessation of NMB is followed by a rapid improvement in oxygenation. It is uncertain why this improvement occurs, but it could be related to improved lung volumes and improved distribution of ventilation relative to perfusion within the lung. For children with RSV disease, prolonged use of NMB may lead to a prolonged duration of mechanical ventilation.

Risk Factors for Upper Gastrointestinal Bleeding in Intensive Care Unit Patients: Role of *Helicobacter pylori*

Ellison RT III, Perez-Perez G, Welsh CH, et al (Univ of Colorado, Denver; Univ of Massachusetts, Worcester; Vanderbilt Univ, Nashville, Tenn; et al)
Crit Care Med 24:1974–1981, 1996   8–30

Objective.—The incidence of acute upper gastrointestinal (GI) bleeding is significant in patients in ICUs. Although GI bleeding has been attributed to gastritis, its exact cause is not known. Within the last 10 years, *Heli-*

cobacter pylori has been found to be a cause of gastritis and peptic ulcer. The association of the presence of *H. pylori* and the increased rate of upper GI bleeding in ICU patients, other risk factors for upper GI bleeding in the ICU, and the effect of immunoglobulin prophylaxis with the frequency rate of bleeding were investigated in a prospective, multicenter, randomized, controlled, cohort study in 6 tertiary care Department of Veterans Affairs Medical Centers.

Methods.—Between 1990 and 1992, immunoglobulin was administered intravenously to prevent GI bleeding in 874 evaluable ICU patients (15 females), average age 63. Serum immunoglobulin A and G antibodies to *H. pylori* were determined by enzyme-linked immunosorbent assay prior to treatment. Multivariate analysis was performed to determine those variables predictive of GI bleeding.

Results.—Of the 9% of ICU patients who had GI bleeding, significantly more died compared with ICU patients who did not have GI bleeding (49% versus 15%). A serum anti-*H. pylori* immunoglobulin A concentration greater than 1.0 was significantly correlated with upper GI bleeding (OR 1.76). There was no such association with anti-*H. pylori* immunoglobulin G. Multivariate predictors of GI bleeding included acute hepatic failure (OR 6.67), duration of nasogastric tube placement (OR 2.59), alcohol abuse (OR 2.23), chronic renal failure (OR 3.03), and a serum anti-*H. pylori* immunoglobulin A concentration greater than 1.0 (OR 1.92). A history of malignancy decreased the incidence of GI bleeding.

Conclusion.—Acute hepatic failure, duration of nasogastric tube placement, alcohol abuse, chronic renal failure, and a serum anti-*H. pylori* immunoglobulin A concentration greater than 1.0 increased the rate of GI bleeding in ICU patients. These findings need to be confirmed in an independent population before they can be generalized.

▶ Some interesting observations (Abstracts 8–29 and 8–30) of a larger national study. The problem with such observations is the question of cause vs. effect. For instance, does prolonged nasogastric intubation cause GI bleeding, or do factors requiring the nasogastric tube predispose to GI bleeding? As the authors point out, these observations must be prospectively confirmed in an independent population before being used for treatment guidelines.

B.A. Shapiro, M.D.

Hepatopulmonary Syndrome With Progressive Hypoxemia as an Indication for Liver Transplantation: Case Reports and Literature Review
Krowka MJ, Porayko MK, Plevak DJ, et al (Mayo Clinic Rochester, Minn; Methodist Hosp, Indianapolis, Ind)
Mayo Clin Proc 72:44–53, 1997   8–31

Background.—Hepatopulmonary syndrome (HPS) is a pulmonary vascular complication of liver disease. In patients with HPS, severe hypoxemia from pulmonary vascular dilation can be very debilitating. Deciding whether liver transplantation should be performed in patients with advanced liver disease and HPS is difficult. Three patients with progressive and severe hypoxemia who underwent successful liver transplantation and resolution of arterial hypoxemia were described, and the literature was reviewed.

Patients and Outcomes.—The patients were 3 women, ages 23, 28, and 47 years. The severity of HPS was considered as an indication for liver transplantation. Hypoxemia was a major factor in recommending liver transplantation because of concerns about the patients' ability to survive the procedure and postoperative course with their deteriorating pulmonary status.

The first patient had a period of clinically stable hepatic dysfunction, followed by a fairly rapid decrease in synthetic function and quality of life at least 4 months before liver transplantation. This surgery was recommended because of hepatic dysfunction and deteriorating arterial oxygenation from HPS. Liver transplantation was recommended to the second patient mainly because of debilitating, severe hypoxemia, necessitating increasing amounts of supplemental oxygen 24 hours a day with stable hepatic abnormality. Adult respiratory distress syndrome complicated HPS in this patient, but she recovered and subsequently underwent a successful liver transplantation. In the third patient, severity of hypoxemia from HPS was the main reason for transplantation. Clinically, the degree of hepatic dysfunction appeared minimal. Oxygenation was normal in this patient 4 months after transplantation.

Literature Review.—A total of 81 children and adults with HPS who underwent liver transplantation have had their cases reported in the literature. Posttransplantation mortality was 16% and was associated with the severity of hypoxemia. The death rate (30%) was significantly higher among those with a pretransplantation PaO_2 of 50 mm Hg or lower, compared with those with a PaO_2 of more than 50 mm Hg.

Conclusions.—In many patients, HPS appears to be reversible after liver transplantation. Progressive hypoxemia may be an indication for liver transplantation. The criteria for patient selection for children and adults may differ. The long-term outcomes of liver transplantation and HPS resolution have yet to be established.

▶ This article reviews 3 cases of HPS in patients with severe end-stage liver disease who underwent liver transplantation and experienced improvement in their oxygenation. Severe hypoxemia often has been considered a contraindication to undergoing liver transplantation. These authors reviewed the cases of 81 patients with HPS (8 cases from the Mayo Clinic and 73 reports from the literature) who subsequently were managed with a liver transplant to correct the severe hypoxemia and treat the hepatic dysfunction. They found that 70% of these patients survived the transplant and were alive 3 months later. Although this may seem to be an extremely high mortality rate, it should be remembered that these patients had severely compromised oxygenation and metabolic status before surgery. Unfortunately, the limits of this study do not allow for the discovery of the true predictors for successful liver transplantation. The investigators concluded that severe hypoxemia (manifested as a $PaO_2 < 50$ mm Hg and an inability to increase the $PaO_2 > 400$ mm Hg on 100% oxygen in the supine position) was a predictor of increased mortality.

This observation needs to be evaluated prospectively in a multicentered, randomized, controlled clinical trial to assess the effectiveness of this guideline for making decisions regarding the utility of liver transplantation as a treatment for HPS. The good news is that despite the severe degree of hypoxemia that existed in this cohort of patients, the mortality rate at 3 months was only 30%. These results would suggest that there may be a defined benefit for this group of patients with a properly timed liver transplantation.

R.A. Balk, M.D.

Retrieval of Organs for Transplantation: Experience of the Australian National Liver Transplantation Unit
Thompson JF, Liew SCC, Chui AKK, et al (Royal Prince Alfred Hosp, Camperdown, Australia; Children's Hosp, Camperdown, Australia; Univ of Sydney, Australia)
Med J Aust 165:375–378, 1996   8–32

Background.—Liver transplantation has been performed in Australia since 1985, and liver transplantation programs in Australia now have 81% and 73% 1- and 5-year patient survival rates, respectively, figures very satisfactory by world standards. In addition to an adequate availability of cadaveric organs, liver transplantation programs rely upon the efficient coordination and participation of a large number of skilled professionals. The experience of the Australian National Liver Transplantation Unit (ANLTU), in Sydney, in procuring multiple donor organs and the outcome of recipient patients were reviewed.

Donor Organ Procurement.—The time required for organ retrieval varied with distance between the donor and recipient hospitals, with year of operation, and with the number of organs retrieved. Retrieval was fastest (1.9–7.5 hours) when the donor hospital was in the Sydney metropolitan area, and slowest (11.2–13.8 hours) when donors were in New Zealand. The mean operation time for liver and kidney retrieval was 3.5 hours in 1986 and decreased progressively to 1.5 hours in 1993. Retrieval of the heart or heart and pancreas in addition to the liver and kidneys increased operation time to approximately 4 hours in 1993. The mean time between donor aortic cross-clamping and reperfusion of the liver in the recipient was 4.75 hours in 1986, but increased to 8 hours in 1989 and subsequently to 10 hours because of the realization that longer cold ischemia times were safe when University of Wisconsin solution, rather than an albumin-based solution, was used as a preservative. Efficient organ retrieval required a highly coordinated effort of several surgical teams. The average cost of liver transplantation in Australia is approximately $130,000, of which $8,000, or 6%, is spent on retrieval of the organ.

Patient Outcome.—One-year graft survival and 1-year patient survival rates achieved by the ANLTU between 1986 and 1995 were 70.3% and 77.1%, respectively, for 337 transplanted livers, including transplants in 89 high-risk patients. Primary nonfunction of the graft occurred in only 1 transplanted organ (0.3%).

Discussion.—The 1-year graft survival of 70.3% achieved by the ANLTU exceeds that reported in other countries, including the United Kingdom (60% from 1988 to 1993), France (61% from 1981 to 1991), and the United States (70% for adult patients from 1987 to 1992). The rate of primary nonfunction of 0.3% was considerably lower than the 4% to 15% reported from most units, possibly because of an early revascularization technique used by the ANLTU, but only possible as a result of high-quality donor organs and efficient organ retrieval. Because successful organ transplants are only possible when the quality of the donor organ is high, it appears well justified to spend 6% of the total cost of the liver transplantation procedure on organ retrieval.

▶ This is a report of the experience of organ retrieval in Australia where primary nonfunction of a transplanted organ is 0.3% vs. a rate of 4% in the United States. The reason for the lower rate in Australia is not clear but could be related to better organ quality, or their routine use of early temporary arterialization of the donor liver's portal vein via a femoral artery shunt while the hepatic artery anastomosis is made.

L.C. Casey, M.D., Ph.D.

A New Method for Continuous Intramucosal P_{CO_2} Measurement in the Gastrointestinal Tract

Knichwitz G, Rötker J, Brüssel T, et al (Westfälische Wilhelms-Universität, Münster, Germany)
Anesth Analg 83:6–11, 1996

8–33

Introduction.—The problem of P_{CO_2} instability in the tonometric fluid can be solved by finding the direct determination of P_{CO_2} using a fiberoptic P_{CO_2} sensor, which can continuously measure P_{CO_2} in blood. A fiberoptic P_{CO_2} sensor would determine the P_{CO_2} of certain fluid better than conventional tonometry. Such a sensor would determine P_{CO_2} continuously and would avoid equilibration times. Variations in arterial and mesenteric venous P_{CO_2} would have good correlation to the P_iCO_2.

Methods.—A thermocouple for determining temperature, a minaturized Clark electrode for determining P_{CO_2} and 2 modified optical fibers for measuring P_{CO_2} and pH are the components of the fiberoptic P_{CO_2} sensor. The device is 0.5 mm in diameter and has a length of 600 mm. The in vitro experiment determined the P_{CO_2} of water and humidified air with predefined PCO_2 values using the fiberoptic PCO_2 sensor and a nasogastric tonometer. The function of the fiberoptic PCO_2 sensor was determined in fluids comparable to the medium within the gastrointestinal track in an in vitro experiment. The performance of the fiberoptic PCO_2 sensor was evaluated in the gastrointestinal tract of 6 female pigs in the in vivo experiment. Determinations were made on cardiac index, arterial PCO_2, mesenteric venous PCO_2, and intramucosal PCO_2 after preparation and 60 minutes of steady state conditions. Variables also were measured after 10 minutes of hypoventilation and after 10 minutes of hyperventilation.

Results.—After 30, 60, and 90 minutes of equilibration for the 3 different gas concentrations, absolute PCO_2 differences between predefined and measured PCO_2 values were made. After 9 minutes of equilibration, with a maximum deviation less than 3.5%, predefined CO_2 values of 35, 42, 49 mm Hg could be assessed in water and humidified air. Tonometry PCO_2 had greater differences from the predefined PCO_2 than it did with the fiberoptic PCO_2 sensor. In the in vivo experiment during hypoventilation, the intramucosal PCO_2 increased from 53.8 ± 2.0 mm Hg to 66.5 ± 4.9 mm Hg. Arterial PCO_2 went from 39.8 ± 1.4 mm Hg to 52.7 ± 31 mm Hg. Mesenteric venous PCO_2 increased from 48.7 ± 2.7 mm Hg to 62.4 ± 5.7 mm Hg. With hyperventilation, the intramucosal PCO_2 decreased from 46.8 ± 2.5 mm Hg. The coefficient of correlation (r^2) was 0.82 between intramucosal PCO_2 and arterial PCO_2. It was 0.94 between intramucosal PCO_2 and mesenteric venous PCO_2.

Conclusion.—Intramucosal PCO_2 can be determined in a precise and reliable manner with the fiberoptic PCO_2 sensor. Fast intraluminal changes of CO_2 in the ileum caused by ventilatory changes can be continuously recorded with this sensor. In the gastrointestinal tract, the fiberoptic PCO_2 sensor appears to be a more reliable monitor of intramucosal PCO_2.

▶ The ability to accurately and "noninvasively" assess impaired gastrointestinal perfusion would be clinically useful, especially if alterations prognosticate survival.[1] Nasogastric tonometry is currently available to assess perfusion of the gastrointestinal tract by measuring intraluminar PCO_2. Methodologically, problems include delayed equilibration; consistent underestimation, even at 90 minutes; and difficulty in injecting and aspirating airless saline. A phosphate-buffered solution instead of saline appears to have eliminated the inaccuracy of PCO_2 determination by blood gas analyzers.

The fiberoptic PCO_2 sensor does appear, both in pigs and glass beakers, to measure PCO_2 with greater accuracy than nasogastric tonometers, which are used currently. Like the fluid-filled tonometer, there appears to be a consistent offset with the fiberoptic PCO_2 sensor. In this case, the sensor consistently overestimated the mesenteric venous PCO_2. Although systemic offsets can be accounted for, the main advantage of the fiberoptic sensor over the nasogastric tonometer is the rapid equilibration time. It appears that the fiberoptic sensor accurately measures PCO_2 within 10 minutes, compared with 30–90 minutes for the fluid-filled nasogastric tonometer. In critically ill patients with variable perfusion, the ability to rapidly determine at the tissue level, the effect of volume, vasopressor or ionotropic support could be quite useful. For physicians currently using nasogastric tonometers, the fiberoptic sensor may provide them with intramucosal P_{CO_2} information more quickly. Other physicians not currently monitoring gastric P_{CO_2} may prefer to await clinical studies demonstrating improved clinical outcomes as a result of monitoring and responding to measured gastric P_{CO_2}.

M.R. Silver, M.D.

Reference

1. Gutierrez G, Palizas F, Doglio G, et al: Gastric intramucosal pH as a therapeutic index of tissue oxgenation in critically ill patients. *Lancet* 339:195–199, 1992.

N-Acetylcycsteine Improves Indocyanine Green Extraction and Oxygen Transport During Hepatic Dysfunction

Devlin J, Ellis AE, McPeake J, et al (King's College School of Medicine and Dentistry, London)
Crit Care Med 25:236–242, 1997

8–34

Background.—Patients with sepsis complicating liver disease have systemic hemodynamic derangements similar to those seen in other forms of critical illness, but often more severe. Pharmacologic manipulation of hemodynamics in severely ill patients should ideally use an agent that improves systemic and regional oxygen delivery without stimulating cellular metabolism. In patients with fulminant hepatic failure, N-acetylcysteine increases cyclic guanosine monophosphate (cGMP) concentration. This study examined the effects of N-acetylcysteine in other liver disorders, including its effect on the hepatic-splanchnic circulation.

Methods.—The study included 15 patients with hepatic dysfunction who were on mechanical ventilation. Eight were studied after liver transplantation and 7 during an acute or decompensated chronic liver disorder. All received prostacyclin at a continuous infusion rate of 5 ng/kg/min for 60 min. After a washout period, the patients received a 15 minute infusion of N-acetylcysteine at 150 mg/kg in 250 mL of 5% dextrose in water; then a 45 minute infusion of N-acetylcysteine at 50 mg/kg in 250 mL of 5% dextrose, at a rate of 62.5 mL/hr. The hemodynamic effects of these infusions were compared.

Results.—N-acetylcysteine infusion was followed by an increase in oxygen delivery, from 667 to 751 mL/min/m². Oxygen consumption improved in 13 of 15 patients, from 150 to 169 mL/min/m². A fiberoptic physiologic monitoring system showed improvement in indocyanine green clearance in 13 of 15 patients, from 7.3% to 11.8%. The 40% of patients whose oxygen consumption increased more than 10% from baseline were considered systemic hemodynamic responders. Baseline oxygen consumption in this group was 133 mL/min/m², compared with 162 mL/min/m² in nonresponders. The increase in oxygen consumption was not significantly related to the increase in indocyanine green clearance. Systemic oxygen delivery was moderately improved by prostacyclin, and indocyanine green

elective AAA patients. The response to unopsonized zymosan was 3 times greater in patients with ruptured AAA than in elective AAA patients (899.8 versus 299.7). The response to complement opsonized zymosan with C5a significantly reduced oxidative burst in phagocytes of patients with ruptured AAA. The response to PMA stimulation was significantly increased in these patients compared with patients with elective AAA (8769.1 vs. 3508.8). C3a des arg levels were similar for both groups.

Conclusion.—Phagocyte priming is involved in the systemic inflammatory response in patients with a ruptured AAA. Oxidative activity is increased during the postoperative period in patients with elective AAA. Phagocyte priming can occur via a receptor-mediated or receptor-independent mechanism.

▶ This article studied phagocyte oxidative burst in patients undergoing either elective or emergent AAA repair. Phagocytes from patients with ruptured aortas requiring emergent repair had increased oxidative burst activity even prior to the surgery. The mechanism for this observation is unclear, but it might contribute to the high incidence of multi-system organ failure seen in patients with ruptured aortas.

L.C. Casey, M.D., Ph.D.

Renal

Predicting Mortality in Intensive Care Patients With Acute Renal Failure Treated With Dialysis
Douma CE, Redekop WK, van der Meulen JHP, et al (Academic Med Ctr, Amsterdam; The Found of Home Dialysis Midden-West Nederland, Utrecht, The Netherlands)
J Am Soc Nephrol 8:111–117, 1997   8–37

Introduction.—Aside from technical improvements, there has been little improvement in the mortality of patients with acute renal failure in an ICU. Many patients even die with dialysis treatment, and it would be useful to know whether it is possible to predict the likelihood of mortality of a patient with acute renal failure before dialysis is initiated. In ICU patients on dialysis for acute renal failure, existing prognostic methods were compared for their ability to predict mortality. It also was hoped that 1 of these models could identify the patients who would not benefit from dialysis because of near 100% certainty of death.

Methods.—There were 238 adult patients who received a first dialysis treatment for acute renal failure in the ICU in this retrospective study. Seven general ICU mortality prediction models and 4 mortality prediction models developed for patients with acute renal failure were examined for their performance, ability to discriminate mortality from survival, and ability to calibrate the observed mortality rate with the expected mortality rate.

Results.—In this patient group, the observed in-hospital mortality rate was 76%. The observed mortality in the highest quintiles of risk was 97%

with the Acute Physiology and Chronic Health Evaluation (APACHE) III model, and it was 98% with the Liano model.

Conclusion.—Excellent discrimination between those patients who died in-hospital and those who did not was found in any of the models. However, the Liano model and the APACHE III model identified a group of patients with a near 100% chance of mortality. To support the decision not to initiate dialysis in a subgroup of patients, these models may have some use. These 2 models can be considered an adjunct to the clinician's informed, but subjective, opinion.

▶ This retrospective study demonstrates that the APACHE III and Liano scoring systems identify a group of patients who, when they develop acute renal failure, have an in-hospital mortality close to 100%. They suggest that this mortality risk estimate may function as a decision support method regarding whether or not to institute dialysis. However, as with similar studies predicting mortality, this may not be any more useful in making predictions for the individual patients than the judgment of the experienced clinicians.

Y. Friedman, M.D.

Haemodialysis Without Anticoagulant: Haemostasis Parameters, Fibrinogen Kinetic, and Dialysis Efficiency
Ramão JE Jr, Fadil MA, Sabbaga E, et al (Univ of São Paulo, Brazil)
Nephrol Dial Transplant 12:106–110, 1997   8–38

Introduction.—For patients at high-risk of bleeding, systemic anticoagulation with heparin has the potential for serious complications. Hemodialysis without anticoagulant has been used in these patients, but there are concerns about the possibility of blood defibrination and fibrin deposition in the dialytic membrane, leading to reduced dialyzer efficacy. Hemostasis parameters, fibrinogen kinetics, and dialysis efficiency were studied in patients undergoing hemodialysis without anticoagulant.

Methods.—Ten patients with chronic uremia undergoing hemodialysis were studied. The patients were studied during 2 consecutive 4-hour dialysis sessions, once with heparin anticoagulation and once without. During each session, hemostasis parameters, ^{125}I-fibrinogen turnover, ^{125}I-fibrinogen deposition in the dialyzer membrane, and dialytic efficiency were studied.

Results.—Mean platelet count, plasma fibrinogen, prothrombin time, and antithrombin III were no different for hemodialysis with vs. without anticoagulation. During hemodialysis without anticoagulation, mean activated partial thromboplastin time was significantly shortened from baseline. Conventional dialysis was associated with no change in fibrin-fibrinogen degradation products. These values were significantly increased after 30 minutes of hemodialysis without anticoagulation, but remained in the range of normal. The biological half-life of ^{125}I-fibrinogen fell from 5 days before hemodialysis to 2.5 days during hemodialysis without anticoagulation; there was no significant change during hemodialysis with anticoagulation. Mean ^{125}I-fibrinogen deposition in the dialyzer membranes was greater during hemodialysis without anticoagulation than during conventional hemodialysis. However, this made no difference in dialyzer efficiency, whether assessed in terms of serum urea, creatinine, potassium, or bicarbonate or by hematocrit. Mean Kt/V was 0.873 for hemodialysis without anticoagulation and 0.870 for hemodialysis with anticoagulation.

Conclusions.—Compared to conventional hemodialysis, hemostasis parameters are unchanged during hemodialysis without anticoagulation. However, hemodialysis without anticoagulation is associated with some activation of the coagulation system. Iodine-125 fibrinogen half-life is reduced and fibrin deposition on dialyzer membranes is increased during hemodialysis without anticoagulation, but dialyzer efficiency is unchanged.

▶ Critically ill patients often have coagulopathies or are prone to hemorrhagic complications. This study evaluated the efficiency of dialysis without the use of heparin in 10 stable patients with chronic uremia. Although there was an increase in fibrinogen deposition on the dialysis membrane, there was no adverse effect or alteration in the efficiency of dialysis. This study substantiates that the performance of dialysis without the use of anticoagulation is an acceptable alternative for patients with chronic renal failure who are at risk for bleeding complications or in whom heparin should be avoided.

R.A. Balk, M.D.

Effect of Continuous Venovenous Hemofiltration With Dialysis on Lactate Clearance in Critically Ill Patients
Levraut J, Ciebiera J-P, Jambou P, et al (Centre Hospitalo-Universitaire de Nice, France)
Crit Care Med 25:58–62, 1997   8–39

Introduction.—Continuous venovenous hemofiltration with dialysis would appear to be well suited for management of acute renal failure in the ICU. Previous studies, however, suggest that because a large amount of plasma lactate is filtered with this technique, the blood lactate concentration fails to reflect tissue oxygenation status. A prospective study was designed to determine the effect of continuous venovenous hemofiltration with dialysis on lactate elimination in critically ill patients.

Methods.—The study group included 10 patients with acute renal failure and stable blood lactate concentrations. All were receiving continuous venovenous hemofiltration with dialysis. In a 2-stage investigation, lactate clearance by the hemofilter was calculated by measuring lactate concentrations in samples of serum and ultradiafiltrate. Total plasma lactate clearance was evaluated by infusing sodium L-lactate (1 mmol/kg of body weight) over 15 minutes. Arterial lactate concentration was determined before, during, and after the infusion.

Results.—Patients had a median ultrafiltration rate of 714 mL/hr. The blood lactate concentration did not significantly alter hemofilter clearances of urea and lactate. Median filter clearance of urea was 23.8 mL/min, and median filter clearance of lactate was 24.2 mL/min. The lactate concentration in the ultradiafiltrate did not differ significantly from the lactate concentration in the blood. Thus, the lactate-sieving coefficient was not significantly different from 1. Filter lactate clearance showed a close correlation with the filter urea clearance. The median blood lactate concentration increased from 1.4 to 4.8 mmol/L at the end of the infusion, then returned to 1.6 mmol/L 60 minutes later.

Discussion.—Filter lactate clearance was found to account for less than 3% of total lactate clearance. Because the lactate removed by continuous venovenous hemofiltration with dialysis is negligible, compared with the overall plasma lactate clearance, blood lactate concentration is minimally altered with the technique and remains a reliable marker of tissue oxygenation.

▶ The authors demonstrate that venovenous hemofiltration with dialysis does not mask the overproduction of lactate. This suggests that the technique can be used in acute renal failure in multiorgan failure without sacrificing the ability to monitor tissue oxygenation.

J. Samuel, M.D.

Predictive Factors for High Mortality in Hypernatremic Patients
Mandal AK, Saklayen MG, Hillman NM, et al (Wright State Univ Dayton, Ohio)
Am J Emerg Med 15:130–132, 1997   8–40

Introduction.—The causes of high mortality in patients with hypernatremia (serum sodium level above 145 mEq/L) are not completely understood. An analysis was conducted to determine the relationship of serum sodium, blood pressure (BP), cognitive function, and therapeutic interventions to high mortality in patients with hypernatremia.

Methods.—Medical records of 116 patients admitted over a 12-month period with a diagnosis of hypernatremia were reviewed for data regarding the following: age and gender; serum sodium levels; whether hypernatremia was first detected in the emergency department, during a clinic visit, or in the hospital; whether hypernatremia led to hospital admission; primary diagnosis; status of cognitive functioning; gastrointestinal symptoms; use of diuretics or nonsteroidal anti-inflammatory drugs; BP; and type of fluid therapy.

Results.—Of 116 patients, 77 (66%) died and 39 (34%) survived and were discharged from the hospital. There were no significant differences in the following factors between nonsurvivors and survivors: gender or age

(70.9 vs. 66.4 years), mean admission sodium level (154.9 vs. 155.1 mEq/L), or mean peak serum sodium level (157.5 vs. 156.8 mEq/L). Nonsurvivors had significantly higher mean late serum sodium levels than nonsurvivors (151.2 vs. 143.1 mEq/L). Nonsurvivors had lower systolic and diastolic BP at admission and throughout the hospital course than survivors. Cognitive abnormalities (confusion, obtundation, and speech abnormality) were significantly higher in nonsurvivors than they were in survivors. Normal saline solution was used significantly more frequently in nonsurvivors than survivors.

Conclusion.—These findings are consistent with earlier reports and confirm that hypernatremia is associated with a high probability of mortality in patients older than 65 years. Higher mean late sodium levels, lower BP throughout hospitalization, higher cognitive abnormalities, and use of normal saline infusions were predictive of high mortality.

▶ Dr. Mandal, et al analyzed 116 patients with hypernatremia at 2 large university-affiliated teaching hospitals to identify factors that predict high mortality. They present new information about the relationships between hypernatremic death, serum sodium levels, hypotension, and the type of fluid administered. Hypernatremic patients who were hypotensive did poorly, compared with those who were normotensive. The type of fluid administered seemed to correlate with mortality, since administration of normal saline solution was associated with a poor prognosis. The authors appropriately point out that this relationship may be due to the fact that patients with hypotension and hypernatremia did tend to receive saline solution. It also is important to note that hypernatremic patients who corrected their serum sodium levels had a lower mortality than those who had persistent late hypernatremia. It is possible that hypotension and late hypernatremia may be signs of patients who are more severely ill.

These studies emphasize the already reported high mortality rate in patients with hypernatremia and identify circumstances associated with a poor prognosis. This retrospective study, however, does not give us new insight into the best methods for treating these patients.

R.V. Rege, M.D.

Therapeutic Recommendations for Management of Severe Hyponatremia: Current Concepts on Pathogenesis and Prevention of Neurologic Complications
Soupart A, Decaux G (Free Univ of Brussels, Belgium)
Clin Nephrol 46:149–169, 1996

8–41

Introduction.—If untreated or treated inappropriately, severe hyponatremia—defined as a serum sodium level of less than 120 mEq/L—can have serious neurologic complications. The hyponatremia causes brain edema, increasing intracranial pressure and possibly leading to neuropathologic complications or death. If the sodium level is excessively corrected, demyelinating lesions, such as central pontine or extrapontine myelinosis, can occur, leading to major disability or death. To understand these events, the clinician must understand the way in which the brain adapts to changes in osmolality. The pathogenesis and management of severe hyponatremia were reviewed.

Pathogenesis.—In the presence of low serum sodium levels, the brain tries to prevent swelling by extruding electrolytes and organic osmolytes. This process is nearly complete by 48 hours. When serum sodium increases again, intracerebral osmolytes are re-established, although their reuptake takes about 5 days. At either stage, brain damage can occur if these mechanisms become overwhelmed.

Management.—Acute hyponatremia (hyponatremia lasting less than 48 hours) usually occurs in the hospital. It generally develops postoperatively and/or after excessive fluid administration. Seizures, respiratory arrest, and coma—sometimes very sudden—can occur after abrupt declines in serum sodium values. It is essential to recognize and promptly treat even minor symptoms of hyponatremia. Patients with acute hyponatremia are generally not at risk of brain myelinosis. Female sex, hypoxia, and younger age may aggravate the prognosis of hyponatremic encephalopathy.

Chronic hyponatremia (hyponatremia lasting longer than 48 hours) usually develops outside the hospital and is usually not as serious. For these patients, a correction level of no greater than 15 mEq/L/24 hr will help to reduce the risk of brain myelinosis. However, as long as the final correction is less than this level, the initial rate of correction can be faster. The rate of correction should be slower still—less than 10 mEq/L/24 hr—for patients with risk factors for myelinosis, i.e., hypokalemia, liver disease, poor nutritional status, or burns.

Correction of Hyponatremia.—Demyelinization can occur in hypernatremia, but generally only when the serum sodium level increases by more than 50% over baseline. Hyponatremic saline (3%) infusion can achieve rapid correction in patients with symptomatic hyponatremia. Urea can also be given, orally or IV. This treatment quickly lowers the brain edema and intracranial pressure, thus permitting correction of hyponatremia. Treatment with urea may also reduce the risk of myelinosis. Patients who have hyponatremia but are asymptomatic do not need rapid correction. They should receive conservative treatment, with close monitoring of the serum sodium level. If indicated, correction can be stopped and diuresis interrupted with desmopressin acetate. Recent studies suggest that hypotonic fluids and desmopressin acetate can rapidly reduce serum sodium—thus decreasing the risk of myelinosis—in patients with overcorrection of hyponatremia.

Discussion.—The article includes detailed guidelines for the correction of severe hyponatremia whether acute and symptomatic, chronic and symptomatic, or asymptomatic.

▶ The information presented in this article is critical for anyone working in the ICU. Although there are still major gaps in our understanding of how to deal with hyponatremia, the article goes a long way toward putting all the available information into 1 very complete work. The flow sheets presented in the original article should be part of any intensivist's treatment plan for this disorder.

E. Gluck, M.D.

Effect of Bicarbonate Administration on Plasma Potassium in Dialysis Patients: Interactions With Insulin and Albuterol

Allon M, Shanklin N (Univ of Alabama, Birmingham; VA Med Ctr, Birmingham, Ala)

Am J Kidney Dis 28:508–514, 1996

8–42

Introduction.—Hyperkalemia with electrocardiographic changes in patients with end-stage renal disease is a medical emergency requiring acute hemodialysis. Temporizing measures are required because of the inevitable delay in initiating dialysis and interventions that decrease plasma potassium are required; this can be achieved by the administration of insulin and albuterol. Another temporizing measure that is recommended is IV administration of sodium bicarbonate, but studies have shown this to be ineffective. For the acute management of hyperkalemia in dialysis patients,

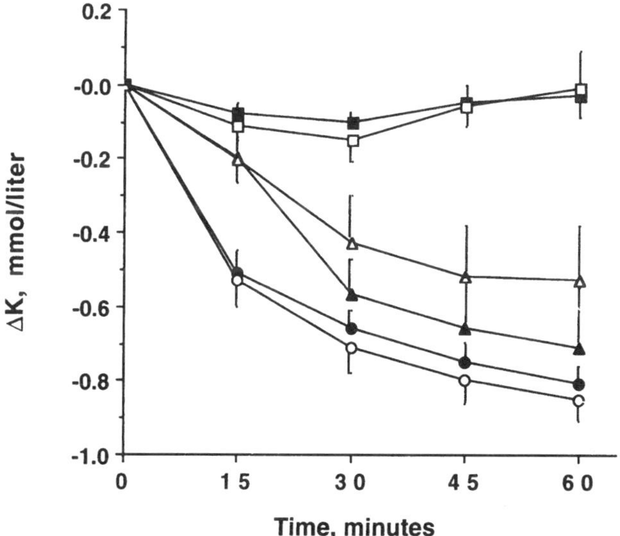

FIGURE 1.—Effect of 6 treatment protocols on plasma potassium. After obtaining a baseline blood sample, treatment was initiated with 1 of six experimental protocols: protocol 1, isotonic sodium bicarbonate (*solid squares*); protocol 2, isotonic saline (*open squares*); protocol 3, IV insulin with dextrose plus isotonic bicarbonate (*solid circles*); protocol 4, IV insulin with dextrose plus isotonic saline (*open circles*); protocol 5, nebulized albuterol plus isotonic bicarbonate (*solid triangles*); and protocol 6, nebulized albuterol plus isotonic saline (*open triangles*). Data are presented as mean values ± SE. Effects of protocols 1 and 2, P = NS; effects of protocols 3 and 4, P less than 0.001 vs. baseline; effects of protocols 5 and 6, P less than 0.01 vs. baseline. (Courtesy of Allon M, Shanklin N: Effect of bicarbonate administration on plasma potassium in dialysis patients: Interactions with insulin and albuterol. *Am J Kidney Dis* 28: 508–514, 1996.)

there has not been a systematic investigation of the value of bicarbonate administration in conjunction with other treatment modalities.

Methods.—In 8 nondiabetic hemodialysis patients, the acute effects of insulin and albuterol on plasma potassium, as well as blood bicarbonate and pH, were investigated with the following protocols: isotonic bicarbonate, isotonic saline, insulin plus bicarbonate, insulin plus saline, albuterol plus bicarbonate, and albuterol plus saline. Plasma potassium was measured every 15 minutes over 1 hour after a baseline blood sample had been taken.

Results.—Plasma potassium was not decreased significantly by isotonic bicarbonate or by isotonic saline (Fig 1). At 60 minutes, neither isotonic bicarbonate (-0.03 ± 0.06 mmol/L) nor isotonic saline (-0.01 ± 0.10 mmol/L) decreased plasma potassium significantly. At 60 minutes, plasma potassium was decreased by a similar level with IV insulin with bicarbonate (-0.81 ± 0.05 mmol/L) and with IV insulin with saline (-0.85 ± 0.06 mmol/L). At 60 minutes, plasma potassium was decreased by a similar degree with nebulized albuterol with bicarbonate (-0.71 ± 0.16 mmol/L) and with nebulized albuterol with saline (-0.53 ± 0.15 mmol/L). Significant increases in blood bicarbonate resulted with the 3 protocols that included clinical trials; the role of cortisol replacement therapy in septic shock with high-output circulatory failure has to be clarified.

▶ Dialysis with removal of excessive potassium is the definitive treatment for patients with acute renal failure and hyperkalemia. Insulin and/or calcium have been used as temporizing measures while awaiting initiation of dialysis. Administration of sodium bicarbonate has also been suggested to lower serum potassium. This study clearly demonstrates that the administration of sodium bicarbonate does little to serum potassium levels in chronic nondiabetic hemodialysis patients. Not only is its effect minimal when given alone, it did not enhance the effectiveness of insulin and glucose. Whether bicarbonate administration is equally ineffective in diabetic patients, patients with acute renal failure, or patients with significant metabolic acidosis is still not known. For patients without these conditions, bicarbonate does change the serum pH, but it does little to serum potassium.

M.R. Silver, M.D.

Alkalinization Is Ineffective for Severe Hyperkalemia in Nonnephrectomized Dogs

Kaplan JL, and the Hyperkalemia Reseach Group (Albert Einstein Med Ctr, Philadelphia; Temple Univ, Philadelphia; Philadelphia College of Osteopathic Medicine, Philadelphia)

Acad Emerg Med 4:93–99, 1997 8–43

Objective.—Many textbooks recommend alkalinization with sodium bicarbonate ($NaHCO_3$) for hyperkalemia. However, clinical studies do not support this recommendation. The results showed only modest or slow lowering of potassium (K) level, and included patients with only slightly elevated K levels. The effects of emergency alkalinization with $NaHCO_3$ in dogs with severe hyperkalemia causing cardiac conduction abnormalities were studied.

Methods.—Dogs were anesthetized and given KCl in a dose sufficient to induce sustained idioventricular or relative junctional bradycardic dysrhythmias. They were then placed on a maintenance dose of KCl. Forty-five minutes later, they received 1 of 3 treatments; each animal received 3 treatments in separate experiments performed at least 1 week apart. The treatments were infusion therapy, consisting of 1.05% $NaHCO_3$ given over 60 minutes; bolus therapy, consisting of 8.4% $NaHCO_3$ over 5 minutes, followed by 14 mL/kg of sterile water over 55 minutes; and saline therapy, consisting of 8.4% NaCl given over 5 minutes, followed by 14 mL/kg of sterile water over 55 minutes.

Results.—In all experiments, the dogs had a mean pretreatment K level of 9.06 mmol/L. A greater reduction in K level was achieved after saline therapy than after bolus therapy. However, for the first 30 minutes of treatment, the differences were neither statistically nor clinically significant. The means of the differences in reductions, calculated as saline minus bolus, were 0.26 at 15 minutes and 0.16 at 30 minutes. One of the 5 dogs studied had a shorter duration of dysrhythmia with bolus therapy than with saline therapy.

Conclusions.—In this canine model of life-threatening hyperkalemia, plasma K is lowered as effectively in the first 30 minutes after hypertonic saline bolus as with $NaHCO_3$ bolus. On its own, alkalinization is unlikely to achieve a clinically important reduction in K level within this time frame. The findings indicate the need for further study of $NaHCO_3$ as first-line therapy for severe hyperkalemia.

▶ This study is very provocative. Generally, alkalinization has been widely recommended for the treatment of hyperkalemia. In this study, hypertonic saline was as effective as $NaHCO_3$ to reverse the hyperkalemia in this model. This was a controlled study making it unique among previous studies of this question. Other potential mechanisms for the effects of hypertonic saline were not studied and can only be speculated. This study would suggest that the clinical efficacy of $NaHCO_3$ may be related to the Na and water load. More studies really are necessary to support or refute clinical recommendations regarding the use of $NaHCO_3$ for treating hyperkalemia.

J.E. Calvin, Jr., M.D.

J.E. Parrillo, M.D.

Hemostatic Disorder of Uremia: The Platelet Defect, Main Determinant of the Prolonged Bleeding Time, Is Correlated With Indices of Activation of Coagulation and Fibrinolysis

Mezzano D, Tagle R, Panes O, et al (Catholic Univ, Valdivia, Chile; Univ of Chile, Santiago; Austral Univ, Valdivia, Chile)
Thromb Haemost 76:312–321, 1996

8–44

Background.—Patients with chronic renal failure (CRF) also suffer an increased bleeding tendency and an increased incidence of thrombotic events. The authors hypothesize that these defects of hemostasis are the result of continuous exposure of platelets, endothelial cells, and/or von Willebrand factor to low doses of thrombin and/or plasmin.

Objectives.—The purpose of this study was to identify hemostasis defects in patients with CRF that might prolong bleeding time; to detect biochemical evidence for activation of coagulation and fibrinolysis; and to relate the hemostasis defects to abnormalities in coagulation and fibrinolysis.

Methods.—The subjects were 48 patients with severe CRF (creatinine clearance less than 20 mL/min) who were not on dialysis and had no disease or drug therapy affecting hemostasis. Blood samples were analyzed and compared with samples from healthy control subjects. Bleeding time was determined for up to 20 minutes.

Results.—Plasma markers of thrombin and plasmin were increased in these patients, and there was evidence of increased plasmin activity. Bleeding time was prolonged in 52% of patients. Prolonged bleeding time was positively correlated with abnormal platelet aggregation–secretion and with severity of renal failure. It was negatively correlated with hematocrit reading and age. The only platelet structural defect that correlated with the platelet dysfunction was a decrease in adenine nucleotide content. Levels of platelet adenosine triphosphate and adenosine diphosphate were negatively correlated with indices of activation of coagulation and fibrinolysis.

Conclusions.—Accelerated generation of thrombin and plasmin in these patients is initial evidence that primary hemostasis in CRF is linked to activation of coagulation and fibrinolysis. This and the other findings suggest that in uremic patients, prolonged bleeding time and increased thrombotic risk may have a common mechanism.

▶ This study evaluated the potential mechanism(s) surrounding the prolongation of the bleeding time observed in the setting of CRF. The study was well structured to avoid patients who were on continuous dialysis, as well as those patients who could have other co-existing coagulation abnormalities. Sophisticated analyses of both procoagulation and anticoagulation pathways were conducted. The findings demonstrated that there was low-grade, regulated activation of both coagulation and fibrinolysis, as evidenced by the accelerated generation of both plasmin and thrombin. Subsequent thrombotic effects are explainable by this excess generation of thrombin, whereas in the setting of relatively low amounts of thrombin and plasmin, there was a reduction in the levels of platelet ADP and ATP, which were associated with defects in platelet aggregation and secretion. This observation was believed to be the main determinant of platelet dysfunction and responsible for the prolongation in the bleeding time that is present in a majority of patients with CRF. Thus, the intricate balance between thrombin and plasmin may be instrumental in thrombotic complications and the prolonged bleeding time noted in patients with CRF.

R.A. Balk, M.D.

Hematology

Does Transfusion Practice Affect Mortality in Critically Ill Patients?
Hébert PC, for the Transfusion Requirements in Critical Care (TRICC) Investigators and the Canadian Critical Care Trials Group (Ottawa Gen Hosp, Ont, Canada)
Am J Respir Crit Care Med 155:1618–1623, 1997   8–45

Background.—The fear of HIV and other transfusion-related infections has prompted a re-evaluation of transfusion practices. These evaluations have generated recommendations and guidelines by the American College of Physicians and other organizations. The guidelines, however, do not specifically address patients who are critically ill. Recommendations derived from studies in other patient populations may not apply to patients who are critically ill because of the complex metabolic and cardiovascular changes that occur in the latter. There is little information regarding the clinical consequences of anemia and transfusion practice in such patients.

Methods.—There were 4,470 patients enrolled in a study of the impact of transfusion or mortality rates in critically ill patients. There were 2,660 enrolled at the time of ICU admission and 1,810 identified by a retrospective review of medical records. All patients were older than 16 years. All hemoglobin values and the number and timing of allogeneic red cell transfusions were included in the analysis. The main outcome measure was ICU mortality.

Results.—Patients who died in the ICU had lower hemoglobin values and received red cells more frequently than patients who did not. In patients with cardiac disease, mortality was higher in those with hemoglobin values less than 95 g/L compared with patients with anemia and other diagnoses (Fig 1). Significantly lower mortality was seen in patients with anemia, high Acute Physiology and Chronic Health Evaluation II scores, and cardiac disease when they received 1 to 3, or 4 to 6 units of allogeneic red cells. The adjusted odds ratio predicting survival was 0.61 after transfusion of 1 to 3 units, and 0.49 after transfusion of 4 to 6 units, compared with anemic patients who had no transfusion. In a subgroup of patients with cardiac disease, higher hemoglobin values in patients with anemia correlated with better survival.

Discussion.—In critically ill patients with cardiac disease, anemia increases the risk of death. The risk of death appeared to be decreased by

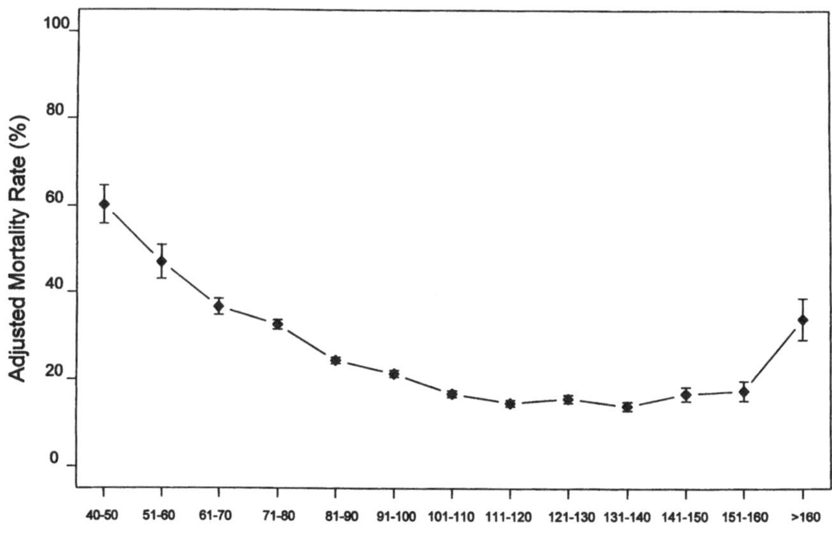

FIGURE 1.—Probability of death in all patients at various pretransfusion hemoglobin values. This figure illustrates an increasing probability of death as hemoglobin values decrease below 100 g/L, whereas mortality rates remain stable between hemoglobin values of 101 g/L and 159 g/L. The probability and 95% confidence interval from each hemoglobin range were derived from logistic models that included gender, institution, diagnosis, institution and diagnosis interaction, Acute Physiology and Chronic Health Evaluation II score, transfusion levels, and pretransfusion hemoglobin in all 4,470 critically ill patients. (Courtesy of Hébert PC, for the Transfusion Requirements in Critical Care (TRICC) Investigators and the Canadian Critical Care Trials Group: Does transfusion practice affect mortality in critically ill patients? *Am J Respir Crit Care Med* 155:1618–1623, 1997. Official Journal of the American Thoracic Society. Copyright 1997 American Lung Association.)

blood transfusion. In patients who are critically ill, the decision to transfuse red cells should include cardiovascular evaluation.

▶ The emotional backlash of the AIDS epidemic included an irrational logic that withholding transfusion of red blood cells from critically ill patients was justified to avoid the risk of transmitted viral diseases. The facts are that red blood cell transfusions are safer than driving to the hospital, and withholding this therapy from critically ill patients with less than normal heart function is not justified.

Diminished oxygen-carrying capacity will significantly increase myocardial work when oxygen demand is greater than normal. This physiologic axiom speaks to the simple truth reflected in the results of this study.

B.A Shapiro, M.D.

Erythropoietin Response Is Blunted in Critically Ill Patients

Rogiers P, Zhang H, Leeman M, et al (Middelheim Gen Hosp, Antwerp, Belgium; Free Univ of Brussels, Belgium)
Intensive Care Med 23:159–162, 1997   8–46

Background.—Erythropoietin is a hormone primarily released by the kidneys that stimulates the production of red blood cells. Decreased arterial oxygen content associated with anemia or hypoxia is the main stimulus for the production of erythropoietin, which results in a rapid exponential increase in erythropoietin synthesis. It has recently been suggested that rheumatoid arthritis, solid tumors, sickle cell anemia, and other disorders can blunt this relation between hematocrit and plasma erythropoietin. In these disease states, granulocyte macrophage colony-stimulating factor, tumor necrosis factor, interleukins, interferon, prostaglandins, and other mediators can interfere with red blood cell formation. Patients who are critically ill often have anemia, which is sometimes caused by sepsis. The role of erythropoietin in the development of anemia in these patients has not been determined.

Methods.—There were 36 critically ill patients, 22 with sepsis and 14 without sepsis, who were in the ICU more than 7 days. Serum erythropoietin levels were determined serially by enzyme-linked immunosorbent assay. Serum erythropoietin levels were also determined in a control group of 18 patients with anemia.

Results.—In the control research subjects, there was a significant inverse relationship between serum erythropoietin and hematocrit levels. This was not found in the study patients, except in a subgroup of patients without sepsis and without renal failure.

Discussion.—These findings indicate that the erythropoietin response to anemia is blunted in patients who are critically ill. In these patients, inadequate erythropoietin levels may be involved in the development of anemia. This effect is significantly stronger in patients with acute renal failure or sepsis, perhaps because of the effect of proinflammatory mediators. A cost-benefit analysis of exogenous administration of erythropoietin to critically ill patients is needed.

▶ Normally, erythropoietin (EPO) levels are inversely proportional to the hematocrit levels. There are a number of studies that have shown that EPO production is blunted by cytokines. This study demonstrated that the EPO response to anemia is severely blunted in critically ill patients (notably those with sepsis and those with acute renal failure). The authors recommend that EPO administration be considered in the management of critically ill patients. Considering the very high cost of EPO, the benefit of giving it to all patients with anemia should be studied further.

J. Samuel, M.D.

Early Changes in Hemoglobin and Hematocrit Levels After Packed Red Cell Tranfusion in Patients With Acute Anemia

Elizalde JI, Clemente J, Marín JL, et al (Univ of Barcelona)
Transfusion 37:573–576, 1997

8–47

Introduction.—During the last 50 years, the clinical use of blood components has increased substantially. There has been some controversy regarding how useful it is to monitor the effect on hemoglobin and hematocrit levels of the administration of packed red blood cells. It was determined whether early measurements of hemoglobin after blood transfusion adequately reflected levels after prolonged equilibration periods in

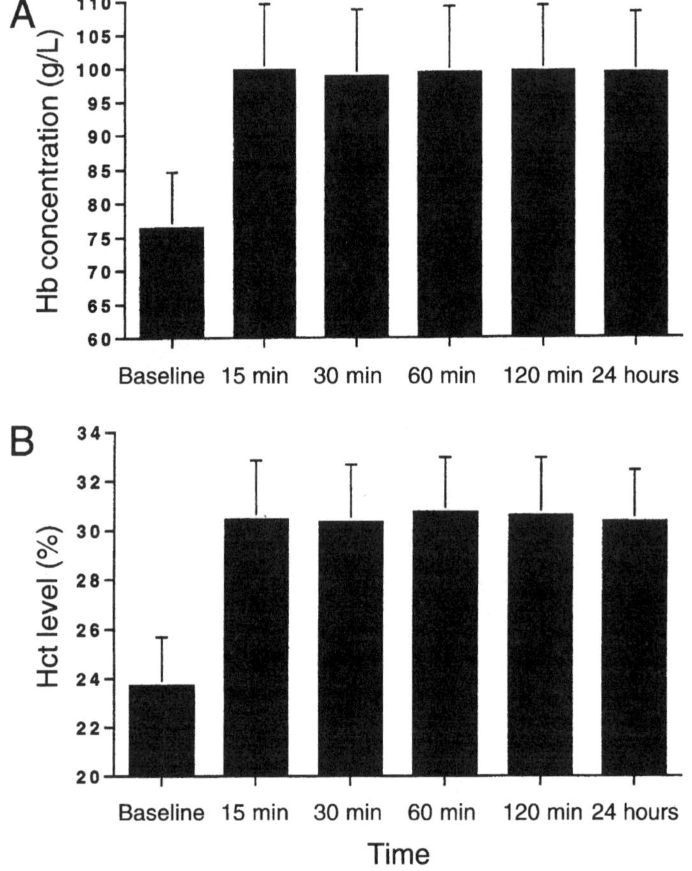

FIGURE 1.—**A,** hemoglobin concentration at baseline and at various intervals after the transfusion of 2 units of packed red blood cells. Results are expressed as mean ± 1 SD. **B,** hematocrit values at baseline and at various intervals after the transfusion of 2 packed red blood cell units. Results are expressed as mean ± 1 SD. (Reprinted by permission from *Transfusion*, courtesy of Elizalde JI, Clemente J, Marín JL, et al: Early changes in hemoglobin and hematocrit levels after packed red cell transfusion in patients with acute anemia. *Transfusion* 37: 573–576, 1997. Published by the American Association of Blood Banks.)

patients with acute anemia. Also determined was whether hematocrit values reflect such changes and whether the calculated increase in hemoglobin differed from that revealed in the observed data.

Methods.—The study included 32 normovolemic patients recovering from an acute bleeding episode who were no longer thought to be bleeding. They received a 2-unit red cell transfusion. Hemoglobin concentration and hematocrit values were measured at baseline and at 15, 30, 60, and 120 minutes and 24 hours after transfusion.

Results.—In hemoglobin concentration, the administration of 2 units of packed red cells elicited a 24-hour increase of 22.4 ± 6.8 g/L. At any of the defined posttransfusion times, hemoglobin values were not different. Over time, hematocrit levels had similar changes. As only 6% of patients were shown to have a clinically significant difference (greater than 6 g/L) between the hemoglobin measurements, agreement between 15-minute and 24-hour values was excellent (Fig 1).

Conclusion.—In normovolemic patients who are recovering from an acute bleeding episode, hemoglobin and hematocrit values rapidly achieve equilibration after transfusion. In patients remaining at risk, this fact would allow a rapid assessment of the effects of transfusion and of the recurrence of bleeding. This concept extends to patients with acute anemia, even when transfusion time is as short as that usually used in a clinical practice.

▶ One reason for continuing medical education is so that we can unlearn "medical facts" that are eventually discovered to be erroneous. If you entered medical school before 1985, you were taught that the hemoglobin level took 24 hours to reach a steady state after red blood cell transfusion. If you, like myself, have been practicing critical care medicine in the last 10 years, you have probably questioned the truth of that 24-hour time line. Some of us have changed our practice as to when we obtain a hemoglobin measurement to evaluate the effect of red blood cell transfusion in an acutely anemic patient who is no longer bleeding. However, most of us have been reluctant to openly champion an earlier time line because credible data regarding adults were not available.

This article presents a well-designed prospective study demonstrating that in adult patients with acute anemia in whom there is no active bleeding present, clinically relevant hemoglobin equilibration occurs within 15 minutes of completion of red blood cell transfusion. Although my clinical practice may not change because of this study, my teaching and consultation practices definitely will change.

B.A. Shapiro, M.D.

Pharmacology and Toxicity

Use of 2% Propofol to Produce Diurnal Sedation in Critically Ill Patients

McLeod G, Wallis C, Dick J, et al (Dundee Med School, Scotland; Univ of St Andrews, Scotland)
Intensive Care Med 23:428–434, 1997

8–48

Introduction.—Major sleep disturbance occurs in critically ill patients in ICUs and is considered to be one of the most dislikeable features of an intensive care stay. Sleep promotes tissue growth and stimulates release of anabolic hormones, whereas sleep deprivation stimulates release of catabolic hormones and increases loss of body nitrogen. Critically ill patients can lose diurnal rhythmicity of the sleep-wake cycle because of the disease suppressing the endogenous pacemaker or because of exogenous factors such as constant sedation for ventilation, lack of natural light, and continuous feeding. A circadian sedation pattern may be achieved by imposing a sleep-wake rhythm by altering consciousness. Propofol may be used for diurnal sedation. The feasibility of producing a diurnal sleep-wake cycle by additional night sedation with propofol 2% in critically ill patients after admission to intensive care was examined.

Methods.—Thirty patients expected to be sedated for more than 50 hours were randomized into 2 groups. A constant background infusion of morphine and a variable infusion rate of propofol was given to all patients. Constantly light sedation over 50 hours that aimed for a Ramsay score of 2–3 was given to 1 group of patients. Constant light sedation between 6 AM and 10 PM was given to the second group of patients, with additional night sedation of propofol between 10 PM and 6 AM aiming for a sedation score of 4–5. Heart rate, blood pressure, sedation scores, and propofol and morphine infusion rates were recorded each hour. Each patient received an Acute Physiology and Chronic Health Evaluation (APACHE) II score.

Results.—Significantly better rhythmicity of sedation levels was found in the additional night sedation group. With respect to age, sex or APACHE II score, there were no differences in the 2 groups. Diurnal sedation was achieved by 9 of 15 patients in the additional night sedation group. Diurnal rhythmicity of sedation was achieved by 3 patients in the constant light sedation group, which was attributed to natural sleep. A deep constant sedation pattern was seen by 5 patients in the constant light sedation group and 3 in the additional night sedation group; these patients had high APACHE II scores, with a median of 21.5. They also had an obtunded conscious level on admission as the result of severe sepsis.

Conclusion.—In critically ill patients, propofol can safely provide diurnal sedation when titrated against the Ramsay score. In some severely ill patients, sedation levels cannot be manipulated.

▶ Although there has always been proper respect given to the physiologic realities of circadian rhythmicity, little real concern has been apportioned to the effects of sleep deprivation in the critically ill patient. This is especially true in patients who are being sedated. This study is interesting because it shows that very sick patients do not have a diurnal cycle, and the least sick patients have a diurnal cycle despite a constant sedation regimen. The study shows that in some patients, the diurnal cycle can be preserved by titrating a propofol infusion to 2 different Ramsey Scale end points for night and day. However, we have no evidence that preserving the circadian cycle in critically ill patients will positively affect morbidity or mortality.

B.A. Shapiro, M.D.

Overnight Sedation With Midazolam or Propofol in the ICU: Effects on Sleep Quality, Anxiety and Depression

Treggiari-Venzi M, Borgeat A, Fuchs-Buder T, et al (Univ Hosp of Geneva)
Intensive Care Med 22:1186–1190, 1996 8–49

Background.—Several factors can lead to high levels of anxiety and depression for patients in the ICU. The effects of overnight sedation with midazolam or propofol on anxiety, depression, and sleep quality in ICU patients were investigated.

Methods.—The open, randomized trial included 40 conscious, nonintubated patients. All were expected to stay in the ICU for 5 days or longer because of trauma or elective surgical procedures. All patients were randomized to receive nightly sedation with midazolam or propofol by infusion, starting at 10:00 p.m. and ending at 6:00 a.m. The Hospital Anxiety and Depression scale was used to assess these symptoms in each patient; a score greater than 10 indicated severe anxiety or depression. Each patient also underwent monitoring of heart rate, pulse oximetry, and blood gases.

Results.—The final evaluation included 32 patients. After their first night of sedation, 31% of patients in the midazolam group and 26% of those in the propofol group had severe anxiety. This situation was little changed in subsequent days. High levels of depression were recorded for 54% of patients receiving midazolam and 16% of those receiving propofol. The quality of sleep tended to improve during the study, but not significantly so. None of the clinical parameters monitored were significantly affected by sedation.

Conclusion.—About half of patients have severe anxiety and depression during their first 5 days in the ICU after surgery or trauma. Sedation with midazolam or propofol has some benefit in terms of sleep quality but does not improve anxiety and depression. Still, better sleep could help these patients to re-establish a physiologic circadian rhythm.

▶ Attempting to study anxiety, depression, and sleep quality in the ICU is an admirable goal because scientific data on these important matters are lacking. This study involved a considerable amount of work and dedication but, unfortunately, provides no new information.

B.A. Shapiro, M.D.

Prolonged Sedation of Critically Ill Patients With Midazolam or Propofol: Impact on Weaning and Costs

Barrientos-Vega R, Sánchez-Soria MM, Morales-García C, et al (Hosp Virgen de la Salud, Toledo, Spain)
Crit Care Med 25:33–40, 1997

8–50

Purpose.—Patients undergoing mechanical ventilation in the ICU usually require sedation, the most commonly used sedatives being midazolam and propofol. Propofol is more expensive than midazolam but has a shorter sedative effect. This could permit quicker extubation, a shorter ICU stay, and decreased costs. Midazolam and propofol were compared for effectiveness of sedation, time to weaning, and costs of prolonged sedation in critically ill, mechanically ventilated patients.

Methods.—The prospective, randomized trial included 108 medical, surgical, and trauma patients admitted to the ICU who required mechanical ventilation for more than 24 hours. They were randomized to receive either midazolam (dose range, 0.1 to 0.5 mg/kg/hr) or propofol (dose range, 1 to 6 mg/kg/hr). Individual patients received the lowest dose that permitted adequate patient-ventilator synchrony. Morphine chloride, 0.5 mg/kg/24 hr, was given to all patients. The Ramsay scale was used to assess level of sedation every 2 hours from the start of mechanical ventilation to weaning. Patients who could not be adequately sedated by the highest dose of either drug were considered treatment failures. Patients receiving propofol underwent measurement of serum triglycerides every 72 hours. When it was time for weaning, sedation was halted abruptly. Time was measured from interruption of sedation to the first T-bridge trial and to extubation. The costs of intensive care were compared for the 2 groups.

Results.—The mortality rate was 28% in the midazolam group and 20% in the propofol group. The therapeutic failure rate was 20% with midazolam and 33% with propofol. The percentages of patients subjected to a T-bridge trial were 52% and 46%, respectively. None of these differences was significant. The mean duration of sedation was about 140 hours in both groups. The costs attributed to sedation were $378 with midazolam vs. $794 with propofol—a significant difference. Time from discontinuation of sedation to extubation was 98 hours with midazolam (49 hours to the first disconnection and 49 hours to extubation) vs. 35 hours with propofol (4 hours to the first disconnection and 31 hours to extubation). The 63 hour difference in weaning time was significant. Cost per patient, including ICU treatment and sedation, was approximately $10,800 in the midazolam group vs. $9,500 in the propofol group.

Conclusion.—For critically ill patients requiring long-term sedation for mechanical ventilation, midazolam and propofol are equally effective. However, propofol is associated with a significantly shorter weaning time. Thus, propofol has a more favorable economic profile, even though it is the more expensive drug. The cost advantage of propofol increases with increasing ICU cost per hour and decreases as the duration of sedation or the mortality rate increases.

▶ Comparing ICU costs between hospitals within the United States involves so many variables that any data are open to serious criticism. Attempting to translate costs in Spain to costs in the United States is even more suspect. The assumption that propofol's added expense may be more than made up for in lower ICU costs is a leap of faith. In the case of midazolam, the prolonged emergence time from continuous sedation administered for more than 24 hours is well known and is the main reason why the SCCM practice guidelines suggest lorazepam.[1]

B.A. Shapiro, M.D.

Reference

1. Shapiro BA, Warren J, Egol AB, et al: Practice parameters for intravenous analgesia and sedation for adult patients in the intensive care unit: An executive summary. *Crit Care Med* 23:1596–1600, 1995.

A Prospective Study of Simplified Omeprazole Suspension for the Prophylaxis of Stress-related Mucosal Damage
Phillips JO, Metzler MH, Palmieri TL, et al (Univ of Missouri, Columbia; Keesler Med Ctr, Keesler AFB, Mo; Univ of Missouri, Kansas City)
Crit Care Med 24:1793–1800, 1996   8–51

Background.—Significant physiologic stress places patients at risk for gastric mucosal damage and subsequent upper gastrointestinal bleeding. The development of stress-related mucosal damage has been associated with mechanical ventilation, coagulopathy, extensive burns, head injuries, and organ transplants. The effects of a simplified omeprazole suspension in patients receiving mechanical ventilation who were critically ill and who had at least 1 additional risk factor for stress-related mucosal damage were studied.

Methods.—Seventy-five adults receiving mechanical ventilation in a surgical intensive care and burn unit were included in the prospective, open-label study. The patients were initially given 20 mL of a simplified omeprazole suspension, containing 40 mg of omeprazole, followed by a second 20-mL dose 6–8 hours later, then 10 mL daily. The suspension was delivered through a nasogastric tube, followed by 5–10 mL of tap water. The tube was clamped for 1–2 hours after each administration.

Findings.—None of the patients had clinically significant upper gastrointestinal bleeding after receiving the omeprazole suspension. Four hours after omeprazole administration, the mean gastric pH was 7.1. The mean gastric pH was 6.8 after beginning omeprazole, and the mean lowest pH after starting omeprazole was 5.6. Pneumonia developed in 12% of the patients. None had any adverse events or a drug interaction from omeprazole.

Conclusions.—A simplified omeprazole suspension is effective, safe, convenient, and cost-effective in the prophylaxis of stress-related bleeding.

A randomized clinical comparison of the simplified omeprazole suspension and continuous-infusion H_2-antagonist is currently under way.

▶ This is a well-done prospective study. The authors did a pharmacoeconomic evaluation and analyzed the stability of the simplified suspension in 75 patients receiving mechanical ventilation who also had at least 1 risk factor. They showed that a simplified omeprazole suspension of 40 mg followed by another 40 mg and then 20 mg daily was safe and effective therapy for the prevention of clinically significant stress-related mucosal bleeding in critically ill patients. The cost of sucralfate would have decreased significantly if pH monitoring were not included (which is not necessary when sucralfate is used). The study was only single arm in design and must be done head to head with sucralfate using the same criteria for both arms.

J. Samuel, M.D.

Pain and Satisfaction With Pain Control in Seriously Ill Hospitalized Adults: Findings From the SUPPORT Research Investigations
Desbiens NA, for the SUPPORT Investigators (Marshfield Clinic and Marshfield Med Research, Wis)
Crit Care Med 24:1953–1961, 1996   8–52

Introduction.—Pain control is frequently not adequate for seriously ill patients. Methodologic problems abound in earlier reports that have found associations between pain and other factors such as depression, anxiety, age, cancer, gender, and race. The pain experience of seriously ill hospitalized patients and their satisfaction with pain control was evaluated in a large, well-defined cohort of seriously ill hospitalized patients with common diagnoses and short life expectancies.

Methods.—Of 9,105 patients enrolled in the Study to Understand Prognoses and Preferences for Outcomes and Risks of Treatment (SUPPORT), 3,624 were able to be interviewed. Patients or family members were questioned about the patient's experience with pain and pain control.

Results.—Pain was reported by 49.9% of patients or family members; 14.9% reported extremely severe pain of any frequency or moderately severe pain occurring at least half of the time. Of patients with pain, 14.9% were dissatisfied with their pain control. Patients who were older and sicker reported less pain. The patients who reported more pain had more dependencies in activities of daily living, comorbid conditions, depression, anxiety, and poor quality of life. Of all disease categories, patients with colon cancer reported the most pain. Levels of reported pain report varied among the 5 hospitals participating in SUPPORT and by physician specialty.

Conclusion.—Pain is a common and severe symptom in hospitalized patients who are severely ill, and many patients are dissatisfied with their pain control. Better pain management is needed for patients who are seriously ill.

▶ Largely as a result of the SUPPORT investigation and the United States Supreme Court decision on assisted suicide, pain control in the ICU is receiving greater attention. This study finds a great deal of room for improvement. No surprise there. Although the article does not elaborate on strategies to effect better pain control, it is clear that physicians and nurses working primarily in the ICU need better training in that aspect of management. Also, an implicit message of the study is that greater resort to consultants with expertise in pain control would be of immense benefit.

C.M. Franklin, M.D.

A Pharmacoeconomic Analysis of Neuromuscular Blocking Agents in the Operating Room

Loughlin KA, Weingarten CM, Nagelhout J, et al (Wayne State Univ, Detroit)
Pharmacotherapy 16:942–950, 1996   8–53

Purpose.—The available nondepolarizing neuromuscular blocking agents (NMBAs) vary significantly in onset, duration, metabolic pathway, and adverse effect profile. The additional cost of the more recently introduced drugs remains to be justified as to their improvements in pharmacokinetics and adverse effects. A pharmacoeconomic analysis was performed to compare the direct costs of different NMBAs for patients undergoing surgical procedures of varying duration.

Methods.—Two groups of patients were selected by estimated length of surgical procedure: group 1, 55 patients whose procedures were estimated to take less than 2 hours, and group 2, 55 patients whose procedures were estimated to take from 2 to 4 hours. The patients were randomly assigned to receive an intermediate-acting NMBA: either atracurium, vecuronium, or rocuronium. Information on anesthetics given in the operating room was obtained from review of anesthesia records, and data on cost was obtained from hospital drug acquisition costs. Patient charges were used to estimate postanesthesia care unit (PACU) costs. The study did not consider costs incurred by patients in all treatment groups, or those that were unrelated to the use of NMBAs. The time-adjusted costs of neuromuscular blockade per hour and of total anesthesia costs per hour were calculated.

Results.—In patients undergoing short-duration procedures, there were no differences in terms of NMBA cost per hour, anesthesia cost per hour, or PACU times or costs. In group 2, however, mean NMBA cost per case was $54 with atracurium vs. $32 with vecuronium. Neuromuscular blockade cost per hour was $22 with atracurium, compared with $14 for vecuronium and $16 for rocuronium. Anesthesia costs per hour were $29, $23, and $23, respectively. The 3 groups were similar in PACU times and costs.

Conclusion.—For surgical procedures estimated to last 2 to 4 hours, vecuronium or rocuronium is a more economical choice than atracurium. For shorter procedures, there are no apparent cost differences among these 3 NMBAs. The pharmacoeconomic analysis techniques used in this study can be applied to other drugs for which economic as well as clinical data are required.

▶ It is unfeasible to directly compare pharmacologic data obtained from patients receiving general anesthesia in the operating room with data obtained from patients receiving mechanical ventilation in the ICU. Further, the operating room studies have the advantage of looking at PACU times as a clinical indicator of faster discharge, whereas ICU studies do not demonstrate that faster recovery from the paralyzing agent is translated into faster discharge from the ICU. However, this article strongly emphasizes the general principle that when relatively intermediate-acting agents are used to provide relatively long-acting effects, the impact of the price differential among the agents will be magnified.

B.A. Shapiro, M.D.

The Impact of Practice Guidelines on Prescribing Patterns of Nondepolarizing Neuromuscular Blocking Agents
Tschida SJ, Hoey LL, Vance-Bryan K (Univ of Minnesota, Minneapolis; St Paul-Ramsey Med Ctr, Minn)
Pharmacotherapy 16:899–904, 1996   8–54

Background.—Despite the growing appreciation of the potential benefits of treatment guidelines, little is known about their performance in everyday clinical practice. In a recent review of nondepolarizing neuromuscular blocking agent (NNMBA) use in their ICU, the authors found that atracurium was the agent of choice for paralysis, with little attention given to clinical value or cost. Subsequently, guidelines were developed to suggest pancuronium as the agent of choice for patients who have adequate renal function and are able to tolerate increases in heart rate, blood pressure, or cardiac output. The guidelines recommended vecuronium for patients who did not meet these criteria and for whom hepatic function was normal, and atracurium for those who did not meet either criteria. A follow-up study was done to assess the effect of the guidelines on prescribing patterns and costs.

Methods.—The analysis included 24 adult patients receiving continuous infusion of an NNMBA in the authors' ICU. All patients were treated at least 7 months after implementation of the new guidelines for NNMBA selection. The findings in terms of NNMBA choice and cost were compared with those of 25 patients evaluated before implementation of the guidelines.

Results.—Before the guidelines were implemented, 68% of patients received atracurium, 24% received vecuronium, and 8% received pancuronium. According to criteria of organ function and hemodynamic stability, atracurium was used inappropriately in 88% of patients, vecuronium in 83%, and pancuronium in none. After the new guidelines were implemented, atracurium was prescribed in 33% of patients, vecuronium in

21%, and pancuronium in 46%. The rates of inappropriate use of these drugs were 38%, 60%, and 0%, respectively. The new guidelines reduced the overall prevalence of inappropriate NNMBA prescription from 80% to 25%. The change saved an estimated $8,400 per year.

Conclusion.—Practice guidelines for NNMBA use have reduced the inappropriate use of these agents for paralysis in the authors' ICU. Significant cost reductions can accrue from more appropriate prescribing practices. The authors call for prospective studies to see how practice guidelines can affect NNMBA prescribing patterns and patient outcomes, particularly adverse effects.

▶ Resistance to clinical practice guidelines has traditionally come from physicians who consider such protocols an unnecessary encroachment on their rights as independent practitioners. As excellently demonstrated in this study, when such guidelines serve the purpose of assuring more appropriate clinical use of an agent or therapy, the "independence" argument becomes indefensible.

B.A. Shapiro, M.D.

Postal Survey on the Long-term Use of Neuromuscular Block in the Intensive Care

Appadu BL, Greiff JMC, Thompson JP (Leicester Royal Infirmary, England)
Intensive Care Med 22:862–866, 1996   8–55

Introduction.—A recent United States survey found that neuromuscular blocking (NMB) drugs were routinely given by "anesthesiologist-intensivists" for a wide range of indications but with few guidelines or recommendations. There are questions regarding which is the best NMB agent to use in the ICU, how monitoring should be performed, how completely patients should be paralyzed, and whether there is some limit to the length of time that these drugs can safely be given. British intensivists were surveyed regarding their use of NMB drugs, with special reference to their long-term use in the ICU setting.

Methods.—A questionnaire regarding use of NMB drugs was mailed to 409 British ICUs. The response rate was 58%.

Results.—Eighty-six percent of the responding ICUs were led by an anesthetist; only 2% were staffed by full-time intensivists. Major indications for prolonged neuromuscular blockade were to facilitate mechanical ventilation and to treat increased intracranial pressure. Eighty-three percent of ICUs used intermediate-duration NMB drugs. Sixty-one percent of ICUs gave these drugs by continuous infusion only, 24% by a bolus dose followed by continuous infusion, and 14% by bolus dose only. The respondents' major reasons for using vecuronium or stracurium were the pharmacokinetics and hemodynamic stability of these drugs. Ninety-two percent of ICUs used clinical monitoring of neuromuscular blockade; only 8% used peripheral nerve stimulation. All responding ICUs used sedatives and/or opioids in combination with NMB agents. The main sedatives used were propofol/midazolam, alone or in combination (89% of respondents), whereas the main opioids used were morphine, fentanyl, or alfentanil (75% of respondents).

Conclusion.—British ICUs vary considerably in their patterns of NMB drug use. It is generally agreed that long-term use of these drugs can have benefits in the ICU setting. However, there are few data to show that outcomes are improved by their use. Many respondents believed that NMB drugs should be used only as a last resort and then for as short a time as possible. The challenge is to identify and manage the subgroup of patients whose outcome depends on judicious use of NMB agents.

▶ Our constant striving to practice evidence-based medicine places an ever-growing responsibility on the investigator, the journal, and the reader to recognize when data is being used to espouse a particular bias. These authors sent a questionnaire asking the respondents what they did and why they did it. However, the article poses and discusses the following questions: (1) which is the best NMB drug for use in the ICU?, (2) should the degree of paralysis be monitored?, (3) how completely should the patients be paralyzed?, and (4) is there a limit to the duration that these drugs can be safely administered? Although I have no significant quarrel with the opinions and biases stated by the authors, I take umbrage at the fact that they have inappropriately presented the results from a postal survey as a pretense for stating their opinions.

B.A. Shapiro, M.D.

Dose Response, Recovery, and Cost of Doxacurium as a Continuous Infusion in Neurosurgical Intensive Care Unit Patients

Prielipp RC, Robinson JC, Wilson JA, et al (Wake Forest Univ, Winston-Salem, NC)
Crit Care Med 25:1236–1241, 1997   8–56

Introduction.—To guide selection and use of neuromuscular blocking drugs in ICU patients, little information is available. For patients with traumatic brain injury, experience is even more limited in the selection of neuromuscular blocking drugs. The most potent neuromuscular blocking agent is doxacurium chloride, a mixture of 3 stereoisomers which is devoid of autonomic, cardiovascular, or histamine-releasing side effects. For treatment of neurosurgical patients, continuous infusions of neuromuscular blocking drugs may be ideally suited to facilitating mechanical ventilation and reducing intracranial pressure. The safety and optimal dosing of continuous infusion of doxacurium in neurosurgical patients with traumatic brain injury were determined.

Methods.—There were 8 critically ill, mechanically ventilated patients with traumatic head injury and normal renal and hepatic function who were given a bolus injection of doxacurium (0.05 mg/kg). This was followed by a continuous infusion (0.015 mg/kg/hr) adjusted to maintain 1 twitch during Train-of-Four nerve stimulation of the adductor pollicis muscle.

Results.—The heart rate, blood pressure, and intracranial pressure were not altered by bolus injections of doxacurium. After infusion of the doxacurium was discontinued, recovery of the fourth twitch occurred in 118 ± 19 minutes. Patients were paralyzed for 66 ± 12 hours. No incidences of myopathy, prolonged weakness, or other adverse events were seen.

Conclusion.—Stable neuromuscular blockade for neurosurgical patients with traumatic brain injury is provided by continuous infusion of doxacurium. Doxacurium is less costly than other neuromuscular blockers used in the ICU and is devoid of clinically important interactions with heart rate, blood pressure, or intracranial pressure.

▶ The clinical need for long-term paralysis in the ICU should be best achieved by a long-acting agent that is devoid of autonomic, cardiovascular, and histamine-releasing side effects. Doxacurium is such a neuromuscular blocking agent. This study demonstrates that doxacurium can provide satisfactory muscle blockade without affecting vital signs or intracranial pressure in head injury patients. The authors suggest that doxacurium's potency allows for economic feasibility. This is a good study that, hopefully, will stimulate further investigations.

B.A. Shapiro, M.D.

A Prospective, Randomized, Controlled Evaluation of Peripheral Nerve Stimulation Versus Standard Clinical Dosing of Neuromuscular Blocking Agents in Critically Ill Patients
Rudis MI, Sikora CA, Angus E, et al (Henry Ford Health System, Detroit)
Crit Care Med 25:575–583, 1997   8–57

Introduction.—It has been suggested that monitoring with a peripheral nerve stimulator reduces neuromuscular blocking agent doses and decreases the risk of prolonged paralysis. Outcomes of critically ill, mechanically ventilated medical patients whose vecuronium doses were individualized by peripheral nerve stimulation vs. standard clinical assessment were compared in a prospective, randomized, controlled investigation.

Methods.—Seventy-seven patients were randomized to the treatment arm (dosing by peripheral nerve stimulation) or the control arm (dosing adjusted by standard clinical assessment). All patients received a loading dose and maintenance infusions of vecuronium. Doses of vecuronium were adjusted to 90% blockade (Train-of-Four of 1/4) in the treatment group. The medical team was blinded to the Train-of-Four results and made dosing adjustments individualized to clinical response.

Results.—There were 35 and 42 patients, respectively, in the control and treatment groups. There were no between-group differences in initial doses and time to reach 90% blockage or clinical response. Significantly less

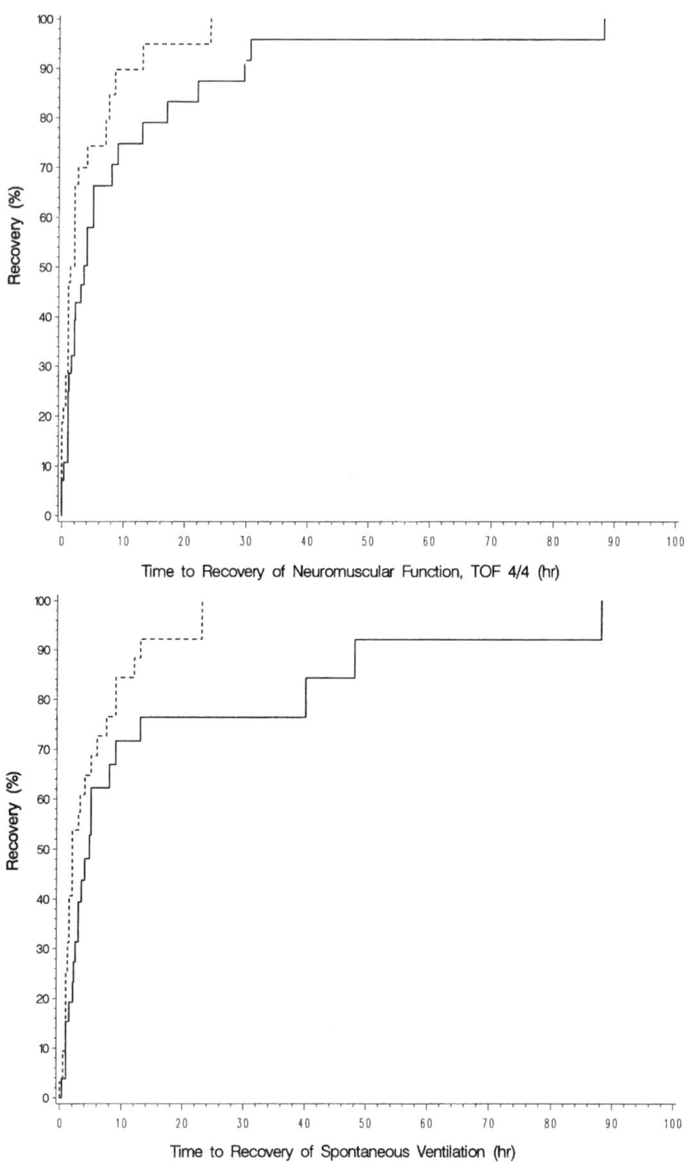

FIGURE 1.—Kaplan-Meier survival analysis curves for time to recovery of neuromuscular function (**top**) and time to recovery of spontaneous ventilation (**bottom**) for the peripheral nerve stimulation group (*dashed lines*) vs. the standard clinical dosing group (*solid lines*). TOF 4/4, 4 switches out of 4 on a Train-of-Four stimulation. (Courtesy of Rudis MI, Sikora CA, Angus E, et al: A prospective, randomized, controlled evaluation of peripheral nerve stimulation versus standard clinical dosing of neuromuscular blocking agents in critically ill patients. *Crit Care Med* 25(4):575–583, 1997.)

drug was used in the treatment group, compared with the control group. The total cumulative amount of vecuronium for the episode of paralysis was 285.8 for the control group vs. 137.1 mg for the treatment group. Compared with control, patients in the treatment group recovered neuromuscular function and spontaneous ventilation significantly faster (Fig 1). Patients with combined renal and liver failure had a quicker recovery when they were in the treatment group.

Conclusion.—Vecuronium dosing of mechanically ventilated critically ill medical patients by peripheral nerve stimulation resulted in smaller effective doses, lower cumulative drug doses, and improvement in the rate of recovery of neuromuscular function and spontaneous ventilation, compared with standard clinical dosing. Use of higher doses has cost and recovery ramifications that could be avoided by use of peripheral nerve stimulation.

▶ A well-done study demonstrating that neuromuscular blockade administered by nerve stimulator criteria requires less drug and produces faster recovery compared with empiric administration of the agent. There is need for investigations to demonstrate that monitoring techniques used to provide the minimal level of paralysis necessary to meet clinical goals will reduce the drug dosage further and produce even faster recovery.

B.A. Shapiro, M.D.

Is Hartmann's the Solution?

White SA, Goldhill DR (Royal London School of Medicine and Dentistry)
Anaesthesia 52:422–427, 1997   8–58

Introduction.—Anesthesiologists routinely use Hartmann's solution for rehydration and maintenance in the operating room. However, knowledge of the constituents, purpose, and metabolism of this solution vary. Anesthetists were surveyed regarding their knowledge of Hartmann's solution.

Methods.—Eighty-two anesthesiologists attending an educational meeting of the Royal College of Anaesthetists were surveyed. Their median time in anesthetic practice was 3.5 years. The study questionnaire asked about the constituents of Hartmann's solution and their concentrations, as well as the reason for and metabolism of the lactate in Hartmann's solution. Information on Hartmann's solution in standard anesthetic textbooks was evaluated as well.

Results.—All 82 anesthesiologists responded. Only 4% correctly noted the constituent electrolytes of Hartmann's solution and their concentrations. Sixty-three believed that lactate served as a source of bicarbonate, and 21% believed that it was a source of glucose. None of the respondents completely described the metabolism of lactate in Hartmann's solution. Most gave an imprecise explanation of lactate metabolism, and 29% gave no explanation. Few of the textbooks examined gave any information on the metabolism of lactate from Hartmann's solution.

Discussion.—Anesthesiologists have a low level of knowledge regarding Hartmann's solution. This widely used solution is designed to match the constituents and concentrations of plasma, leading to reduced ion and fluid shifts after transfusion. Lactate metabolism occurs through both oxidation and gluconeogenesis. Lactate metabolism takes place mainly in the liver and results in bicarbonate generation within 1 to 2 hours. Although Hartmann's solution is appropriate for use in most patients, there are some contraindications to remember.

▶ It is important to remind ourselves that without a working knowledge of fundamentals, complicated and sophisticated techniques have little chance of making a difference. This report is sobering.

B.A. Shapiro, M.D.

Preventable Adverse Drug Events in Hospitalized Patients: A Comparative Study of Intensive Care and General Care Units
Cullen DJ, Sweitzer BJ, Bates DW, et al (Harvard Med School, Boston; Brigham and Women's Hosp, Boston; Harvard School of Public Health, Boston; et al)
Crit Care Med 25:1289–1297, 1997   8–59

Introduction.—Medications are the most common cause of injuries related to medical care, and many adverse drug events are preventable. Human error may be a particularly likely cause of adverse drug errors in the ICU. Systems factors may increase the chances of making a medication error and decrease the chances of detecting the error. The rate and preventability of adverse drug events is compared in the ICU and general care unit. Systems factors related to adverse drug events in various practice settings is assessed as well.

Methods.—The prospective cohort study included 4,031 adult patients admitted to a stratified, random sample of 11 medical and surgical units over a 6-month period. The units—including 2 medical and 3 surgical ICUs and 4 medical and 2 surgical general care units—were located in 2 tertiary care hospitals. Approaches used to identify medication-related incidents included self-report by nurses and pharmacists and daily chart reviews. Each incident was independently classified as an adverse drug event or potential adverse drug event. The severity and preventability of each event was evaluated as well. For each preventable adverse drug event and potential adverse drug event, detailed interviews were conducted with the individuals involved. The different types of units were compared for the frequency and preventability of drug events. Systems factors involved in adverse drug events—including individual care givers, care unit teams, and patients—were compared for ICU vs. non-ICU settings and for medical vs. surgical ICUs.

Results.—Preventable adverse drug events and potential adverse drug events occurred at a rate of 19 events/1,000 patient-days in ICUs vs. 10

events/1,000 patient-days in non-ICUs. The rate was 25 events/1,000 patient-days in medical ICUs vs. 14 events/1,000 patient-days in surgical ICUs. However, after adjustment for numbers of drugs used or ordered, there was no significant difference in drug event rates between ICUs and non-ICUs. The ICUs and non-ICUs differed significantly in patient acuity, length of stay, and adverse drug event severity. These factors were not significantly different between medical and surgical ICUs. In interviews, the patient, care team, systems, and care giver characteristics involved in the drug events were very similar between the ICUs and non-ICUs.

Conclusion.—Preventable adverse drug events and potential adverse drug events are twice as likely in ICUs vs, non-ICUs. However, this difference disappears after adjustment for differences in the number of drugs ordered in these 2 settings. The findings suggest that preventable and potentially adverse drug events are not necessarily related to workload, stress, or the practice environment. Rather, such events can occur in normally functioning units involving care givers under reasonably normal circumstances. The systems factors involved are not significantly different between ICUs and non-ICUs.

▶ Human error is an integral part of any patient care environment. This study shows that the frequency of preventable adverse drug events correlates with the number of drugs ordered and does not correlate with the caregivers' workload. The study is not justifying the errors, but rather helping us to realize that they are always with us and we must always be vigilant.

B.A. Shapiro, M.D.

Interrater Agreement in the Measurement of QRS Interval in Tricyclic Antidepressant Overdose: Implications for Monitoring and Research
Buckley NA, O'Connell DL, Whyte IM, et al (Univ of Newcastle, Australia; Newcastle Mater Misercordiae Hosp, Australia)
Ann Emerg Med 28:515–519, 1996   8–60

Objective.—For patients with tricyclic antidepressant (TCA) overdose, predictions about seizure and arrhythmia risk and decisions about treatment are based on measurement of the QRS interval. However, there have been no studies of observer variation in this situation, particularly as it relates to the suggested cutoff points for treatment and monitoring. Intraobserver variation in measurement of QRS intervals in patients with TCA overdose was evaluated, including the clinical implications of any disagreement.

Methods.—Three investigators with experience in the management of TCA poisoning participated in the study. Each observer independently and manually measured QRS intervals from the admission ECGs of 231 patients with TCA poisoning. The measurements were made without knowledge of the patients' outcomes or the measurements made by other raters.

Agreement among the raters was assessed, particularly in terms of the clinical cutoff points for treatment and disposition.

Results.—The observers showed good agreement on measurement of QRS intervals, with intraclass correlation coefficients of .60 for transformed data and .82 for raw data. The observers agreed on patient classification by category of QRS interval in 73% of patients. However, in about 20% of cases, they did not agree as to whether the QRS interval was more or less than 100 msec, a clinical cutoff point for seizure risk.

Conclusions.—In patients with TCA overdose, experienced observers vary considerably in their assessments of whether the QRS interval falls above or below the clinical cutoff point of 100 msec. Because of this intraobserver variation, manual measurements of QRS interval should not be considered reliable in making treatment decisions. However, agreement is good enough for use in overall assessments of toxicity.

▶ The results of this study suggest the need of on-line computer-assisted measurements of QRS and other ECG measurements. The point should be made that the correct threshold of QRS duration on which to base treatment decisions is still debated.

J.E. Calvin, Jr., M.D.

J.E. Parrillo, M.D.

Arterial and Venous Cocaine Plasma Concentrations in Humans: Relationship to Route of Administration, Cardiovascular Effects and Subjective Effects
Evans SM, Cone EJ, Henningfield JE (NIH, Bethesda, Md)
J Pharmacol Exp Ther 279:1345–1356, 1996   8–61

Purpose.—Cocaine that is smoked—either free-base or as "crack"—is thought to have greater addictive potential than cocaine taken by other routes. One possible explanation is the very short time it takes smoked cocaine to reach the brain—7 to 9 seconds. The physiologic and behavioral effects of smoked drugs should be closely related to the arterial plasma drug concentrations. Arterial and venous cocaine plasma concentrations after smoking and IV injected cocaine were compared.

Methods.—The study included 9 otherwise healthy men who were current users of IV and smoked cocaine. In the initial phase of the study, subjects were tested under all dosing conditions to determine their ability to tolerate each cocaine dose to be used in the study. In the second phase, they were tested with an arterial catheter in place. On 2 separate days, the subjects took part in 4 smoked-cocaine sessions, with a sham session and cocaine doses of 12.5, 25, and 50 mg; and 4 IV cocaine sessions, in doses of 0, 8, 16, and 32 mg. The doses were given in ascending order and 90 minutes apart. Arterial and venous blood samples were obtained before, during, and after administration of the 2 highest doses by each route. The cardiovascular and subjective effects of the drug were assessed at the same times.

Results.—Both routes of administration produced higher arterial than venous cocaine concentrations. Arterial cocaine concentrations peaked within 15 seconds by both routes, whereas it took 4 minutes for venous concentrations to peak. The cardiovascular and subjective effects also occurred quickly and were more closely related to the arterial cocaine concentrations than to the venous concentrations. Smoked cocaine was associated with lower arterial and venous concentrations than IV cocaine. However, there was no significant difference in the cardiovascular and subjective effects, suggesting that smoked cocaine may have a greater effect despite a similar concentration.

Conclusions.—The greater effects of smoked vs. IV cocaine do not appear to result from the drug reaching the brain faster, as measured by peripheral arterial blood samples. Smoked cocaine has greater cardiovascular and subjective effects at blood concentrations similar to those produced by IV cocaine. Nonpharmacologic factors, such as ease of administration, may account for the reportedly greater addictiveness of smoked vs. IV cocaine.

▶ This carefully performed study suggests that smoked cocaine produces similar effects as IV cocaine but at lower arterial concentrations. This may be because of limitations in the experimental design, including the use of arterial catheters. Arterial concentrations better predict both objective and subjective effects.

J.E. Calvin, Jr., M.D.

J.E. Parrillo, M.D.

Psychoactive Substance Use Disorders Among Seriously Injured Trauma Center Patients
Soderstrom CA, Smith GS, Dischinger PC, et al (Univ of Maryland, Baltimore; Johns Hopkins Univ, Baltimore, Md; Natl Inst on Drug Abuse, Baltimore, Md)
JAMA 277:1769–1774, 1997   8–62

Objective.—Substance abuse has been linked to injury to self and others. A standardized diagnostic interview was used to investigate the incidence of psychoactive substance use disorders (PSUDs) in a large, unselected cohort of trauma center patients.

Methods.—The Structured Clinical Interview (SCID) from the *Diagnostic and Statistical Manual of Mental Disorders, Revised Third Edition* was administered to 1118 trauma patients (312 female), age 18 or older, who had stays 2 days or longer. Demographic and injury data were collected, and toxicology screens were performed on all patients. Results were analyzed statistically.

Results.—Men had significantly higher blood alcohol levels than women (36.6% versus 21.4%). Those age 21 to 59 had higher blood alcohol levels than younger or older patients (35.8% versus 13.8% versus 19.2%). Of the 718 patients tested for drugs, 15.6% were positive for opiates, 14.0% for cocaine, 10.9% for phencyclidine, and 0.1% for amphetamine. One or more lifetime abuse or dependence PSUD were found in 54.2% of patients. There were 24.1% of patients who were currently alcohol dependent with men having a significantly higher incidence than women (27.7% versus 14.7%). Drug dependence was found in 17.7% of patients with men again having a significantly higher incidence than women (20.2 versus 11.2%). Whereas alcohol dependence did not differ between races, lifetime and current drug dependence was significantly higher among nonwhites than whites and higher in intentional than in unintentional injury patients. Of patients with positive screening tests, 54.3% were currently alcohol dependent and 38.7% were currently drug dependent. Among patients with negative screening tests, 11.7% were currently alcohol dependent and 3.9% were currently drug dependent.

Conclusion.—PSUDs were diagnosed in a high percentage of trauma patients. These patients should be identified and referred for treatment.

▶ This study suggests that many patients suffering serious trauma may be current alcohol or drug abusers. The authors emphasize the need for follow-up care. I would like to emphasize the need to include this possibility in our routine evaluation criteria for seriously injured patients. It could make a significant difference in matters of sedation and analgesia.

B.A Shapiro, M.D.

9 Socioeconomic Issues, Outcomes, and Ethics

Socioeconomic Issues

The Experiences of Families With a Relative in the Intensive Care Unit
Jamerson PA, Scheibmeir M, Bott MJ, et al (Univ of Kansas, Kansas City)
Heart Lung 25:467–474, 1996
9–1

Introduction.—When a family member is admitted to the ICU, there is an immediate impact on the family. It is crucial that families' needs be addressed. The experiences of families with members in the ICU were assessed to determine the best approach to meeting their needs.

Methods.—Focus groups and individual unstructured interviews were audiotaped and transcribed to identify, code, and categorize themes of families' experiences.

Results.—Four categories, as follows, were used to create a model of family experiences in the ICU (Fig 1): hovering, information seeking, tracking, and garnering resources. In the hovering stage, relatives are confused, stressed, and uncertain. Through information seeking, families help themselves to move out of the hovering stage and identify the patients' progress. Families use tracking to observe, analyze, and evaluate patient care and status and the family's satisfaction with the environment and the care givers. When family members garner resources, they are acquiring what they perceive is needed by their relative or by themselves.

Conclusion.—Family members go through 4 stages when a relative is admitted to the ICU. Health care professionals can minimize the stress of ICU stay by intervening in ways that anticipate and address family needs for information and resources.

▶ This is a good article for anyone who is involved in the administration of an ICU or anyone concerned about making the often overwhelming ICU experience easier for patients' family members to endure. The authors (all of whom are nurses) have prepared a nice table of suggested interventions for nurses and their institutions to adopt.

C.M. Franklin, M.D.

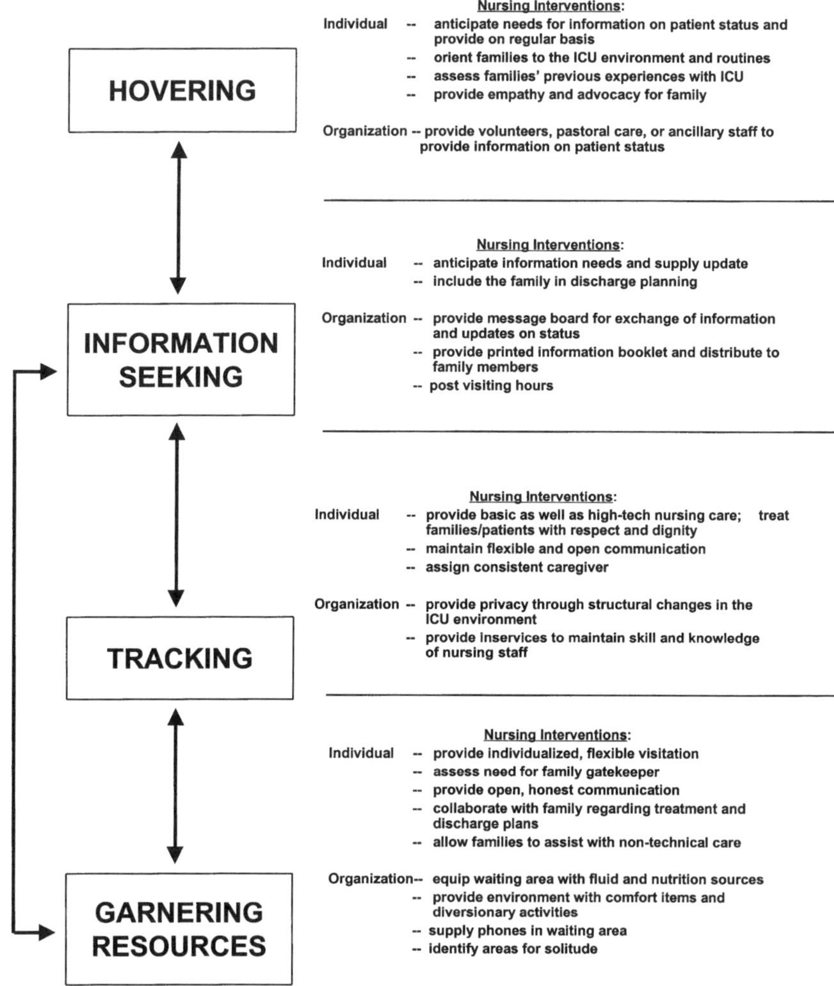

FIGURE 1.—Model of families' experiences in the ICU. For each stage, suggested interventions by nurses and the institution are listed. (Courtesy of Jamerson PA, Scheibmeir M, Bott MJ, et al: The experiences of families with a relative in the intensive care unit. *Heart Lung* 25:467–474, 1996.)

Method of Medicare Reimbursement and the Rate of Potentially Ineffective Care of Critically Ill Patients

Cher DJ, Lenert LA (Stanford Univ, Calif)
JAMA 278:1001–1007, 1997

9–2

Introduction.—A slow, painful death, in which the patient's and family's suffering are extended through impotent medical interventions, may be the worst outcome of critical care. The authors have used potentially ineffective care (PIC) as a proxy of this "worst" outcome in assessing the quality of critical care. Given the incentives of physicians in managed care settings to limit critical care, it might be expected that PIC rates would be lower for patients treated in these settings. Medicare data were analyzed to see if PIC was less likely for HMO patients than fee-for-service patients.

Methods.—The study used Medicare data for patients in California ICUs during fiscal year 1994. The study definition of PIC was death in the hospital or within 100 days of hospital discharge in the face of total hospital costs above the 90th percentile. The treatment cost model adjusted hospital costs for institution-specific cost-to-charge ratios and local wage indices, based on Health Care Financing Administration cost reports. Rates of PIC were compared for HMO versus fee-for-service patients, with adjustment for age, sex, race, elective hospitalization, Charlson index diseases, common diagnosis-related groups for death by 100 days, ICU size, and number of residents in the hospital.

Findings.—About 5% of patients received PIC, with this group consuming 22% of all ICU resources. The adjusted odds ratio for PIC among HMO patients was 0.75, with a 95% confidence interval of 0.65 to 0.87. At the same time, the risk of in-hospital death was no greater for HMO patients. The risk of death within 100 days of hospital discharge was only slightly elevated for the HMO group, adjusted odds ratio 1.08.

Conclusions.—The rate of PIC outcomes among Medicare patients is about 5%, these data suggest. These patients consume a disproportionately high share of ICU resources. Medicare patients enrolled in HMOs are less likely to experience PIC outcomes than those enrolled in fee-for-service plans, after adjustment for other factors. Thus HMOs may do a better job of limiting inappropriate use of critical care resources for patients near to the end of life.

▶ This article raises an extremely important question to everyone who works in critical care, namely does managed care do a better job of evaluating when and how to use critical care resources. Although the article suggests this may be true (and there is little in the data to refute that conclusion), this is too complex a question to be answered in a single study. In this respect, this article should be viewed as a starting point to answering that question. Obviously the potential danger posed by badly carried out managed care is that sick patients will not receive services they require, death being cheaper. As one physician suggested, only half in jest, the perfect managed care patient is healthy for thirty years, then develops a terminal illness and dies before anyone can do anything about it.

I'm optimistic enough to believe that there is enough good faith in the system to make those concerns nothing more than theoretical. There is no firm evidence that managed care has done a bad job with critically ill patients, but this article suggests the opposite. We can hope that this article will be read and studied by people in a position to duplicate (or refute) the results, and we will better understand if, as far as critically ill patients are concerned, managed care is an answer or a question.

C.M. Franklin, M.D.

Methods.—The retrospective study analyzed data on patients admitted to the medical ICU of a community teaching hospital before and after the hiring of a medical intensivist as full-time director of critical care. There were 459 patients in the year before the director was hired (BD) and 471 patients in the year after the director was hired (AD). The 2 groups were compared for mortality and lengths of stay. The scores of residents on a standardized critical care examination were compared for the same 2 periods.

Results.—The BD and AD groups were similar in terms of case mix and illness severity scores. Mortality in the ICU was 21% in the BD period versus 15% in the AD period. At the same time, in-hospital mortality dropped from 34% to 25%. For most disease categories, disease-specific mortality was reduced in the AD period (Table 1). More detailed analysis was performed in the subgroup of patients with pneumonia. Again, there were no differences in patient characteristics or severity of illness. Pneumonia-specific mortality decreased from 46% to 31% across illness severity categories.

Mean length of hospital stay decreased from 23 days in the BD period to 18 days in the AD period. Mean ICU stay decreased from 5 to 4 days. The residents' critical care in-service test scores improved from 54% to 68%. For residents at a comparable level of treatment, scores were significantly higher in the AD period than in the BD period.

Conclusions.—Adding a medical intensivist to the staff of a community hospital is linked to improvements in patient and educational outcomes. Though no cause-and-effect conclusions can be drawn, the findings suggest that the costs of providing full-time intensivist coverage may be justified at many hospitals. Reduced mortality most likely results from improved staff education and proficiency in the ICU, or improved ICU organization and coordination between disciplines.

▶ A convincing study demonstrating how the hiring of an intensivist reduced hospital mortality for a group of intensive care patients. The data are impressive, and I certainly believe the cause-and-effect nature of the results. However, one of the first studies that demonstrated similar results in the 1980s is flawed because although the authors demonstrated a lower mortality for intensive care patients after an intensivist was hired, it was also true that the mortality for all hospitalized patients (intensive care and non-intensive care) went up, a fact the previous authors failed to recognize or comment upon. This suggests the possibility that an intensivist may be able to change mortality for intensive care patients by selecting them differently (triage bias), possibly excluding certain types of patients.

In theory, the scoring system employed will screen for this bias (and in this study APACHE II scores were no different), but I am not convinced that the scoring system will necessarily identify a triage bias. To illustrate, what if many patients in the preintensivist era were oncology patients with an APACHE score of 20 and in the intensivist era they were cardiac patients with an APACHE II score of 20 (because the intensivist put in a policy discouraging oncology patients)? It is not clear that the patients would be matched equally, and the oncology patients of the earlier era might simply die in the second era without being admitted to the intensive care unit. Mortality for intensive care patients might be the same or lower, but mortality in all hospitalized patients might be higher leading one to question the true benefit of the intensivist.

I am not suggesting that triage bias was an issue in the current study. In fact, looking at the diagnostic categories suggests that this was not true. (Triage bias could work the other way, leading the intensivist to select sicker patients, in which case their benefit is even greater.) But when studies such as this one are undertaken (and when they are analyzed after publication), it is important to take into account a careful evaluation of the case-mix and how it may have changed from one period to the next. It is also important to measure total hospital mortality for all patients in the intervals considered to ensure that sick patients who do not come to the intensive care unit are not being neglected in the results.

C.M. Franklin, M.D.

Prediction of Outcome From Intensive Care: A Prospective Cohort Study Comparing Acute Physiology and Chronic Health Evaluation II and III Prognostic Systems in a United Kingdom Intensive Care Unit
Beck DH, Taylor BL, Millar B, et al (Queen Alexandra Hosp, Portsmouth, England; St George's Hosp Medical School, London)
Crit Care Med 25:9–15, 1997   9–5

Introduction.—Prognostication of outcome from critical illness continues to be a focus in this era of escalating health care costs. The Acute Physiology and Chronic Health Evaluation (APACHE) II and III systems are 2 predictive models. APACHE III was created in 1991 as a revision of APACHE II and consists of a numerical score ranging from 0 to 299, reflecting the weights assigned to the variables of 3 principal data categories: physiologic measurements, chronic health status, and chronological age. These 2 prognostic systems used to predict hospital mortality in adult ICU patients were evaluated and compared.

Methods.—There were 1,144 patients who had APACHE II and APACHE III prognostic systems applied to assess the probabilities of their hospital mortality and to compare results with the actual outcome. Both models were assessed for overall goodness-of-fit.

Results.—There was a strong positive correlation between the 2 systems according to risk estimates. For all decision criteria applied, the total correct classification of APACHE III was greater. For APACHE III, the best overall total correct classification rate was 80.6% and for APACHE II, it was 77.9%. Trauma patients had the highest mortality ratios for both models, and those with respiratory disease had the lowest mortality ratios for both models. There were significantly better predictions for patients with gastrointestinal disease with APACHE II. The older model also had superior risk estimates for surgical admissions. For medical patients, both models were similar.

Conclusion.—A similar degree of overall goodness-of-fit was demonstrated in both predictive models. Better calibration was shown with APACHE II, but APACHE III had better discrimination. Both models underestimated hospital mortality, but APACHE III was worse. There was considerable variation across the disease spectrum of ICU patients in the risk estimates of both models. In the comparison of the 2 models, the performance of APACHE III was not found to be superior to APACHE II, and, in some instances, the newer version was worse.

▶ This study again confirms that patients who are "sicker" (i.e., have a higher APACHE III score) have a poorer prognosis. However, it also confirms the fact that the APACHE III score does not discriminate between those who will survive and those who will not. Further, there was a poor correlation between plasma cytokine concentrations, physiologic derangement, and mortality. Additionally, the fluctuations in plasma cytokine levels may explain the lack of effect seen in trials of anticytokine antibodies. This may temper enthusiasm for future anticytokine therapy.

Y. Friedman, M.D.

Basics of Stratifying for Severity of Illness

Gross PA (Hackensack Univ, Newark, NJ)
Infect Control Hosp Epidemiol 17:675–686, 1996   9–6

Introduction.—It is generally accepted that stratification for severity is necessary when assessing health care processes and outcomes. However, severity of illness may not always be the most essential correction; data should be analyzed with and without severity adjustment to be sure that the adjustment is necessary. This article reviews some key areas related to adjustment for severity of illness.

Severity Stratification By Disease.—Patients with cardiac disease may be stratified for severity in several different ways. The New York Heart Association score is the most widely used functional classification. However, the recently described Specific Activity Scale is more specific and sensitive. A weighted scoring system for angioplasty risk has been described as well. Systems of assessing cardiac surgery mortality risk have been developed as well, and these have been used to improve risk-adjusted mortality after coronary artery bypass grafting. In the area of infectious disease, risk stratification systems have been developed for surgical wound infections, ventilator-associated pneumonia, community-acquired pneumonia, sepsis, and AIDS outcomes. The Dukes system is well known for staging of colorectal cancer, and the primary tumor, regional nodes, metastasis system for staging of lung cancer. The Ranson criteria were developed to predict mortality and complications associated with pancreatitis.

Severity Indicators for All Disease Groups.—The diagnosis-related groups (DRGs) were introduced to incorporate severity of illness adjustment into the Medicare prospective payment system. Used with the International Classification of Diseases, ninth revision, Clinical Modification, the DRGs are useful in estimating severity of illness. Many other commercial systems for severity adjustment have been developed, including the Acute Physiology, Age, and Chronic Health Evaluation; the Medical illness severity group system; the computerized severity index; the patient management categories; and the acuity index method.

There have been few independent studies to compare these systems, however, making it difficult to say which are best for assessing quality of care. Though severity of illness accounts for part of the variation in cost and quality, other factors such as small area variation may be more critical. The most recent versions of the DRGs assess illness severity more comprehensively and estimate resource utilization more accurately. Research groups for whom cost is the greatest concern may therefore be able to use the DRGs without additional adjustments for severity of illness.

Discussion.—Systems of stratification for disease severity—disease-specific and general—are reviewed. These systems will continue to be used more often to evaluate the quality of health care delivered than variations in cost. Insurance companies will continue to select hospitals on the basis of cost, but will also start looking at measures of severity and risk-adjusted outcomes as surrogate markers of quality. However, more progress is needed in the science of evaluating quality of care before outcomes data can be reliably used for quality assessment.

▶ This article is a useful review of various risk stratification schemes that are in place for cardiac and infectious disease, cancer and pancreatitis. The author lists the different types of indicators that are used in severity systems and review what comparisons have been made. While acuity adjusters are useful in looking at quality assurance issues, they are not the sole influences on the type of care that patients receive; variations in care can be attributable to patient presentation, the tempo of the disease, and physician and patient preferences, especially in areas where there is no clear-cut evidence for preferred treatments. While this paper is a good introduction into the subject of acuity adjustment, the interested reader will need to consult other texts and articles.

J.E. Calvin, Jr., M.D.
J.E. Parrillo, M.D.

Mortality Predicted by APACHE II: The Effect of Changes in Physiological Values and Post-ICU Hospital Mortality

Goldhill DR, Withington PS (Royal London Hosp)
Anaesthesia 51:719–723, 1996
9–7

Introduction.—The most commonly used scoring system for evaluating outcome in patients admitted to the ICU is the Acute Physiology and Chronic Health Evaluation (APACHE) II. Its methodology may have limitations that do not allow for improvements in physiologic values after intervention. A large intensive care database was used to determine the contribution of physiologic values to the APACHE II score.

Methods.—For the database, the APACHE II scores were calculated from the worst values within 24 hours of ICU admission. The number of points contributed to the APACHE II score by each variable was determined. The data were sorted into 10 bands, based on predicted mortality. The contributions made by the variables in each band were measured. The mortality ratio was plotted for each predicted risk of death band, then data were reanalyzed.

Results.—A review of 100 random charts indicated that there was a 20% likelihood of an inaccuracy in 1 of the 11 physiologic variables. The most frequent error was incorrectly scoring a variable as normal. The 11 physiologic variables contributed a mean of 8.9 points, or 54% of the APACHE II score. The 6 variables judged to be the most easily influenced by treatment were heart rate, mean arterial blood pressure, respiratory rate, pH, oxygenation, and hemoglobin. These selected variables contributed a mean of 6.1 points, or 37% of the total. The mortality ratio was 1.13. The APACHE II scores and post–intensive care mortality were altered to evaluate the effect of the changes on mortality ratio (Table 3). When the scores were increased by 2 or 4 points, mortality ratios dropped to 1.00 and 0.89, respectively. When the scores were decreased by 2 or 4 points to a minimum of zero, mortality ratios rose to 1.27 and 1.44,

TABLE 3.—Mortality Ratios for Actual and Perceived Data

	MR	(95% CI)
Physiological points minus 4 points	1.44	(1.41 to 1.47)*
Physiological points minus 2 points	1.27	(1.25 to 1.30)*
25% more deaths	1.21	(1.19 to 1.23)*
Actual data	1.13	(1.11 to 1.15)*
25% fewer deaths	1.05	(1.03 to 1.07)*
Physiological points plus 2 points	1.00	(0.98 to 1.02)
Physiological points plus 4 points	0.89	(0.88 to 0.91)*

Note: Mortality ratio (MR) is the observed number of deaths divided by the predicted number. Physiologic points are points contributed by physiologic variables.

*P <0.01, observed vs. predicted.

Abbreviation: CI, confidence interval.

(Reprinted from Goldhill DR, Withington PS: Mortality predicted by APACHE II: The effect of changes in physiological values and post-ICU hospital mortality. *Anesthesia* 51:719–723, 1996, by permission of the publisher, WB Saunders Company Limited, London.)

respectively. When post–intensive care hospital rates were increased or decreased by 25%, mortality ratios were 1.21 and 1.04, respectively.

Conclusion.—Physiologic values differ with the timing of collection and the accuracy of recording. Small consistent differences in score may cause potentially significant changes in the mortality ratio. Data collection and effective management before and after intensive care must be standardized, as mortality ratios are inaccurate and misleading.

▶ The authors have presented a practical demonstration of a number of weaknesses of physiology-based scoring systems that have not previously been adequately addressed. In the case of APACHE II, the fact that mortality prediction is heavily dependent on a limited number of variables means that any type of minor variation (e.g., observer variation or error) in 1 of those variables can have an important impact on the predicted mortality. The authors also discuss other factors that influence the mortality ratio (the relationship between predicted and observed mortality) including pre- and post-ICU care. The most important issue in this respect is treatment-influenced variables, where the APACHE II score may be calculated only after the patient has received important therapy.

Scoring system developers have never been able to fully factor the effect therapy has on physiology into the severity of illness concept. Ironically, even the potential for receiving therapy may alter a risk prediction (does a patient in the throes of ventricular fibrillation have the same predicted mortality risk on a city street, where no defibrillator is available, as he would in the coronary care unit?).

C.M. Franklin, M.D.

Plasma Proinflammatory Cytokine Concentrations, Acute Physiology and Chronic Health Evaluation (APACHE) III Scores and Survival in Patients in an Intensive Care Unit
Friedland JS, Porter JC, Daryanani S, et al (St George's Hosp, London; Univ of Michigan, Ann Arbor)
Crit Care Med 24:1775–1781, 1996   9–8

Introduction.—In the pathophysiology of severe illness, proinflammatory cytokines are undoubtedly involved. In patients dying of acute meningococcal sepsis and severe malaria, plasma tumor necrosis factor concentrations have been significantly high. Patients with septic shock also have had high levels of interleukin-1β. The presence of systemic inflammation resulting in derangement of whole body physiology and development of multiple organ failure are the most potent clinical indications of poor prognosis. A quantitative index of disease severity has been developed with several scoring systems, including the Acute Physiology and Chronic Health Evaluation (APACHE) III system. The prognostic significance of plasma concentrations of 4 cytokines in the proinflammatory responses were investigated.

TABLE 4.—Independent Predictors of Survival in Severely Ill Patients, Using a Subtraction Logistic Regression Model of Illness*

	Odds Ratio	95% CI	p Value
APACHE III (ln)	11.4	2.3–55.7	.003
TNF bioactivity in plasma	3.2	1.2–8.5	.022
Predicted mortality	9.1	1.0–83.8	.05

*No other cytokine or physiologic measurement had independent significance in this model.
Abbreviations: CI, confidence interval; *ln,* natural logarithm.
Chi-square (3 degrees of freedom) = 83.25.
(Courtesy of Friedland JS, Porter JC, Daryanani S, et al: Plasma proinflammatory cytokine concentrations, Acute Physiology and Chronic Health Evaluation (APACHE) III scores and survival in patients in an intensive care unit. *Crit Care Med* 24:1775–1781, 1996.)

Methods.—There were 251 patients in an ICU who had calculations of daily APACHE III scores. The following four proinflammatory cytokines also were measured in blood samples: tumor necrosis factor α, interleukin-1β, interleukin-6, and interleukin-8.

Results.—In 42 patients, plasma tumor necrosis factor concentrations were increased. In 15 patients, interleukin-1β was increased. In 194 patients, interleukin-6 was increased; and in 52 patients, interleukin-8 was increased. In patients who died in the ICU, admission plasma interleukin-1β, interleukin-6, and interleukin-8 concentrations were higher when compared with those of the survivors. In patients with a fatal outcome, only admission plasma interleukin-8 concentrations were higher, if all in-hospital deaths were considered. The best predictor of mortality was the APACHE III score. A weak, independent predictor of death was detection of tumor necrosis factor. There was no relationship between plasma cytokine concentrations and the presence of the systemic inflammatory response or of bacteremia. There were 19 patients in the ICU for more than 10 days, and of these, 16 had prolonged increases of plasma cytokines. Daily APACHE III scores and mortality had a variable relation with persistently increased plasma cytokine concentrations.

Conclusion.—In serious illness, plasma cytokine concentrations fluctuate and have a poor correlation with derangement of whole body physiology in seriously ill patients. An independent predictor of mortality was the presence of bioactive tumor necrosis factor (Table 4). Clinical application in the ICU setting is unlikely with daily measurement of plasma proinflammatory cytokine concentrations. However, in specific subgroups of patients, it may be a possibility.

▶ Reports of ICU admissions of AIDS patients have gone through 3 distinct periods. Initial reports showed uniformly grim prognoses. The second period showed significantly improved prognoses, mostly in patients with acute respiratory failure (ARF). Recently, there has been a decrease in the survival of AIDS patients admitted to ICUs.

This study found that mortality was related to physiologic derangement, with the duration of diagnosis before admission being the only direct AIDS-related prognostic factor. However, patients with simple pneumothoraces without ARF were admitted to the ICU, whereas patients with wasting disease and HIV dementia were not, thus possibly reducing this hospital's ICU mortality as a result of selection bias. Their conclusion, with which I agree, is that patients with AIDS should be evaluated for ICU admission on the same basis as any other patients.

Y. Friedman, M.D.

The Glasgow Coma Scale: A Critical Appraisal of its Clinimetric Properties
Prasad K (All India Inst of Med Sciences, New Delhi)
J Clin Epidemiol 49:755–763, 1996   9–9

Background.—The Glasgow Coma Scale (GCS), on its own or in combination with other measures, has been used to assess patients with a wide range of clinical conditions. The uses of this instrument have been expanded with little attention to its clinimetric properties. The clinimetric properties of the GCS were assessed in an analysis of published research.

Methods.—The literature was searched for articles describing or commenting on the clinimetric properties of the GCS. Twenty-nine primary articles on this topic were identified. Clinimetric properties evaluated were clinical function, clinical justification, item selection, item scaling, item reduction, aggregation, reliability, validity, and sensitivity to change.

Results.—The analysis suggested that the GCS had good sensibility and reliability, with an intraclass correlation coefficient of 0.8 to 1.0 when used by trained clinicians. Strong evidence of cross-sectional construct validity was found. A generating sample found that the GCS had good predictive validity in patients with traumatic coma; used in combination with age and brain stem reflexes, it had a sensitivity of 79% to 97% and a specificity of 84% to 97%. There were no reports of testing in an external validation sample, however, nor was there sufficient evidence of longitudinal construct validity.

Conclusion.—The available evidence suggests that the GCS has good clinimetric properties for use as a discriminative instrument. However, its validity as a predictive and evaluative instrument (the latter being the purpose for which it was constructed) remains to be established. It performs best as a predictive instrument if each subscale is treated as a separate variable to be combined with other predictor variables.

▶ Since its introduction in 1974, the GCS has been commonly used to assess patients with traumatic and nontraumatic neurologic disease. The authors evaluated the properties of the GCS for discriminating severity of injury, evaluating changes in the level of dysfunction, and predicting ultimate outcome. They found limitations in all 3 areas. The failure of the aggregate score (especially because of lack of reliability and reproducibility in measuring verbal response) to reliably indicate changes in level of consciousness may require changes in the way neurologic assessment of patients is performed in many ICUs.

Y. Friedman, M.D.

Relationship Between Glasgow Coma Scale and Functional Outcome
Zafonte RD, Hammond FM, Mann NR, et al (Wayne State Univ, Detroit)
Am J Phys Med Rehabil 75:364–369, 1996   9–10

Background.—A major challenge in the treatment and rehabilitation of patients with traumatic brain injuries (TBIs) is the prediction of both long-term and immediate outcome. The Glasgow Coma Scale (GCS) is a commonly used predictor of morbidity and mortality; however, its ability to predict functional outcome has yet to be established for patients surviving TBI and receiving rehabilitation. The relationship between GCS and 4 measures of functional outcome was explored.

Methods.—Data were collected between 1988 and 1993 on 501 patients, 16 years or older, who sustained a TBI within 8 hours of presentation to the emergency department of a participating hospital. The GCS was determined and recorded for each patient at the time of presentation, and the lowest and highest GCS within the 24 hours after the traumatic episode were determined. Functional outcome was predicted at both the time of admission to and discharge from a TBI rehabilitation unit using the Disability Rating Scale (DRS), the Rancho Los Amigos Levels of Cognitive Function Scale (LCFS), and both the cognitive and motor components of the Functional Independence Measure (FIM-COG and FIM-M, respectively).

Results.—The correlations between GCS and all outcome variables were significant but weak, with correlation coefficients of between 0.16 and 0.37. The FIM-COG and LCFS at the time of admission were the functional outcome scales most highly correlated with GCS. Correlations between GCS motor score and the outcome variables were, again, statistically significant but weak, accounting for only 3.2% to 7.3% of the functional outcome variance. The GCS motor score, however, was a superior predictor of functional outcome than was the total GCS score in all but 1 patient. Patient age was also a significant but weak indicator of functional outcome, accounting for 0.4% to 6% of the functional outcome variance.

Conclusion.—Although GCS is a valuable tool in predicting patient mortality after TBIs, the usefulness of the scale in predicting functional and cognitive outcome is limited.

▶ The GCS is the most widely used index of severity of illness in patients with traumatic head injury. However, the GCS has limitations in describing severity of injury and evaluating changes in the patient's level of consciousness. This study further demonstrates limitations of the GCS in predicting functional outcome.

Y. Friedman, M.D.

Survival and Quality of Life After Intensive Care
Capuzzo M, Bianconi M, Contu P, et al (Azienda Ospedaliera S Anna, Ferrara, Italy)
Intensive Care Med 22:947–953, 1996   9–11

Introduction.—The initial goal of ICUs was survival. The Second European Consensus Conference on Intensive Care Medicine has stated, "mortality is an insufficient measure of ICU outcome . . . Future outcome evaluation of intensive care should incorporate quality of life." Reports vary on how quality of life (QOL) is defined. Survival and QOL were evaluated in patients who had been discharged from an ICU.

Methods.—Cooperative patients were interviewed during their ICU stay and 6 months after discharge from the hospital. Patients were questioned regarding residence, change in physical activity, social functioning, oral communication, functional limitations, and perceptions of life after hospital discharge.

Results.—Predicted and actual 1-year survival rates were 84% and 82.4%, respectively. Of patients who died, the mortality rate was 36.3% after urgent neoplastic surgery, 19.4% for medical admission, and 4.9% after nonneoplastic surgery. Of 160 patients interviewed during their ICU stay, 8 were not able to respond to the perceived QOL question at 6 month follow-up. At 6 month follow-up, there was a reduction in physical activity in 31% of patients, social life was worsened in 32%, and functional limitations increased in 30%. There was no change in perceived QOL.

Conclusion.—At 6-month follow-up after an ICU stay, survival was similar to that of the general population and was influenced more by pre-ICU admission conditions than by the ICU course or treatment. Most patients admitted to the ICU maintained their pre-admission physical activity level and social status. Any worsening of these measures was slight and did not affect perceived QOL.

▶ It seems somewhat counterintuitive, but this study showed that survival and QOL were not measurably affected by ICU admission. This is another study I would like to see reproduced by other medical centers before its conclusions are broadly accepted. Nevertheless, for those who care for ICU patients on a daily basis, a measure of optimism is warranted, based on these findings.

C.M. Franklin, M.D.

Why Do Patients Die on General Wards After Discharge From Intensive Care Units?

Wallis CB, Davies HTO, Shearer AJ (Ninewells Hosp, Dundee, Scotland)
Anaesthesia 52:9–14, 1997

9–12

Introduction.—The hospital mortality rate of patients in the ICU averaged 27.7% in the Intensive Care Society's Acute Physiology and Chronic Health Evaluation (APACHE II) investigation. The ICU mortality rate was actually 17.9%; the remaining 9.8% died in hospital wards after ICU discharge. Do deaths on hospital wards after ICU discharge represent a waste of resources in the ICU or a missed opportunity to prevent deaths? The characteristics and causes of death of patients who died on hospital wards after ICU discharge were assessed in a retrospective review of 1,700 patients admitted to the ICU over a 5-year period.

Methods.—Data regarding age, admission APACHE II scores, and duration of stay were collected for 3 patient groups: those who died in the ICU, those who died in the hospital ward after ICU discharge, and those who survived. Patient outcome was predicted at the time of ICU discharge as expected to die, considered at risk of death, or expected to survive. Formal tests of significance were not used in this investigation.

Results.—Of the 1,700 patients, 341 (20%) died in the ICU, 153 (9%) died in the hospital ward after ICU discharge, and 1,206 (71%) were survivors. Using data collected at discharge from the ICU, 54.2% of patients who died were considered at risk of death, 25.5% were expected to die, and 20.3% were expected to survive. The causes of death for patients considered at risk were primarily pneumonia, cerebrovascular accident, malignancy, renal failure, multi-organ failure, and myocardial infarction. The major causes of death in patients expected to die were effects of hypoxia and structural brain damage. Of the 20.3% of patients expected to live, causes of death were usually pneumonia, sepsis, malignancy, myocardial infarction, thromboembolism, and cerebrovascular accident.

Conclusion.—The major causes of death on hospital wards after discharge from the ICU were pneumonia and irreversible brain damage. Some deaths were inevitable, but most occurred in patients who remained at risk on ICU discharge or were expected to survive. An important concern is that patients are being discharged from the ICU too early in response to demand for beds.

▶ In general, the sickest group of hospitalized patients are those in the ICU and the second sickest group are those who have been discharged from the ICU. This study showed a 9% hospital mortality rate post ICU discharge. Past studies have documented similar numbers as well as a statistically higher incidence of cardiac arrest in patients discharged from the ICU. As more attention is devoted to "appropriate" lengths of stay in the ICU, we need to focus more on negative outcome variables such as post ICU deaths (and readmissions). Although some of these are to be expected, this study suggests that a significant percentage may be avoidable.

C.M. Franklin, M.D.

Five-Year Survival After Intensive Care—Comparison of 12,180 Patients With the General Population

Niskanen M, and the Finnish ICU Study Group (Univ of Kuopio, Finland; Turku Univ, Finland; Tampere Univ, Finland; et al)
Crit Care Med 24:1962–1967, 1996   9–13

Background.—Intensive care outcomes are usually measured by in-unit or in-hospital mortality. Determining life expectancy after intensive care may be a better way to assess the efficacy of intensive care.

Methods.—Twenty-five ICUs at 17 hospitals in Finland participated in the prospective study. The participating ICUs included 13 in 5 tertiary care centers. Data on 12,180 consecutive adults admitted to the ICUs in 1987, divided into 7 diagnostic subgroups, were obtained.

Findings.—The 5-year mortality in this cohort was 3.3 times greater than that of the Finnish general population. The survival rate of patients in the ICU paralleled that of the general population at 2 years, whereas the relative survival rate of the patients at 5 years was 66.7%. In a multivariate analysis, cancer was a strong determinant of a poor outcome (relative risk,

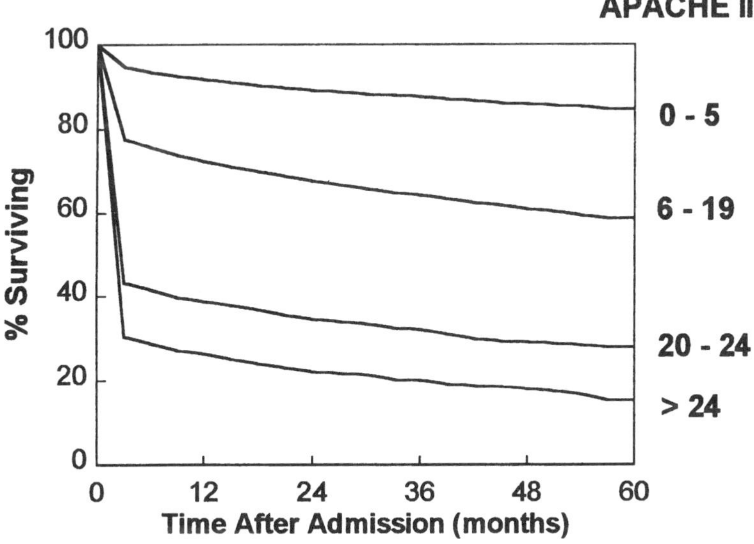

FIGURE 2.—The 5-year survival rates of 12,180 patients in the ICU stratified by the severity of illness at the time of ICU admission. *Abbreviation: APACHE II,* Acute Physiology and Chronic Health Evaluation II score. (Courtesy of Niskanen M, and the Finnish ICU Study Group: Five-year survival after intensive care—comparison of 12,180 patients with the general population. *Crit Care Med* 24:1962–1967, 1996.)

TABLE 2.—Factors Contributing to 5-yr Mortality of Intensive Care Unit Patients (n=11,817)

Variable	Relative Risk	(95% Confidence Interval)	p Value
Age (yr)	1.03	(1.03–1.03)	<.0001
Male gender (0.1)	1.16	(1.09–1.23)	<.0001
APS at admission	1.07	(1.07–1.08)	<.0001
Chronic Health Evaluation score	1.06	(1.05–1.08)	<.0001
Admission after elective surgery (0.1)	0.56	(0.52–0.61)	<.0001
Cardiovascular disease (0.1)	1.22	(1.12–1.34)	<.0001
Respiratory failure (0.1)	1.37	(1.23–1.53)	<.0001
Gastroenterologic disease (0.1)	1.45	(1.30–1.62)	<.0001
Trauma (0.1)	0.96	(0.82–1.13)	NS
Intoxication (0.1)	0.75	(0.62–0.89)	<.01
Cancer	3.17	(2.86–3.51)	<.0001
Postcardiac arrest (0.1)	1.70	(1.50–1.93)	<.0001

Note: By Cox's regression analysis. (0.1) refers to a dichotomous variable.
Abbreviation: APS, Acute Physiology Score.
(Courtesy of Niskanen M, and the Finnish ICU Study Group: Five-year survival after intensive care-comparison of 12,180 patients with the general population. *Crit Care Med* 24:1962–1967, 1996.)

3.17). The 5-year mortality of the patients in the ICU compared with the general population was greatest among patients admitted to the ICU after intoxication. Trauma victims and patients with a cardiovascular disease reached the general population's risk of death in the shortest time (Fig 2 and Table 2).

Conclusion.—On average, patients in the ICU achieve a life expectancy comparable with that of the general population 2 years after admission. However, the diagnostic category influences the time at which survival parallels that of the general population.

▶ The findings here are not exactly the same as those in the study by Capuzzo,[1] but the message is the same—patients who are successfully discharged from the ICU tend to do better than many people believe. Although initial mortality in the first 2 years was significantly higher for ICU discharges than it was for the general population, it quickly reverted to normal after that. It will be interesting to do a cost–benefit analysis of ICU care with this type of data, especially if the data are carried out to 5-year intervals. The costs and life-years saved may be favorable when compared with other therapies.

J. Samuel, M.D., and C.M. Franklin, M.D.

Reference

1. Capuzzo M, Bianconi M, Contu P, et al: Survival and quality of life after intensive care. *Intensive Care Med* 22:947–953, 1996.

Prediction of Outcome for Critically Ill Patients With Unexplained Hypotension

Heidenreich PA, Foster E, Cohen NH (Univ of California, San Francisco)
Crit Care Med 24:1835–1840, 1996   9–14

Background.—Patients who are critically ill and who have hypotension have a poor prognosis. Various scoring systems have been developed to help determine the prognosis of hospitalized patients in the ICU. These scales are useful in comparing patient groups but may have limited value in predicting the outcome of individual patients. Because of this, scoring systems for specific diseases have been developed. However, these scoring systems for specific diseases require a diagnosis or data from invasive hemodynamic monitors.

Methods.—In a prospective study, data from an initial derivation group of 50 patients with sustained unexplained hypotension were analyzed and used to develop a prognostic scoring system that was validated in the next 51 patients with sustained unexplained hypotension. The main outcome measures were hospital discharge or death.

Results.—In the derivation and validation groups combined, overall mortality was 58%. Multivariate analysis identified 3 independent predictors of hospital mortality: the Acute Physiology and Chronic Health Evaluation (APACHE) II score at the time of hypotension, time from admission to the hypotensive episode, and admission for surgery or treatment of the malignancy. The Hypotension Score was developed by weighing and combining these variables. The Hypotension Score separated all 101 patients into 3 prognostic groups: (1) a Hypotension Score of less than 40 and a mortality of 7%, (2) a Hypotension Score of 40–64 and a mortality of 70%, and (3) a Hypotension Score of 65 or greater and a mortality of 92%. For the APACHE II score alone, the area under the receiver operating characteristic curve was 0.85 for the derivation group, and it was 0.83 for the validation group.

Discussion.—This Hypotension Score to predict survival in patients with unexplained hypotension uses variables from the time of hypotension. Its predictive power was unchanged when tested in an independent patient group. The Hypotension Score is simple to calculate and includes the length of stay before hypotension and the indication for admission, thereby improving on the APACHE II score.

► This study examines 101 adult patients in the ICU who were admitted with sustained, unexplained episodes of hypotension. The first 50 patients were used to develop a prognostic score, and the formula was then tested on the next 51 patients. Three independent prognostic predictors of hospital mortality were identified: the APACHE II score at the time of hypotension, the time from admission to the hospital to the hypotensive episode, and a hospital admission for surgery or treatment of a malignancy. The utility of the Hypotension Score would be in its comparison of mortality rates for ICUs. Essentially, the formula developed was designed to determine a severity of

these reactions. It does point out the need for post-discharge intervention and support services, a place where the ICU staff may have a role.

C.M. Franklin, M.D.

Outcome Prediction in Intensive Care: Results of a Prospective, Multicentre, Portuguese Study

Moreno R, Morais P (Hosp de Santo António dos Capuchos, Portugal)
Intensive Care Med 23:177–186, 1997   9–17

Purpose.—The Acute Physiology and Chronic Health Evaluation (APACHE) II score and Simplified Acute Physiology Score (SAPS II) are measures of severity of illness in critically ill patients. Before broad application, these scoring systems must be evaluated in the target population. An evaluation and comparison of the performance of the SAPS II and APACHE II scores in the Portuguese population—a completely separate population from those used in the development of the scores—is reported.

Methods.—The prospective, multicenter study included 1,094 consecutive patients admitted to 19 Portuguese ICUs over a 4-month period. As in the original criteria for both scores, the study excluded patients less than age 18, readmitted patients, patients with acute myocardial infarction, patients with burns, post-coronary artery bypass graft patients, and patients with ICU stays of less than 24 hours. This left 982 patients for

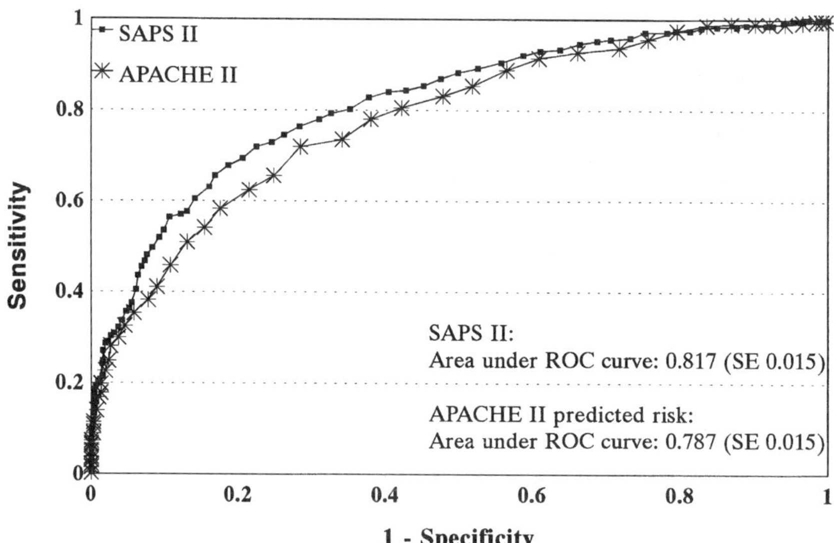

FIGURE 1.—Receiver operating characteristic (*ROC*) curves for SAPS II and APACHE II. The relationship between true positives *Sensitivity* and false positives *1 minus sensitivity*, is shown for both models. (Courtesy of Moreno R, Morais P: Outcome prediction in intensive care: results of a prospective, multicentre, Portuguese study. *Intensive Care Med* 23:177–186, 1997. Copyright 1997 by Springer-Verlag.)

analysis. Admission data necessary for calculation of the SAPS II and APACHE II scores were collected. Manpower utilization during the study period was evaluated using the Therapeutic Intervention Scoring System (TISS) and the Simplified TISS. The presence or absence of organ dysfunction was also assessed. Vital status at hospital discharge was evaluated.

Results.—The SAPS II showed better discrimination than the APACHE II score, with areas under the receiver operating characteristic curve of 0.817 and 0.787, respectively (Fig 1). However, calibration was poor with both models, showing significant differences between observed and predicted mortality. A stratified analysis revealed no clear pattern of association between the models' poor performance and specific patient subgroups. The exception was patients in the most severe categories of illness, for whom both the SAPS II and APACHE score overestimated mortality.

Conclusion.—In an independent population, the SAPS II better predicts the outcomes of ICU patients than does the APACHE II score. However, the SAPS II is not currently adequate to analyze the quality of care or performance among ICUs in the target population. It might be possible to customize the SAPS II for this purpose. Future severity scores should consider not only patient variability but also variability among ICUs.

▶ International literature continues to support the view that standardized scoring systems perform fairly well in predicting intensive care outcome but not well enough to use for global quality of care analysis. It is becoming clear that the major scoring systems will require modification or customization for specific populations if these goals are to be met in the near future. This well-done study emphasizes that point.

C.M. Franklin, M.D.

Assessing the Impact of Patient Characteristics and Process Performance on Rural Intensive Care Unit Hospital Mortality Rates

Jiang HJ, Fielselmann JF, Hendryx MS, et al (Virginia Commonwealth Univ, Richmond; Univ of Iowa, Iowa City; Washington State Univ, Spokane; et al)
Crit Care Med 25:773–778, 1997   9–18

Background.—A growing number of studies have assessed the quality of ICU care. These studies have focused on outcome analysis, particularly hospital mortality. Most of these studies have been done in urban hospitals; there are few data on the quality of care in rural ICUs. Associations among patient characteristics, care processes, and risk of hospital mortality were assessed in a retrospective study of data from rural Iowa ICUs.

Methods.—The study used data on 214 patients receiving mechanical ventilation for more than 96 hr in 19 rural Iowa ICUs between 1992 and 1994. The analysis included 138 survivors and 76 nonsurvivors. Relationships between patient characteristics, selected processes of care, and hospital mortality were assessed by logistic regression analyses. The care processes addressed were laboratory work, nursing assessment, stress ulcer protection, immobilization protection, nutritional management, ventilator management, and weaning.

Results.—Factors associated with an increased risk of death included patient age, odds ratio (OR) 1.03; elevated Acute Physiology and Chronic Health Evaluation (APACHE) II score, OR 1.06; and longer pre-ICU length of stay, OR 1.14. The hospitals varied significantly in terms of carrying out processes of care. Performance was greatest for nursing management and ventilator weaning, and worst for stress ulcer protection and complications of immobilization. After adjustment for patient characteristics, mortality risk was lower with better performance in ulcer protection (OR 0.1) and ventilator management (OR 0.03). Predictive accuracy was greater for a model incorporating both patient characteristics and processes of care than for a model including only patient characteristics. Area under the receiver operating characteristic curve was 0.80 versus 0.70, respectively.

Conclusion.—Factors affecting the quality of care in rural ICUs were studied. Differences in patient physiology and demographics account for most of the variation in mortality in this study. The data suggest that improving performance in certain processes of care—notably ulcer protection and ventilator management—could significantly reduce mortality risk. Useful predictors of mortality in the rural ICU setting include age, timing of ICU admission, and APACHE II score.

▶ This study examined outcomes in rural intensive care units as they were related to patient characteristics and processes of care (a vague term referring to specific ICU tasks). The most important finding is probably that the hospital length of stay prior to ICU transfer had a significant impact on mortality risk suggesting that early recognition of how sick patients are on presentation deserves greater attention in analysis of ICU care.

C.M. Franklin, M.D.

Anaylzing Intensive Care Unit Length of Stay Data: Problems and Possible Solutions
Weissman C (Columbia Univ, New York)
Crit Care Med 25:1594–1600, 1997

9–19

Objective.—Length of ICU stay is frequently reported as a mean value. However, because some patients have extended lengths of stay, this value may not adequately describe the typical length of stay or central tendency. Other descriptors are needed, including ways of identifying outliers with shorter or longer stays than the rest of the data. New approaches to analyzing length of stay patterns in the ICU were investigated.

Methods.—The retrospective study included all 4,499 patients admitted to the surgical ICU of a university hospital over a 6-year period. The patients were considered in diagnostic groups representing either a surgical procedure or, in the absence of any predominant procedure, a surgical

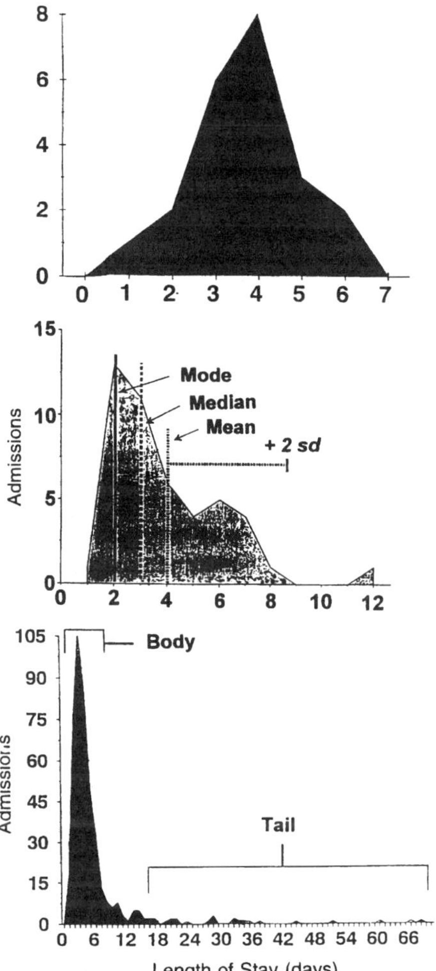

FIGURE 1.—**Top:** An example of a diagnostic group (thymectomies, Year 3) that had a nearly "normal" (symmetric) length of stay distribution. **Middle:** Frequency distribution of patients who had undergone urologic procedures (Year 1). Note the rightwardly skewed distribution. **Bottom:** Frequency distribution for all patients admitted in Year 1 plotted. In addition to a rightwardly skewed distribution, there are many outliers. The distribution can be divided into a "body" that includes the majority of patients who stayed for a week and a "tail." (Courtesy of Weissman C: Analyzing intensive care unit length of stay data: problems and possible solutions. *Crit Care Med* 25:1594–1600, 1997.)

discipline. The data were analyzed to determine how best to evaluate the typical length of stay for various patient groups and to identify patients with extended stays. The uses of these data in assessing critical care resource utilization are examined as well.

Measurements.—Most of the frequency distributions were skewed to the right. The "body" of the distribution included most of the patients and described the "typical" behavior; the "tail" provided information on outliers (Fig 1). For all diagnostic groups, the average of the mean lengths of stay was 3.9 days, compared with 2.7 days for the average of the medians and 2.1 days for the average of the modes. This was consistent with the right skewness of the length-of-stay distributions. Seventy-five percent of patients had a length of stay equal to the median plus or minus 1 day, thus, the median was the best descriptor of central tendency.

A number of different techniques were assessed for identification of outliers, including visual identification of histograms of the frequency distributions. On conventional analysis, outliers were identified as those patients with lengths of stay more than 2 standard deviations from the mean. However, with right-skewed distributions, this underestimated the number of outliers. Methods defining outliers according to a specific length of stay or percentage of patients resulted in differing numbers of patients identified as outliers.

Conclusion.—A visual examination of the frequency distribution is essential when analyzing length-of-stay data on ICU patients. Because of characteristic right skewness, traditional statistical concepts such as mean and standard deviation are not ideal for describing the typical length of ICU stay. The median, mode, and harmonic mean are more useful values. Some indication of the characteristics of the data is needed when reporting length of stay, such as a graph of the frequency distribution or reporting the mean, median, and range.

▶ This is an important paper that takes a common problem, length of stay, and looks at it in a useful new way. Length of stay does not behave according to gaussian distribution; therefore, graphing frequency distribution and describing data in a different mathematical way, using more complicated analysis of trends and outliers, make sense and have a great deal of potential value. I suspect that diseases we see in the intensive care unit (ICU) will have characteristic frequency distributions that will allow easier comparison between different ICUs. All of this is a result of our ubiquitous computer power and is theoretically available to anyone in the near future who has access to ICU data and a willingness to explore this area. While the math employed here is a little beyond those of us who gave up serious math around junior year in high school, it should not be a deterrent. I highly recommend this article. I believe it should stimulate a good deal of thinking.

C.M. Franklin, M.D.

Can Clinical Interventions Change Care at the End of Life?
Hanson LC, Tulsky JA, Danis M (Univ of North Carolina, Chapel Hill; Veterans Affairs Med Ctr, Durham, NC)
Ann Intern Med 126:381–388, 1997   9–20

Background.—Several different types of interventions have been studied in an attempt to alter care for patients at the end of life. The goals of these interventions have included increasing the use of patient preferences, minimizing pain and suffering, reducing the inappropriate use of life-sustaining treatments, and reducing costs. The results have varied, with some studies claiming success but others failing to meet their goals. A detailed review of clinical interventions to change care at the end of life was performed.

Methods.—The investigators searched for clinical trials of interventions designed to change medical care at the end of life. Nonclinical studies and studies performed outside the United States were not included. The interventions were classified as being targeted at patients and physicians or both. They were then assessed for their impact on the clinical goals of increased use of patient preferences, minimization of pain and suffering, reduced use of life-sustaining treatments, and reduced costs. Successful and unsuccessful trials were compared in terms of differences in intervention, target group, and strength of study methods.

Results.—Most educational interventions led to increased expression of treatment preferences by patients. Interventions were more likely to be successful if they targeted more severely ill patients and combined written materials with repeated conversations in clinical encounters. Use of patient preferences was increased by educational interventions directed toward physicians. However, getting physicians to change their behavior required sophisticated educational approaches. Some studies suggested that educational interventions for physicians reduced the use of life-sustaining treatments. However, none of the interventions tested was effective in reducing pain, suffering, or the cost of medical care.

Conclusion.—The best approaches to changing care at the end of life seem to be intensive educational interventions for physicians and broad institutional initiatives. These types of interventions are more effective than advance directives, the available evidence suggests. The authors call for more research into changing physician practice patterns, reducing the costs of end-of-life care, and improving such patient-centered outcomes as pain control and satisfaction.

▶ This article is essentially a metaanalysis of studies of clinical interventions at the end of life. It concludes that intensive educational interventions for physicians and broad institutional programs are more promising than advance directives. I'm not sure that isn't simply a function of the methodology, i.e., the publication bias that is the weakness of metaanlaysis. In any event, this is not an either-or question. Unfortunately, advance directives have not been used as much as hoped. In this respect, effective educational programs should be complementary, rather than used in place of advance directives.

C.M. Franklin, M.D.

Mortality Among Appropriately Referred Patients Refused Admission to Intensive-Care Units

Metcalfe MA, Sloggett A, McPherson K (London School of Hygiene and Tropical Medicine)

Lancet 350:7–12, 1997

9–21

Introduction.—Emergencies or prebooked surgical patients constitute the majority of referrals to ICUs. Some patients are refused admission because the units may be full, because there are insufficient trained nurses, or because the admitting clinicians deem the patients to be too well or too ill. Because there is a concern that refusals have higher attributable risk of death, how mortality rates were affected by refusals of admission to an ICU was investigated.

Methods.—During a 3-month period, referrals to ICUs with different numbers of beds were monitored. For all patients known to be alive at hospital discharge, data on mortality were obtained from family physicians 90 days after first referral. Adjustments were made for bed provision, surgery and emergency categories, disease severity, appropriateness of referral age, and sex. For patients who were refused admission and for those admitted, multivariate analysis by multiple logistic regression was conducted to compare the adjusted 90-day mortality rates.

Results.—There were 165 of 480 patients who were refused admission. Among the admitted group, there had been 178 deaths (37%) 90 days after referral, and there were 75 (46%) among the refused group. When compared with the group of appropriately admitted patients with medium Acute Physiology and Chronic Health Evaluation (APACHE) II scores for disease severity, there was a 1.6 relative risk of death for 113 patients appropriately referred for intensive care but refused admission to their first-choice ICU. Differences in mortality among all referrals were also attributed to age, the assessed need for treatment or monitoring interventions, and emergency status. Excess mortality was not significantly affected by bed provision.

Conclusion.—In patients who were refused intensive care, particularly for an emergency, there was a higher rate of attributable mortality. The provision of more beds alone may not be the solution, but there is an urgent need for more appropriate admission and discharge criteria.

▶ This article provides insights into the triaging of critically ill patients in the United Kingdom. The initial hypothesis was that patients referred to ICUs but refused admission would experience a twofold increase in morality after controlling for severity of illness and other factors affecting mortality. The 90-day mortality rate among those patients referred and admitted (178 deaths/480 patients or 37%) was less than the death rate among those patients referred but refused admission (75 deaths/165 patients or 46%). The relative risk of death for patients appropriately referred but refused admission was 1.6. Over 30% of patients refused admission were deemed inappropriate referrals, and 17% of patients who were admitted were also deemed inappropriate referrals.

Subsets of patients had markedly different outcomes. Refused surgical patients had a generally lower risk of death than refused nonsurgical patients. The number of interventions performed, APACHE II score, and surgical and emergency patient status all affected mortality. Of 129 patients refused admission, 72 patients were too well, whereas 55 patients were too sick. Lack of beds was responsible for nearly 2/3 of the patients being refused admission. Lack of nurses accounted for most of the other refusals.

This study is hampered by several factors that the authors recognized but were unable to control for. First, data such as APACHE score and need for interventions were not known for the refused cases. Second, the indications for referral to an ICU were variable, uncontrolled, and not ascertainable. Subsequent to this paper, guidelines for admission and discharge have been promulgated.[1] In this setting, it is difficult to conclude much about mortality, especially as it was not possible to adjust for case mix data for refused cases. Increasing the number of ICU beds might have a modest effect on survival, but it would be difficult to justify that outlay based entirely upon these data.

M.R. Silver, M.D.

Reference

1. Working Group. Guidelines on admission to and discharge from intensive care and high dependency units. London: Department of Health, 1996.

Evaluating Laboratory Usage in the Intensive Care Unit: Patient and Institutional Characteristics That Influence Frequency of Blood Sampling
Zimmerman JE, Seneff MG, Sun X, et al (George Washington Univ, Washington, DC; Univ of Virginia, Charlottesville)
Crit Care Med 25:737–748, 1997   9–22

Introduction.—Overuse of laboratory testing can increase the cost of patient care and result in iatrogenic anemia, with the subsequent need for transfusion and its associated risks. Recent economic and federal regulatory developments have mandated re-examination of laboratory use. The number of blood samples drawn for laboratory testing within a large and diverse population of patients admitted to ICUs was evaluated to identify patient and institutional characteristics influencing the frequency of blood drawing.

Methods.—A consecutive sample of 17,440 patients admitted to ICUs was used and 14,043 blood samples obtained for laboratory testing on ICU days 2–7 were evaluated. On ICU day 1, data on patient demographics and physiology were recorded. Information was collected on the type and number of blood samples taken for laboratory testing. Using only data from ICU day 1, the subsequent number of samples drawn on ICU days 2 and 2–7 were predicted.

Results.—In the 42 ICUs participating, the mean number of blood samples drawn on ICU days 2–7 was 16.2 per patient. The mean was 23 in teaching ICUs and 9.9 in nonteaching ICUs. The most significant determinants of the number of blood samples drawn on ICU days 2–7 were the ICU day 1 Acute Physiology Score and admission diagnosis. After controlling for patient variables, hospital teaching status, number of beds, and location of hospitals in the East and South were significantly associated with increased blood sampling on ICU day 2 and ICU days 2–7. There was an association between increased blood sampling, more frequent use of arterial cannula, and mechanical ventilation.

Conclusion.—This method of adjusting for patient and institutional variables and being able to predict the number of blood samples drawn for laboratory tests allows ICUs to compare their practices with those of other ICUs. In the present environment of concern regarding cost of medical care, this information can be useful.

▶ This well-researched paper provides statisticians with a veritable banquet, but leaves clinicians sniffing for a few morsels. Using old data (1988–1990), the authors perform a plethora of statistical gymnastics to prove that sicker patients in teaching hospitals with easy access (arterial lines) get more blood samples drawn. The discussion section, however, is worthwhile reading, emphasizing the need for discrimination in testing as a means of achieving cost reduction and blood conservation. Helpful suggestions for achieving these goals are proposed in the form of benchmarking and process improvement projects.

This work is really 2 different presentations: boring study and excellent editorial. It is difficult to tell whether the 2 parts are related in any clinically significant fashion.

H. Nearman, M.D.

Racial Variation in Predicted and Observed In-hospital Death: A Regional Analysis

Gordon HS, Harper DL, Rosenthal GE (Case Western Reserve Univ, Cleveland, Ohio; Cleveland Health Quality Choice Coalition, Ohio)
JAMA 276:1639–1644, 1996   9–23

Background.—Important questions remain about the relationships between race and health care delivery. This article compares observed, predicted, and risk-adjusted hospital mortalities in white and black patients.

Methods.—Thirty hospitals in northeast Ohio contributed data on a total of 88,205 patients discharged consecutively between 1991 and 1993 with diagnoses of acute myocardial infarction, congestive heart failure, obstructive airways disease, gastrointestinal hemorrhaging, pneumonia, or strokes. Predicted risks of death at admission were measured for each diagnostic group, and in-hospital mortality was adjusted in white and black patients for predicted risk of death and other covariates.

Findings.—The predicted risks of death were lower in black patients with 4 of the 6 diagnoses. The adjusted odds of hospital death were lower in blacks with congestive heart failure and obstructive airways disease and similar in those with the other diagnoses. For all diagnoses in aggregate, the adjusted odds of hospital death were 13% lower in black patients than in white patients. After further adjustments for differences in length of stay, site of hospitalization, and discharge triage practices, findings were similar.

Conclusion.—The predicted risks of death and risk-adjusted mortality in this study were generally lower in black patients. This unexpected finding may reflect racial differences in hospital admission practices or in access to outpatient care. However, once hospitalized, black patients appear to have outcomes similar to or better than those of white patients, as determined by hospital mortality.

▶ The findings of the study run counter to what most observers believe. It is a fairly extensive and well-performed study, so it is not easy to dismiss the findings. There is a suggestion in the data that a major reason black predicted risk of death was lower was because there may have been a lower threshold of admission for these patients, and this in turn may have been because of a number of factors related to access to primary care. Studies like this that challenge conventional wisdom are especially useful in leading to new avenues of thought. It is hoped that the work done here is being carried further by the Cleveland Health Quality Choice, one of the national leaders in outcomes research.

J. Samuel, M.D. and C.M. Franklin, M.D.

Assessing the Efficiency of the Admission Process to a Critical Care Unit: Does the Literature Allow the Use of Benchmarking?
Kennan SP, Doig GS, Martin CM, et al (Univ of Western Ontario, London, Canada)
Intensive Care Med 23:574–580, 1997   9–24

Objective.—Cost control issues have forced the health care industry to improve the efficiency of the admission process, especially for critical care units. Peer hospitals can be compared using benchmarks if sufficient data are available. The ability of the literature to provide useful references for benchmarks for the admission process of a multidisciplinary critical care unit was retrospectively reviewed.

Methods.—Demographic data, admission diagnosis, and daily Therapeutic Intervention Scoring System (TISS) scores as "active" or "nonactive" treatment variables, and Acute Physiology and Health Evaluation (APACHE) II scores were collected. The proportion of patients receiving active care at the 30–bed multidisciplinary critical care index unit was compared with similar information about other critical units found in the literature.

Results.—Of the 614 patients admitted to the index critical care unit during the 6-month study period, 97.7% received active treatment compared with 20% to 66.5% of patients at other institutions. There was a significantly larger proportion of patients requiring active treatment in the index institution than in institutional studies reported in the literature. Reasons for these differences other than efficiency could include low critical care bed availability, availability of intermediate care units, an extended-role recovery room, different patient populations, and heterogeneity in hospitals represented.

Conclusion.—The literature does not supply sufficient data to compare the critical care admission process in different hospitals.

▶ The authors point out several important problems with benchmarking. First, reliance on published data that were collected for different reasons has inherent selection biases. Second, important pieces of information are often missing that affect how resources are used. We agree that there is a need for large multicenter databases that are designed especially for the purpose of benchmarking. The National Registry for Acute Myocardial Infarction is a good example of what can be done. Hopefully, initiatives such as Project Impact will serve a similar purpose.

J.E. Calvin, Jr., M.D.

J.E. Parrillo, M.D.

How to Use Diagnostic Test Articles in the Intensive Care Unit: Diagnosing Weanability Using f/Vt

Jaeschke RZ, Meade MO, Guyatt GH, et al (McMaster Univ, Hamilton, Ont, Canada; Univ of Toronto; Univ of Western Ontario, London, Canada)

Crit Care Med 25:1514–1521, 1997   9–25

Introduction.—Generating a set of hypotheses and obtaining information that modifies these hypotheses are the basis for making medical diagnoses. It is useful to use diagnostic test studies in addition to the history, physical examination, and laboratory investigations of the patient. A critical appraisal of a diagnostic article should include the following determinations: whether the results of the study are valid; whether there was an independent, blind comparison with a reference standard; whether the patient sample included an appropriate spectrum of patients; and whether the results of the test influenced the decision to apply the reference standard.

Determining results.—The test properties of the study should be examined. Is there a presentation of the test's sensitivity, specificity and likelihood ratios? The properties of a diagnostic test in patients in who the clinical condition of interest is absent or present constitute the sensitivity and specificity of results. Likelihood ratios should be analyzed.

Helping patients.—The value of the diagnostic test in the management of the patients must then be determined. It must be determined whether the methods for performing the test are described in sufficient detail to permit replication. It must also be determined whether the reproducibility of the test results and its interpretation would be satisfactory in another setting. Are the results applicable to your patients? Will management of patients change because of the result? Finally, it must be determined whether patients will be better off as a result of the test.

Conclusion.—When the performance and interpretation of the test is similar in study and clinical settings, study results will be more easily applicable. To improve the process of patient care and patient outcome, diagnostic tests are conducted, and test ordering behavior ideally reflects these goals. Serial modifications of the probabilities of diseases or conditions occur in the diagnostic process.

▶ This is an interesting analysis of the pitfalls in applying single tests (e.g., f/Vt) to complex issues (weanability).

B.A. Shapiro, M.D.

Influence of Multiple Organ Dysfunction Syndrome on Duration of Critical Illness and Hospitalization

Barie PS, Hydo LJ (Cornell Univ, New York)
Arch Surg 131:1318–1324, 1996   9–26

Background.—Care of critically ill patients is often extended and costly, and there is no agreement on the definition of a prolonged hospital stay in the general surgery ICU or how to determine costs. Infection is a major risk factor for multiple organ dysfunction syndrome (MODS), which is the leading cause of death in critically ill surgical patients. The effect of MODS in patients with less severe illness is less certain. MODS may be an important predictor of length of stay in patients with short stays in the surgical intensive care unit and likely survival.

Methods.—In a prospective study, 2,646 consecutive patients were analyzed; 115 of these patients stayed in the surgical ICU for more than 21 days. APACHE II and III scores were determined after 24 hours. Daily and cumulative multiple organ dysfunction scores were also determined. The relation between modest degrees of MODS and length of stay in the surgical ICU was determined. It was also determined if daily multiple organ dysfunction scores could distinguish survivors from nonsurvivors before the surgical ICU stay became prolonged.

Results.—Follow-up was carried out until discharge or death. The mean patient age was 65 years. The mean APACHE II score was 13.8. The mean APACHE III score was 44.2. The incidence of MODS was 44.3% (1,173 patients). Hospital mortality was 9.2%. In survivors, there was a close correlation between cumulative multiple organ dysfunction score and length of stay in the surgical ICU, especially when the stay was less than 10 days. There were similar correlations between prevalence of MODS and longer length of stay in the surgical ICU, and between length of hospital stay and cumulative multiple organ dysfunction score. In patients who stayed in the surgical ICU more than 21 days, daily multiple organ dysfunction scores distinguished survivors from nonsurvivors by day 2 of the stay.

Discussion.—These results show that modest degrees of MODS are closely correlated with length of care in patients who are not critically ill. It may be possible to identify patients at risk for extended illness and death by determining multiple organ dysfunction scores early.

▶ This is an interesting case of a cohort of surgical ICU patients who were not thought to be extremely ill and who manifested modest APACHE II and III scores. The overall mortality rate was 9%. Using a daily MODS score the authors were able to determine which patients were destined to have a prolonged stay in the surgical ICU. This difference was manifested early in this retrospective study.

The value of this MODS score and the ability to determine the prolonged hospitalization group remains to be determined. As of this time there is no uniformity in MODS scores or even in the exact definition of what is individual or multiple organ dysfunction. This scoring system weights all organs equally and doesn't differentiate between dysfunction of selected organ systems. Not all researchers believe that all organs are created equally or that all dysfunctions carry the same risk for survival and prolongation of hospital stay once they are manifest. Finally, as with most scores, the impact of prior or preexisting organ dysfunction/failure poses a difficulty as does the impact of the treatment of some organ failures while other organ dysfunction/failures are merely supported or ignored. The results of this trial are interesting and provoke a desire to prospectively evaluate the MODS score in additional ICU patient populations with the goal of ascertaining its ability to distinguish who may be at greater risk for mortality or whose length of stay may be effectively shortened by specific interventions.

R.A. Balk, M.D.

Clinical Features and Outcome of Patients Admitted to the Intensive Care Unit After Plastic Surgical Procedures: Implications for Cost Reduction and Quality of Care
Talmor M, Hydo LJ, Shaikh N, et al (New York Hosp-Cornell Med Ctr)
Ann Plast Surg 39:74–79, 1997   9–27

Background.—Previous studies have identified criteria for identification of surgical patients who can benefit from care in an ICU vs. a "step-down" unit (SDU). However, few of these studies have addressed patients undergoing plastic surgery. Close monitoring is needed for patients undergoing major reconstructive surgical procedures. Toward defining the appropriate perioperative management of patients undergoing major plastic and reconstructive surgery, a series of patients admitted to the surgical ICU were analyzed.

Methods.—The retrospective study included 2,805 consecutive patients admitted to the surgical ICU during a 6-year period. Of those, 42 (1.5%) had undergone major plastic or reconstructive surgery. Outcomes evaluated included mortality, length of ICU and hospital stay, and degree of organ dysfunction. The findings were compared with those of a group of patients undergoing vascular surgery, matched for severity of illness, and a matched population of ICU patients. A case-control study was also performed to compare the plastic surgery group of ICU patients with a group of patients admitted to the postanesthesia care unit for at least 24 hours of postoperative monitoring.

Results.—The patients undergoing plastic surgery were 33 men and 9 women, mean age 54 years. Most had major reconstruction with free microvascular tissue transfer, usually after cancer surgery. Mortality in this group was 9.5%, compared to 0% in the random sample of ICU patients. Twenty-four percent of the plastic surgery group had organ dysfunction. In the case-control study, Acute Physiology and Chronic Health Evaluation (APACHE II) score was 11 for the case-patients vs. 7 for controls. The severity of illness scores and mortality findings suggested that patients admitted to the ICU after major reconstructive surgery were appropriately selected. The reconstructive procedures lasted an average of nearly 10 hours, after which the patients required an average of 48 hours of mechanical ventilatory support.

Conclusions.—Patients undergoing major reconstructive surgery can be appropriately monitored in the surgical ICU. Factors to consider in deciding which patients will benefit from ICU care include premorbid condition, medical history, immune and nutritional status, and operative stress. On the other hand, patients admitted to the postanesthesia care unit may be overmonitored. A specialized unit with a dedicated nursing staff might be developed specifically to manage such patients.

▶ The authors claim that the purpose of this study is to evaluate the clinical features, management, and outcome of patients undergoing plastic surgery admitted to the ICU postoperatively. They wanted to test the hypothesis that most such patients can be safely monitored in areas outside of the ICU. Unfortunately, this hypothesis never gets tested in an appropriate fashion, and in the end the reader is left wondering what the answer is. This is a retrospective analysis that tries to match study and cohort groups on the basis of both APACHE II and APACHE III scores. These severity of illness scoring systems are felt by some not to be reliable in assessing postoperative surgical patients, which may thus weaken the assumption of comparability of groups. In addition, no consistent clinical criteria for ICU admission were followed, and bed availability seemed to be given as much weight in the admission decision process as severity of underlying illness. Finally, in evaluating ICU mortality and length of stay, it would be helpful to know whether each group's attending surgeons were responsible for patient management while in the ICU, or whether there was an intensivist directing an ICU team.

There are 2 worthwhile points that the authors reinforce concerning patient care and resource utilization: (1) the cost of an overnight stay in the postanesthesia care unit may be more than in an ICU because of the more concentrated resource dedication required; and (2) appropriately staffed, less costly intermediate-care units can provide needed postoperative care for a significant number of patients otherwise admitted to an ICU.

H. Nearman, M.D.

How Should Multiple Organ Dysfunction Syndrome be Assessed? A Review of the Variations in Current Scoring Systems

Bertleff MJOE, Bruining HA (Univ Hosp, Rotterdam, The Netherlands)
Eur J Surg 163:405–409, 1997   9–28

Introduction.—The scoring systems used to evaluate multiple organ dysfunction syndrome (MODS) vary enough to make it difficult to compare trial results. A summary of variables used to describe dysfunction of various organs was presented.

Variables Used to Describe Organ Dysfunction

There are 3 subgroups used to describe pulmonary dysfunction: 1 describes pulmonary dysfunction as a function of time and degree of mechanical ventilation; 1 uses respiratory rate, partial pressure of carbon dioxide, and alveolar-arterial oxygen diffusion; and 1 uses the definition of adult respiratory distress syndrome to describe pulmonary dysfunction.

Cardiovascular dysfunction.—Several variables are used to describe cardiovascular dysfunction: arrhythmia, acute myocardial infarction, cardiac tamponade, cardiogenic shock, and endocarditis.

Renal dysfunction.—Nearly all scoring systems describe renal dysfunction as an increased creatinine concentration. Need for hemodialysis or peritoneal dialysis are other criteria that have been used.

Hepatic dysfunction.—presence of ascites, unexplained hypoglycemia, or clinical jaundice.

Gastrointestinal dysfunction.—presence of symptoms (bleeding from stress ulcers, acalculous cholecystitis, pancreatitis, enteral intolerance, ileus, nasogastric drainage, malabsorption, and acute perforations).

Nervous system dysfunction.—Glasgow Coma Scale (most commonly used), coma, diffuse neuropathy, intracranial hemorrhage, cerebral infarction, or sudden onset of confusion or psychosis.

Metabolic dysfunction.—need for insulin or the presence of diabetes mellitus with associated acidosis or hypocortisolism.

Immunologic dysfunction.—delayed hypersensitivity skin testing (1 group; this is not widely accepted for routine use) to determine immunologic integrity.

Conclusion.—There is quite a bit of variability regarding use of scoring systems, which variables should be scored, and which variables are most appropriate. Scoring systems have limits, but they could be used to provide better patients stratification and follow-up in clinical research.

▶ This review summarizes all the variables used in a variety of scoring systems and provides a brief critique of why some are used.

J.E. Calvin, Jr., M.D.

J.E. Parrillo, M.D.

Survey of Physicians' Attitudes About Risks and Benefits of Chest Computed Tomography
Renston JP, Connors AF Jr, DiMarco AF (Case Western Reserve Univ, Cleveland, Ohio)
South Med J 89:1067–1073, 1996   9–29

Background.—Computed tomography and high-resolution CT (HRCT) of the chest are used often to assess a variety of intrathoracic abnormalities. However, the specific indications for the appropriate use of CT and HRCT in clinical practice are vague in many circumstances. Furthermore, physicians' attitudes toward and knowledge of the potential risks and benefits of CT and HRCT are not known.

Methods.—A survey was mailed to 1,000 randomly selected board-certified physicians from several medical specialties. Three hundred thirteen questionnaires were returned complete.

Findings.—Computed tomographic ordering practices varied according to specialty. Sixty-four percent of the respondents believed that CT provided new information, and 62% believed that it influenced patient management. However, only 30% of physicians felt that the use of CT improved patient outcomes. More than 90% of the respondents did not know or significantly underestimated the degree of radiation associated with CT (it is equivalent to 100 posteroanterior chest radiographs).

Conclusions.—Although CT and HRCT are unarguably valuable diagnostic tools in the assessment and management of pulmonary disorders, the indications for, benefits of, and potential risks of these imaging modalities have still not been defined prospectively in many circumstances. Physicians in all specialties should carefully consider the anticipated benefits and potential risks of CT and HRCT.

▶ The most interesting thing to come out of this study was the amount of radiation associated with CT. Although this may be common knowledge to radiologists, it is clearly not common knowledge to internists, family practitioners, and chest physicians. Nothing else in this study was particularly striking—any survey of physicians regarding a new diagnostic test, especially one that is noninvasive, will show a wide variation of opinions and enthusiasm. The authors make an appeal for prospective studies to better define indications for chest CT. No one would oppose that, but the reader should not come away thinking that prospective studies alone will definitively answer such a complex question.

J. Samuel, M.D. and C.M. Franklin, M.D.

Ethics

Influence of Alterations in Forgoing Life-sustaining Treatment Practices on a Clinical Sepsis Trial

Sprung CL, and the HA-1A Sepsis Study Group (The Hebrew Univ of Jerusalem, Israel; et al)

Crit Care Med 25:383–387, 1997   9–30

Background.—Various prospective studies in the last 10 years have evaluated new treatment modalities for patients with sepsis. During this time, decisions to forgo life-sustaining treatment in patients in intensive care units have become more common throughout the world. In clinical trials, the timing of forgoing treatment is important because it may affect study results and conclusions.

Methods.—In a prospective, randomized, double-blind, placebo-controlled study, 543 patients had life-sustaining treatment withheld or withdrawn. Among the factors analyzed were the types of disorders, interventions, reasons for and timing of withholding or withdrawing treatment, the treatment's effect on mortality and study results.

Results.—Among the 543 patients, life-sustaining treatment was forgone in 117 patients; this occurred within 72 hours of administration of the study drug in 38 patients. Withholding treatment occurred more frequently than withdrawing treatment. However, in the first 72 hours, withdrawing treatment was more common than withholding treatment. Among all patients, 52% had severe underlying disorders and a poor prognosis. Hospital mortality was 94% of the 117 patients. The mean time from withholding treatment until death was 2.83 days, and the mean time from withdrawing treatment until death was 0.32 days. Mortality rates were higher in the first 72 hours in patients who had treatment forgone in the first 24, 48, or 72 hours after administration of the study drug.

Discussion.—Many patients in sepsis trials have severe underlying diseases. Forgoing life-sustaining treatment often occurs early in the study and affects mortality. In new trials, exclusion criteria should be carefully defined. The enrollment of patients with severe underlying diseases and changes in the practice of forgoing life-sustaining treatment may bias new treatment modality study results.

▶ This important observation confirms what has been suspected by a number of investigators involved in clinical research protocols meant to evaluate new interventions in critically ill patients. It has long been suspected that there are a significant number of patients who are entered into clinical trials only to have the aggressive management strategy reversed after 48–72 hours when there was no visible response to the aggressive therapy. This study does not address the rightness or wrongness of this response, which is often driven primarily by the patient's family. Instead, this study sheds light on the impact this decision ultimately has on the results of the trial and on our ability to fairly evaluate the value of the intervention under investigation. In this review of the HA-1A antiendotoxin trial 22% of the study population had the life-sustaining therapies either withheld or withdrawn. Nearly one third of these episodes took place during the initial 72 hours of the study. 87% of patients who had therapy withheld had a DNR order. While some believe that withholding and withdrawing therapy have the same ends and therefore are not different, many feel that withdrawal of therapy is an active process and likely to result in a predictable outcome. During the first 72 hours of the study active withdrawal of therapy was the most common form of forgoing life-sustaining treatment.

This study clearly points out a potential problem in the conduct of a large prospective, randomized, controlled trial that may have a significant influence on the primary result. In this trial almost a quarter of the study population had life sustaining therapy either withheld or withdrawn. One third of the episodes took place in the initial 3 days of the study. This active interference in the provision of aggressive life-sustaining treatment can be expected to have a dramatic effect on 28 day patient survival, the primary study end point. While this lack of continued aggressive support may accurately reflect common clinical practice, it likely has a profound negative effect on the conduct of a clinical study and our ability to discern a true benefit from a therapeutic intervention.

R.A. Balk, M.D.

Increasing Incidence of Withholding and Withdrawal of Life Support From the Critically Ill
Prendergast TJ, Luce JM (Univ of California, San Francisco; San Francisco Gen Hosp, Calif)
Am J Respir Crit Care Med 155:15–20, 1997   9–31

Introduction.—The decision to withhold or withdraw life support from critically ill patients has increased since the late 1980s. The incidence of recommendations to withhold or withdraw life support from critically ill patients was evaluated in 2 hospital ICUs to determine how often these recommendations are implemented or rejected and to characterize reasons for a recommendation to limit life-sustaining treatment.

Methods.—One-hundred seventy-nine consecutive patients for whom a recommendation was made to withhold or withdraw life support in 1992 and 1993 were prospectively enrolled. Data were compared with information collected in the same ICUs over a similar period in 1987 and 1988.

Results.—In 1992–1993, recommendations were made to withhold or withdraw life support in 179 of 200 deaths (90%), compared with 114 of 224 deaths (51%) in 1987–1988. This difference is significant. Cardiopulmonary resuscitation was initiated in 10% and 49% of deaths in 1992–1993 and 1989–1988, respectively. Ninety percent of patients or surrogates agreed to physicians' recommendations to withhold or withdraw life support within 5 days (61% immediately and 27% within 48 hours); 8 patients or surrogates (4%) refused. When there was conflict, physicians deferred to patients/surrogates with 1 exception. That case, in 1992–1993, concerned a patient who was considered hopelessly ill.

Conclusion.—Ninety percent of the patients who died in 1992–1993 did so after a decision to limit therapy. This indicates a major change in practice in these institutions over a 5-year period. Physicians were willing to override patient/surrogate choice, but only when death was imminent. Concurrent with physicians' requests to limit therapy was patient/surrogate acceptance of the recommendation.

▶ This article illustrates how practice patterns have changed in relation to terminal care at 1 university medical center. The results demonstrate that cardiopulmonary resuscitation was less often applied in the terminal setting in 1992–1993 than it had been 5 years previously. The authors suggest that a reasonable balance is developing between patients and surrogates on 1 side and ICU physicians on the other. As the authors acknowledge, it would be helpful to examine data from other hospitals and medical centers to determine whether this is a national trend.

C.M. Franklin, M.D.

Treatment Decision-making at the End of Life: A Survey of Australian Doctors' Attitudes Towards Patients' Wishes and Euthanasia
Waddell C, Clarnette RM, Smith M, et al (Univ of Western Australia, Nedlands; Osborne Park Hosp, Perth, Western Australia; Silver Chain Hospice Care Services, Perth, Western Australia; et al)
Med J Aust 165:540–544, 1996   9–32

Introduction.—Life can now be maintained beyond the limits of reasonable quality because of advances in medical technology. This has led to more requests for physician-assisted death or euthanasia. Few studies have shown how treatment decisions are made. Advance health care directives have been recently proposed to advise the physician of the patient's wishes regarding care. Physicians were surveyed and presented with clinical scenarios to examine the factors that influence their decisions about treatment for patients with life-threatening or terminal illnesses.

Methods.—A 3-month survey was conducted of 2,172 hospital trainees, physicians, general practitioners, palliative care practitioners, and surgeons. They were asked to prescribe treatment for patients whose characteristics varied in terms of prognosis, illness severity, mental competence, presence of advance directives, sociodemographic factors, and request for assisted death. They were also asked about their own sociodemographic and medical training characteristics.

Results.—The survey resulted in a 73% response rate. There were 3 main findings in this study: physicians generally did not adhere to patients' request for assisted death; physicians generally did adhere to family and patient wishes when they became known; and the decisions of the physicians varied systematically by medical and sociodemographic training factors, and were not consistent. This suggests that there are no uniform guidelines for physicians to make these decisions.

Conclusion.—The individual characteristics of the physician significantly determine the treatment provided. The nature of the medical problem does not solely affect the treatment provided. Variations of treatment related to medical training factors and sociodemographic factors could be reduced by participation in the informed consent process and in the preparation of advance health care directives by practitioners. The basis for an informed euthanasia policy could be provided by stronger empirical data on the way treatment decisions are made.

► This study was performed at a time when the issue of physician-assisted suicide was hotly debated in Australia. The wide variation in decision making by doctors concerning terminally ill patients lends credence to the belief that simple policies in the area of physician-assisted suicide are not possible. Physicians in North America who are interested in the ongoing debate about physician-assisted suicide should follow the parallel debate going on in Australia, where physician-assisted suicide was legally accepted in one territory for a brief period before a national reconsideration.

C.M. Franklin, M.D.

Physician Responses to a Hospital Policy Allowing Them to Not Offer Cardiopulmonary Resuscitation
Swig L, Cooke M, Osmond D, et al (Univ of California, San Francisco; San Francisco Gen Hosp)
J Am Geriatr Soc 44:1215–1219, 1996   9–33

Introduction.—Patients and their surrogates have historically been offered cardiopulmonary resuscitation (CPR), regardless of potential benefit. The resuscitation policy of San Francisco General Hospital grants physicians the right to withhold CPR from patients unlikely to benefit. Attending physicians were interviewed to determine whether they exercised their freedom to write do not resuscitate (DNR) orders for their patients.

Methods.—Physicians were questioned regarding patients admitted over a period of 5 months for whom they wrote DNR orders. Only the first patient for whom each physician wrote a DNR order was assessed.

Results.—During the 5-month evaluation period, there were 7,675 nonnursery admissions to San Francisco General Hospital attended by about 90 physicians. Of these, 71 physicians wrote DNR orders. Sixty-nine physicians were available to answer questions about their first DNR order during the evaluation period. Fifty-seven physicians were aware of the policy. Of the 57, 49 said they generally agreed with the policy. Thirty-three physicians thought CPR should be offered only to patients likely to benefit, and 36 physicians thought CPR should be offered to all patients, regardless of benefit. Physicians offered CPR to 25 of 69 patients (36%) not likely to benefit and 15 of 22 surrogates. No discussion was held regarding CPR in the case of 1 patient because the physician thought the discussion would cause discomfort for both parties.

Conclusion.—Physicians generally offered CPR to patients, regardless of benefit and despite a policy allowing them to write DNR orders. Most physicians thought CPR should be offered to all patients, regardless of benefit. Many physicians seem to hold attitudes inconsistent with policies that allow them to write DNR orders.

▶ This study underlines the need for continued movement toward evidence-based medical practice and outcome studies. Although I am not surprised, I find it remarkable (embarrassing?) that a majority of physicians practicing in a university-affiliated hospital would hold the attitude that CPR should be offered to all patients, regardless of potential benefit. Physician, educate thyself!

B.A. Shapiro, M.D.

Do-Not-Resuscitate Decisions in the Medical ICU: Comparing Physician and Nurse Opinions
Eliasson AH, Howard RS, Torrington KG, et al (Walter Reed Army Med Ctr, Washington, DC; Uniformed Services Univ of the Health Sciences, Bethesda, Md)
Chest 111:1106–1111, 1997   9–34

Objective.—The nursing staff at the medical ICU at Walter Reed Army Medical Hospital contend that physicians frequently disregard do-not-resuscitate (DNR) orders or subject patients to unnecessary resuscitation efforts in the absence of a DNR order, subjecting both the patient and the family to unnecessary ordeals. A quality improvement study addresses 3 questions to determine whether changes in practice were warranted: When do physicians and nurses arrive at the DNR decision? How often do they disagree? How often do patients or surrogates disagree with staff decisions?

Methods.—Demographic data of ICU patients were collected for 10 months. Each physician team and nurse were surveyed daily regarding their DNR opinion. Characteristics of patients with and without DNR orders were compared statistically. Time to DNR decision by the physician team and the nurse and differences in opinion were analyzed statistically.

Results.—Of the 368 consecutive patients (59% male) studied, 84 had a DNR order. Patients with a DNR order were significantly older (66.2 vs. 59.2 years), had a significantly higher Acute Physiology and Chronic Health Evaluation (APACHE) II score (22.6 vs. 12.3), had a significantly lower Glasgow Coma Scale score (10.8 vs. 14.3), and a significantly longer hospital stay (5 vs. 2 days) than patients without a DNR order. There were

6 cases (7%) of DNRs with which nurses did not agree. The average time for physicians to recommend a DNR was 1 day, not significantly different from the nurses' recommendation. In the 284 patients without a DNR, physicians were significantly more likely than nurses to recommend a DNR. Physicians and nurses agreed on a DNR recommendation in 14% of patients and disagreed on a DNR recommendation in 12% of patients. There was no significant difference in survival between patients with a DNR recommendation by physicians or by nurses.

Conclusions.—Physicians and nurses decide in approximately the same amount of time whether a DNR recommendation is appropriate. Both physicians and nurses should have input into the DNR recommendation, and patients and family members should be involved in a discussion of the possibility early in the course of the illness.

▶ Increasingly, DNR orders are having an impact on patient management. While it is fortunate that the agreement between physicians and nurses was high, the fact that some disagreement exists suggests the need for good communication between health care workers.

J.E. Calvin, Jr., M.D.

J.E. Parrillo, M.D.

Do Advance Directives Provide Instructions That Direct Care?
Teno JM, for the SUPPORT Investigators (George Washington Univ, Washington, DC)
J Am Geriatr Soc 45:508–512, 1997   9–35

Background.—Although advance directives are intended to guide the medical treatment of seriously ill patients, it has been reported that these directives are not associated with improved decision-making regarding resuscitation of seriously ill patients. There are 2 forms of advance directives: instructional directives regarding decisions about future care and proxy directives naming a proxy decision-maker. Living wills are the oldest advance directives. A standard living will states that there is a point at which the individual would prefer to die than to continue living through artificial means, but these wills are generally not specific about which efforts to prolong life should cease and when. The content of documented advance directives was examined to determine whether they contained clear instructions for guiding medical care.

Methods.—The Study to Understand Prognoses and Preferences for Outcomes and Risks of Treatments (SUPPORT) enrolled 4,804 patients with at least 1 of 9 serious illnesses after implementation of the Patient Self-Determination Act. A review of the advance directives from hospital medical records through 6 months of follow-up or death noted content, date of completion, and whether the directives had been witnessed and notarized. The content of documents with instructions beyond the standard legal form was analyzed. Charts were reviewed for evidence of clinical decision-making and use of life-sustaining treatment.

Results.—From the 4,804 patients, only 688 documents from 569 patients showed advance directives placed in their medical records. About 66% were durable powers of attorney and 31% were standard living wills or other forms of written instructions. Only 90 documents had additional instructions beyond naming a proxy or stating preferences in a standard living will. Only 36 documents had specific instructions regarding use of life-sustaining treatment, and only 22 indicated that life-sustaining treatment should not be used in the patient's current medical condition. Some patients used terms such as "no advanced life support" and "no CPR, no ventilators, no nasogastric tubes." In 9 of these 22 patients, treatment was consistent with the patient's instructions, and 2 patients may have changed inconsistent instructions after discussion with hospital staff.

Discussion.—The naming of a health care proxy may provide valuable information to clinicians, but this outcome variable was not addressed in this study. In general, the advance directives examined did not provide specific instructions regarding medical treatment. Implementation of the Patient Self-Determination Act has not solved the problem of decision making for seriously ill individuals. This area of health care needs much improvement.

Consensus Statement of the Society of Critical Care Medicine's Ethics Committee Regarding Futile and Other Possibly Inadvisable Treatments
Danis M, Troug R, Devita M, et al (Univ of North Carolina, Chapel Hill; Univ of Pittsburgh, Pa; Commonwealth of Massachusetts, Boston; et al)
Crit Care Med 25:887–891, 1997   9–36

Introduction.—Policies limiting futile treatments are one way to distribute limited medical resources. A consensus statement by the Ethics Committee of the Society of Critical Care Medicine on policies regarding futile and other possibly inadvisable treatments is presented.

Methods and Recommendations.—The committee performed a literature review, data synthesis, and discussion to define futility and to identify principles and procedures for addressing cases in which life-sustaining treatment is futile or inadvisable. The committee defines a futile treatment as one that will not accomplish its intended goal. Inappropriate and inadvisable treatments were defined as those extremely unlikely to be beneficial, extremely costly, or of uncertain benefit; however, such treatments would not meet the definition of futile. The committee concludes that only a small fraction of medical care is futile, and thus that basing treatment decisions on the concept of futility will not lead to major reductions in resource utilization.

The committee acknowledges, however, that limiting inadvisable treatments is a legitimate community interest. The rationale for limiting inadvisable treatments should be explicit, equitable, and democratic. It should not place disabled, poor, or uninsured patients at a disadvantage and should recognize the diverse values and goals of individuals. The committee suggests some characteristics of policies to limit inadvisable treatments, including disclosure in the public record, reflection of the community's moral values, no exclusive basis in prognostic scoring systems, clear mechanisms for appeal, and recognition by the courts. The Committee recommends that health care organizations controlling payment and thus influencing treatment decisions should have formal criteria for identifying inadvisable treatments and should share accountability for those decisions.

Summary.—Recommendations related to futile and inadvisable treatments are reported. A definition of futility is offered. Withholding futile treatments is unlikely to have a significant impact on resource utilization. Policies regarding inadvisable treatment are discussed, including legal requirements and implications for insurers.

▶ A consensus statement that is readable and concise is becoming increasingly rare as the work products of medical consensus conferences grow ever longer and more abstruse. The thrust of this statement concerns the concept of futile care. The committee comes down squarely against using "futility" as a broad argument for denying care or rationing services. The statement is also conservative on the use of scoring systems for individual patients, calling it inappropriate to employ them as the sole guide in making decisions about initiating or continuing care.

C.M. Franklin, M.D.

The Doctor's Role in Discussing Advance Preferences for End-of-Life Care: Perceptions of Physicians Practicing in the VA
Markson L, Clark J, Glantz L, et al (Edith Nourse Rogers Mem Veterans Hosp, Bedford, Mass; Boston Univ)
J Am Geriatr Soc 45:399–406, 1997   9–37

Background.—Although in the United States individuals who are mentally competent have the legal right to make informed decisions about their health care, many individuals do not actually make decisions about life-sustaining treatment until after they have become ill and mentally incapacitated. Studies also indicate that proxy decision makers may not predict the patient's desires accurately. Advance directives are intended to enhance autonomy and facilitate end-of-life decisions about medical treatment. Laws such as the Patient Self-Determination Act require community health care centers to tell patients about their legal right to prepare advance directives. Many surveys report that physicians as well as patients believe that patients should discuss their preferences for medical treatment with their physicians and document their preferences.

Methods.—Data were collected from a national survey of physicians in VA medical centers. Questionnaires were sent to 1,050 physicians. The questionnaire contained 178 items covering the physicians' actual experiences discussing advance directives with patients and following those directives; obligations of their role in helping patients make advance decisions and in complying with those decisions; attitudes toward factors that help or hinder discussion of advance preferences with their patients; and opinions on the content and the format of advance directive forms.

Results.—The response rate was 67%. About 79% of respondents had discussed advance preferences with at least 1 patient in the previous year, and 19% had talked to more than 25 patients. Overall, 73% stated that they had used a written directive to make decisions regarding treatment of at least 1 patient. Independent factors associated with discussing advance directives were younger age, board certification, less time spent in the outpatient setting, and personal experience with advance decision making. Of physicians who had discussed advance preferences with patients, 59% had often initiated the discussion, 55% usually had such discussions in inpatient settings, and 31% usually had such discussions in outpatient settings. About 82% believed that physicians should initiate discussions about advance preferences; 91% would try to persuade a patient to change a decision that was not well-informed; 88% would try to change a decision that was not medically reasonable; and 88% would try to change a decision that was not in the patient's best interest. Only 14% would try to change a decision that conflicted with their own moral beliefs.

When asked about factors that would increase the likelihood of their discussing advance preferences with patients, 80% reported that they expected a discussion of advance preferences to make future decisions easier, and 76% believed that having such discussions was a professional responsibility. When asked about factors that would make it difficult to discuss advance preferences with patients, 34% named discontinuity of care between inpatient and outpatient settings, 23% named pressure to see many patients in a given period, and 21% named scheduling policies as major factors.

Discussion.—These findings show that a large number of physicians in VA ambulatory and hospital centers discuss and carry out advance preferences regarding medical treatment of seriously ill patients. Most of the respondents in this survey believed that physicians should be involved in their patients' decision making regarding future treatment if they became seriously ill. Some have argued that physicians have never had a tradition of sharing information or decisions with their patients. This trend may be shifting because of the greater availability of life-sustaining technology, physicians' serious moral concerns about the use of such treatment at the end of life, and a greater emphasis on death and dying in medical schools in the last 10 years.

▶ The good news is that the vast majority of physicians believe it is part of their responsibility to discuss advance directives with patients and to clarify decisions that may be ill informed or against the patient's best interest. The bad news is that this may not be happening as much as it should. The trend does seem to be positive in that it is occurring much more than in the past, and this type of study should be repeated every several years to observe what physicians' attitudes actually are and what they are doing to carry out their beliefs.

C.M. Franklin, M.D.

Advance Directives for Seriously Ill Hospitalized Patients: Effectiveness With the Patient Self-Determination Act and the SUPPORT Intervention
Teno J, Lynn J, Wenger N, et al for the SUPPORT Investigators (George Washington Univ, Washington, DC; et al)
J Am Geriatr Soc 45:500–507, 1997   9–38

Background.—Under the Patient Self-Determination Act (PSDA), patients must be informed about their rights to make medical treatment decisions and the instruments available to give their advance decisions legal force. However, there are few data on how such advance directives (ADs) actually perform in practice. The Study to Understand Prognoses and Preferences for Outcomes and Risks of Treatments (SUPPORT) is a 5-year hospital project aimed at describing and improving decision-making and outcomes for seriously ill adults. The impact of ADs on resuscitation decisions in seriously ill, hospitalized patients was assessed, including the effects of promotion of ADs by the PSDA and of the SUPPORT intervention.

Methods.—The analysis included 9,015 seriously ill, hospitalized patients at 5 teaching hospitals. An observational cohort study was performed for 2 years before and after the PSDA. This study required that patients be informed about ADs at admission and that ADs be documented in the medical record. In addition, a randomized controlled trial of the SUPPORT intervention to improve clinical decision making was performed after the PSDA. Under the SUPPORT intervention, a nurse acted to enhance communications regarding treatment alternatives and their outcomes and to encourage the use of ADs when appropriate. Patients, their surrogates, and physicians were interviewed about their awareness, the completion, and the impact of ADs. Information on resuscitation preferences, "do not resuscitate" orders, ADs, and the use of resuscitation at the time of death was gleaned from the medical record.

Results.—One fourth of the study patients died during their initial hospitalization and one half died within 6 months. Half of the patients were unconscious for their last 3 days of life. Before implementation of the PSDA, about 60% of patients knew about living wills, and about 20% had an AD. These figures were little changed after the PSDA and the SUPPORT intervention. However, the percentage of ADs mentioned in the medical record increased from 6% before the PSDA to 35% after the PSDA and 78% after the SUPPORT intervention (Table 2). After the PSDA, patients with and without ADs were similar in their rates of documented discussions regarding resuscitation—33% and 38%, respectively. Having an AD also made little impact on the percentage of DNR orders among patients who did not wish resuscitation and the percentage of attempted resusci-

want to. Patients who do not discuss preferences, for whatever reason, will probably have interventions that they do not want.

▶ Again, the Study of Understand Prognoses and Preferences for Outcomes and Risks of Treatment (SUPPORT) warns us of the threat of unwanted resuscitation. This is the underlying theme in a number of articles (hopefully, the point has been made by this time). One thing the data in this article do not demonstrate is whether there were a large number of patients who actually did receive resuscitation who did not want it. With all that the SUPPORT group has published on this topic, it is still unclear whether or not unwanted resuscitation is a large, growing problem.

C.M. Franklin, M.D.

Validation of Preferences for Life-sustaining Treatment: Implications for Advance Care Planning

Patrick DL, Pearlman RA, Starks HE, et al (Univ of Washington, Seattle; Veterans Affairs Puget Sound Health Care System, Seattle)
Ann Intern Med 127:509–517, 1997   9–40

Introduction.—Advance care planning can help patients to think about and communicate their preferences regarding life-sustaining treatments. However, preferences can change, and patients can misunderstand the outcomes of their preferences; thus preferences voiced before the occurrence of a life-threatening illness may differ from actual decisions. Agreement between prospective treatment preferences and ratings of health states is studied as an indicator of the validity of treatment preferences.

Methods.—Seven groups of subjects reflecting a broad range of health states were studied: younger and older healthy adults; patients with chronic diseases, terminal cancer, or AIDS; survivors of stroke; and nursing home residents. Each subject indicated 6 treatment preferences and 5 health state ratings. Logistic regression was used to measure the increase in likelihood of treatment refusal by change in health state ratings. If a subject refused treatments in health states rated as worse than death and accepted treatments in health states rated as better than death, the treatment preferences were considered concordant.

Results.—The subjects' ratings of their own current health were significantly different from their ratings of the hypothetical health states offered (Table 2). Health state ratings had a strong effect on the probability of prospective refusal of treatment. A 1-unit change in health state—that is, a change in health state rating from a little worse than death to somewhat worse than death—was associated with a 70% to 94% increase in the odds of refusing treatment. When asked about the reasons for discordance at the end of the study, the subjects either gave an understandable explanation or changed the discordant health state rating or treatment preference.

Conclusion.—The findings suggest that prospective preferences for life-sustaining treatments have high convergent validity. Most people's treat-

TABLE 2.—Percentage of Participants Who Rated Their Current Health State and Four Hypothetical Health States as Worse Than Death at Baseline*

Health State	Younger Well Adults ($n = 50$)	Older Well Adults ($n = 49$)	Persons with Chronic illness ($n = 49$)	Persons with Terminal Cancer ($n = 48$)	Persons with AIDS ($n = 50$)	Stroke Survivors ($n = 45$)	Nursing Home Residents ($n = 50$)	All Participants ($n = 341$)
					%			
Current health†	0	0	0	2	0	0	2	1
Dementia	24	31	31	29	30	27	18	27
Severe stroke	30	49	39	25	46	29	26	35
Severe pain‡	30	57	43	31	48	33	26	38
Coma‡	66	57	59	44	66	44	28	52

*Includes ratings much worse than death, somewhat worse than death, and a little worse than death.
†P less than 0.001 compared with other states for every group.
‡Preferences differed across groups (P less than 0.02).
(Courtesy of Patrick DL, Pearlman RA, Starks HE, et al: Validation of preferences for life-sustaining treatment: Implications for advance care planning. *Ann Intern Med* 127:509–517, 1997.)

ment preferences appear to be grounded in a consistent belief system. Asking patients about their health state ratings and treatment preferences at the same time can help to identify situations in which treatment is clearly desired or not desired. Noting the concordance or discordance between these preferences and ratings may afford a chance to examine the patients' values and reasoning.

▶ This study clearly documents that some patients feel there are states of health, specifically in this situation permanent coma, that are worse than death. One of the important aspects of this study was that a broad cross-section of patients was surveyed, including both the healthy and the infirm. The data also demonstrated a high level of concordance (essentially a measure of how consistent the patient's treatment wishes are with their perception of a proposed state of health). Physicians and surrogate decision-makers should explore not just patients' treatment wishes but their perceptions about the specific medical situations they may be facing and how it squares with their desire for treatment.

C.M. Franklin, M.D.

AIDS in a Medical Intensive Care Unit: Immediate Prognosis and Long-term Survival

Lazard T, Retel O, Guidet B, et al (Hôpital Saint-Antoine, Paris)
JAMA 276:1240–1245, 1996

9–41

Purpose.—Intensive care can seem futile in a fatal condition such as AIDS. Although studies of patients with AIDS requiring ICU admission have been published, they have included small numbers of patients with no prognostic analysis. Information on in-hospital and long-term prognosis is needed to establish policies on ICU admission. A large case series of patients with AIDS admitted to a medical ICU (MICU) was reviewed.

Patients.—The analysis included 120 consecutive patients with AIDS admitted to an MICU from 1990 to 1992. They were followed for a median of 1 year. There were 104 men and 16 women with a mean age of 38 years. The admission diagnosis was acute respiratory failure in 50% of patients, CNS dysfunction in 22.5%, pneumothorax in 12.5%, shock in 11%, and other conditions in 4%. Eighty-six patients survived to be discharged from the MICU. Factors associated with death before and after MICU discharge were identified.

Findings.—Three factors were associated with a poor MICU outcome: a Simplified Acute Physiology Score greater than 10, longer than 1 year between AIDS diagnosis and MICU admission, and a serum albumin level less than 30 g/L. Relative risks for these factors were 6.1, 6.0, and 4.9, respectively. Mortality in the MICU was unaffected by CD4 cell count, β_2-microglobulinemia, or a history of opportunistic infection. Survival after MICU discharge was 86% at 1 week, 82% at 1 month, 53% at 6 months, and 39% at 1 year. Outcomes after MICU discharge were associated with Karnofsky scale score and number of previous opportunistic infections. Predictive factors associated with survival in the MICU did not affect survival after MICU discharge.

Conclusion.—For patients with AIDS requiring MICU admission, mortality in the MICU is linked to immediate severity, as assessed within 48 hours of admission and the interval between AIDS diagnosis and MICU admission. The severity of the AIDS—not the illness precipitating MICU admission—is the only factor affecting long-term survival after discharge from the MICU. Thus, decisions about admitting patients with AIDS to the MICU should be made on the same basis as for non-AIDS patients.

▶ Many scoring systems have been developed in an attempt to predict the outcome of ICU care. As of today, none of the scoring systems have been shown to be adequate in this respect. The Acute Physiology and Chronic Health Evaluation (APACHE) III score was designed to improve the predictive ability of APACHE II. However, in this study, APACHE III underestimated risk of death to a greater degree than APACHE II. Furthermore, the APACHE systems have been advocated as a means of comparing groups in different ICUs. As this study showed, clinical practice patterns in different institutions may affect APACHE scoring, rendering comparisons difficult. This, coupled with the cost of the APACHE III system, may mitigate the benefits associated with its use.

Y. Friedman, M.D.

Does HIV Status Influence the Outcome of Patients Admitted to a Surgical Intensive Care Unit? A Prospective Double Blind Study
Bhagwanjee S, Muckart DJJ, Jeena PM, et al (Univ of Natal, South Africa)
BMJ 314:1077–1084, 1997   9–42

Background.—The expense associated with intensive care and the limited resources available for health care have compelled physicians to consider rationing of this resource. Frequently, patients not regarded as salvageable are refused admission to the ICU. The role of HIV infection status on outcome, in patients admitted to the ICU for other diseases, is not clear, leading to confusion about the use of HIV status in admission decisions. The impact of HIV status on outcome of patients in an ICU was studied prospectively.

Methods.—Each patient admitted to the ICU at King Edward VIII Hospital, in Durban, South Africa, between September 1993 and February 1994, was tested for HIV by enzyme-linked immunosorbent assay, immunofluorescence, Western blotting, and flow cytometry. The patient population was subdivided into HIV-negative patients, HIV-positive patients, and patients with AIDS. Patient outcomes were recorded.

Results.—Fifty two (13%) of the 402 patients admitted to the ICU during this period were HIV positive. The remaining 350 patients (87%) were HIV negative. None of the patients had AIDS. There were no significant differences in hospital or ICU mortality, survival time, or mean APACHE II score based on HIV status. The incidence of septic shock was significantly greater in HIV-positive (38%) than in HIV-negative patients (15%), as was the incidence of organ failure (71% vs. 49%).

Conclusions.—Although a positive HIV status appears to increase the risk of morbidity in the ICU, the risk of in-hospital or ICU mortality is not similarly increased by HIV infection. Therefore, HIV status should not be used as a criterion for ICU admission.

▶ Less than a decade ago, it was commonly suggested that HIV-infected patients not be admitted to the ICU. Today, no one would assert that patients be excluded from the ICU based solely on a diagnosis of AIDS. Greater clinical perspective and knowledge of important related issues such as the balance between the virus and the immune system allow us to treat AIDS in the same way we treat other chronic diseases in terms of ICU triage. This question must have been raised in South Africa where resource constraints may have prompted this study. The finding that HIV status did not influence mortality is further support of our current thinking. While the study is not especially sophisticated in terms of measuring viral load or CD4 counts, it demonstrates simply but convincingly that there is no rationale for a blanket exclusion of HIV-positive patients in the ICU.

A tangential issue raised by this study was the ethics of obtaining HIV results on patients without their informed consent. It's an interesting question in this particular article, one that the authors address, although not entirely to my satisfaction (an editorial critical of their methods was published next to the article). Readers should determine for themselves whether the clinical implications of the study were important enough for the authors to waive the patients' right to informed consent.

C.M. Franklin, M.D.

Informed Consent for Research Purposes in Intensive Care Patients in Europe: Part II. An Official Statement of the European Society of Intensive Care Medicine

Lemaire F, Blanch L, Cohen SL, et al (Hôpital Henri Mondor, Créteil, France; Hosp de Sabadell, Spain; UCL Med School, London; et al)
Intensive Care Med 23:435–439, 1997   9–43

Introduction.—The present status of informed consent for research purposes in intensive care patients in 16 European countries was examined. A questionnaire ascertained the basis for obtaining consent, the identity of the individual deciding competency of the critically ill patient, the possibility of delegating consent to a surrogate, and the possibility of doing research without informed consent.

Results.—In 8 countries the basis for informed consent is given by law, although in 1 country the law has never been implemented. In most other countries the basis is generally accepted good clinical practices and/or ethical committees or declarations. Most countries require informed consent from the patient or the surrogate under all circumstances. In most countries, competency is judged by the physician or an administrator in consultation with medical or psychiatric staff.

Conclusions.—Whereas half the countries have no legal requirement for informed consent, most countries require it. Competency is judged by the physician in most countries. There is no consensus regarding the use of surrogates.

▶ This statement about informed consent for research on critically ill patients summarizes the legal status of informed consent in 16 European countries. Although significant differences among countries exist, there appears to be significant consensus that informed consent is necessary. There is no consensus about the use of surrogates or who determines mental competency. This appears to be a very ambiguous area at the moment. However, it is a very important area that requires a greater effort at building international consensus.

J.E. Calvin, Jr., M.D.

J.E. Parrillo, M.D.

survival and quality of life after, 333

survival in, and plasma cytokine concentrations and APACHE III scores, 329

thrombosis incidence in, deep venous, 98

pediatric, analysis of costs in, 269

pneumonia in

community-acquired, severe, prospective validation of prognostic score, 112

nosocomial, scoring system for, 103

rural, mortality rates in, 341

sedation in, overnight, with midazolam or propofol, 303

South African, poor discriminatory performance of PRISM score in, 243

surgical

blood cultures in, utilization and diagnostic yield of, 212

effect of HIV status on outcome, 371

infections in, patient-to-patient spread of single strain of *Corynebacterium striatum* causing, 210

ventilation in, mechanical, parameters of, chest x-ray changes in air space disease associated with, 164

Intensivist

medical, effects on patient care in community teaching hospital, 323

Interferon

-gamma level increase in lung by injurious ventilatory strategies (in rat), 173

Interleukin

-1β

level increase in lung by injurious ventilatory strategies (in rat), 173

levels and APACHE III scores and survival in ICU patients, 330

production in sepsis-related multiple organ failure, 62

release, early, in severe intraabdominal infection and sepsis, interleukin-10 prevents (in mice), 71

-1ra levels, circulating, do not predict development of ARDS, 87

-6

levels, bronchoalveolar and systemic, in ARDS, severe pneumonia and cardiogenic pulmonary edema, 116

levels after burns, 196

levels and APACHE III scores and survival in ICU patients, 330

levels and circulating erythropoietin levels in children with sepsis and septic shock, 258

levels in sepsis, correlation with APACHE III and MPM II scores, 55

levels in septic shock, cardiogenic shock, and bacterial pneumonia, 65

production in sepsis-related multiple organ failure, 62

release, early, in severe intraabdominal infection and sepsis, interleukin-10 prevents (in mice), 71

-8 levels

APACHE III scores and survival in ICU patients and, 330

bronchoalveolar and systemic, in ARDS, severe pneumonia and cardiogenic pulmonary edema, 116

after burns, 196

-10

levels, circulating, do not predict development of ARDS, 87

levels, increase in lung by injurious ventilatory strategies (in rat), 173

prevents early cytokine release in severe intraabdominal infection and sepsis (in mice), 69

production in ARDS, 93

-12 levels in sepsis, correlation with APACHE III and MPM II scores, 55

Interventions

clinical, effect on care at end of life, 344

Intoxication

cardiac arrest due to, out-of-hospital, outcome of, 4

Intraabdominal

infection and sepsis, severe, interleukin-10 prevents early cytokine release in (in mice), 69

Intracranial

aneurysm rupture, rebleeding of, and very poor prognosis, 28

pressure

effects of varying levels of PEEP on, 226

monitoring, bedside burr hole performed by intensive care physicians for, 227

waveform analysis, significance after head injury, 228

Intramucosal

P_{CO_2}, new continuous measurement method in gastrointestinal tract (in pig), 282

Workers
  health care, mupirocin treatment of, to
    control methicillin-resistant
    Staphylococcus aureus outbreak in
    burn unit, 189
Wounds
  stab, cardiac, 37

X

X-ray (*see* Radiography)

Author Index